Multiple Myeloma - A New Era of Treatment Strategies

Editors

Klaus Podar

National Center of Tumor Diseases (NCT), University of Heidelberg and German Cancer Research Center (DKFZ), Germany; and Dana-Farber Cancer Institute (DFCI), Harvard Medical School, USA

Kenneth C. Anderson

Dana-Farber Cancer Institute (DFCI), Harvard Medical School, USA

CONTENTS

CHAPTERS

Section 1: MULTIPLE MYELOMA

Section 2: TREATMENT GUIDELINES

Section 3: THE BONE MARROW MICROENVIRONMENT AND THE PATHOGENESIS OF MULTIPLE MYELOMA

Section 4: NEW TREATMENT STRATEGIES

FOREWORD

The pace at which myeloma therapy has evolved in recent years has been nothing short of spectacular. Conventional textbooks can scarcely keep up with the advances. This electronic book edited by Dr. Klaus Podar and Kenneth Anderson is therefore both timely and appropriate. I would like to congratulate the editors for assembling a stellar cast of investigators to author the various chapters in this e-Book. The editors and authors have done a masterful job with the content and organization of the e-Book. I am sure this e Book will be an invaluable resource for physicians worldwide.

S. Vincent Rajkumar,
Mayo Clinic
USA

PREFACE

Multiple Myeloma (MM), the second most common blood cancer in adults, is a clonal plasma cell malignancy within the bone marrow characterized by osteolytic bone lesions, renal disease, and immunodeficiency. The development of MM is a complex multi-step process involving both early and late genetic changes in the tumor cell as well as selective supportive conditions by the bone marrow (BM) microenvironment. It is now well established that MM cell-induced disruption of the bone marrow homeostasis between the highly organized cellular and extracellular compartments supports MM cell proliferation, survival, migration, and drug resistance *via* activation of various signaling (e.g. PI3K/Akt, JAK/ Stat-, Raf/MEK/MAPK-, NFκB-, and Wnt-) pathways. Based on this knowledge prototypic drugs thalidomide, bortezomib, and lenalidomide, which target both MM cells and the BM microenvironment have already fundamentally changed treatment options of this disease. Indeed, their benefit is now not only shown in relapsed and refractory disease but they also improve overall response, duration of response, and progression-free and overall survival when used as part of first-line regimens. However, despite these new insights into MM pathogenesis and exciting derived therapeutic advances, MM still remains incurable. Ongoing studies are therefore aiming to further delineate mechanisms of MM pathogenesis within the bone marrow to identify novel agents with enhanced cytotoxicity and decreased drug resistance to improve patient outcome.

We are very happy having been able to win eminent physician/ scientists to write the chapters of this e-Book which aims to provide readers with a comprehensive account of the most recent developments in the field of MM; a field which we believe represents a paradigm for translational research in general. Our foremost goal was to address a broad audience of readers including clinicians, scientists, students, and interested patients.

After a brief historic review by Drs. Kyle and Steensma, **Section 1** will cover newest insights into the epidemiology and etiology of MM (Drs. Birmann and colleagues), as well as attempts to generate a genetically based classification system (Dr. Tonon).

In **Section 2**, Dr. Podar and colleagues will first give a brief overview of up-to-date treatment strategies both for upfront therapy as well as for therapy of relapsed/ refractory MM. Dr. Harousseau will then specifically focus on the changing role of autologous and allogeneic stem cell transplantation as part of new treatment regimens. Drs Vallet and Raje will review the pathophysiology and treatment options of MM bone disease thereby identifying potential therapeutic alternatives to bisphosphonates. Dr. Lentzsch will then discuss the management of complications in MM and supportive treatment regimens. Finally, Dr. Kumar will summarize promising advanced clinical trials, which are likely to change once more MM treatment regimens in near future. Taken together, Section 2 aims to address the needs of clinicians who are looking for the rationale of up-to-date treatment guidelines in the day-to-day practice.

In **Section 3** exciting new preclinical results will be discussed. Chapters of this section will delineate the pathophysiologic key role of the BM microenvironment in MM (Dr. Roccaro and colleagues), and the role of MM BM angiogenesis (Drs. Ribatti and Vacca), in particular. Moreover, Drs. Fulciniti and colleagues will discuss MM mouse models, their advantages and pitfalls in translational MM research.

Based on mechanistic data presented in **Section 3, Section 4** will finally summarize potential new therapeutic targets and derived new treatment strategies with focus on small molecules (Drs. Podar and colleagues), as well as antibodies (Dr. Tai).

Sections 3 and 4 aim to predominantly address the interests of scientists and clinical investigators in the MM field. However, we hope and believe that our own and other studies of the pathophysiologic role of the tumor microenvironment, the identification of novel therapeutic targets, and the clinical introduction of derived agents in MM also may serve as a paradigm for translational research in other fields of oncology.

Klaus Podar

National Center of Tumor Diseases (NCT), University of Heidelberg and
German Cancer Research Center (DKFZ), Germany;
Dana-Farber Cancer Institute (DFCI),
Harvard Medical School, USA

Kenneth C. Anderson

Dana-Farber Cancer Institute (DFCI), Harvard Medical School, USA

List of Contributors

Kenneth C. Anderson

Kraft Family Professor of Medicine; Medical Director, Kraft Family Blood Center, The LeBow Institute for Myeloma Therapeutics and Jerome Lipper Myeloma Center, Department of Medical Oncology, Dana Farber Cancer Institute, Harvard Medical School, Boston, MA, USA

Brenda M. Birmann

Instructor in Medicine/ Harvard Medical School; Channing Laboratory, Department of Medicine, Brigham and Women's Hospital and Harvard Medical School, Boston, MA USA.

Dharminder Chauhan

Principal Associate in Medicine, The LeBow Institute for Myeloma Therapeutics and Jerome Lipper Myeloma Center, Department of Medical Oncology, Dana Farber Cancer Institute, Harvard Medical School, Boston, MA, USA

Brian C.-H. Chiu

Associate Professor of Epidemiology, Department of Health Studies, University of Chicago, USA

Wendy Cozen

Associate Professor of Preventive Medicine and Pathology, Department of Preventive Medicine and Pathology, Norris Comprehensive Cancer Center, Keck School of Medicine, University of Southern California, Los Angeles, CA, USA

Michela Frenquelli

Postdoctoral Fellow, Division of Molecular Oncology, San Raffaele del Monte Tabor Scientific Foundation, Milan, Italy

Mariateresa Fulciniti

Postdoctoral Fellow, The LeBow Institute for Myeloma Therapeutics and Jerome Lipper Myeloma Center, Department of Medical Oncology, Dana Farber Cancer Institute, Harvard Medical School, Boston, MA, USA

Irene Ghobrial

Assistant Professor of Medicine, Department of Medicine, Harvard Medical School, Kirsch Lab for Waldenstrom Macroglobulinemia, Department of Medical Oncology, Dana Farber Cancer Institute, Harvard Medical School, Boston, MA, USA

Jean-Luc Harousseau

Professor of Medicine, René Gauducheau Cancer Center, Nantes/ St Herblain, France

Teru Hideshima

Principal Associate in Medicine, The LeBow Institute for Myeloma Therapeutics and Jerome Lipper Myeloma Center, Department of Medical Oncology, Dana Farber Cancer Institute, Harvard Medical School, Boston, MA, USA

Jonathan L. Kaufman

Assistant Professor of Medicine, Department of Hematology and Medical Oncology Winship Cancer Institute, Emory University School of Medicine, Atlanta, GA, USA

Shaji Kumar

Associate Professor of Medicine, Department of Medicine, Division of Hematology, Mayo Clinic, Rochester, MN, USA

Robert A. Kyle

Professor of Medicine, Department of Medicine, Division of Hematology, Mayo Clinic, Rochester, MN, USA

Jacob P. Laubach

Instructor in Medicine, Department of Medicine, Harvard Medical School, The LeBow Institute for Myeloma Therapeutics and Jerome Lipper Myeloma Center, Department of Medical Oncology, Dana Farber Cancer Institute, Harvard Medical School, Boston, MA, USA

Suzanne Lentzsch

Assistant Professor of Medicine, Division of Hematology/Oncology, University of Pittsburgh Cancer Institute, Pittsburgh, PA, USA

Sagar Lonial

Associate Professor of Medicine, Vice Chair of Clinical Affairs, Department of Hematology and Medical Oncology Winship Cancer Institute, Emory University School of Medicine, Atlanta, GA, USA

Kristin Muench

Research Associate, Department of Preventive Medicine, Norris Comprehensive Cancer Center, Keck School of Medicine, University of Southern California, USA

Paola Neri

Postdoctoral Fellow, Division of Hematology and Bone Marrow Transplant, University of Calgary, AB, Canada

Klaus Podar

Associate Professor of Medicine, Principal Investigator and Group Leader at the National Center for Tumor Diseases (NCT), University of Heidelberg and German Cancer Research Center (DKFZ), Germany; Visiting Professor at The LeBow Institute for Myeloma Therapeutics and Jerome Lipper Myeloma Center, Department of Medical Oncology, Dana Farber Cancer Institute, Harvard Medical School, Boston, MA, USA

Noopur Raje

Associate Professor of Medicine, Division of Hematology-Oncology, Massachusetts General Hospital Cancer Center, Harvard Medical School, Boston, MA, USA

Paul G. Richardson

Associate Professor of Medicine, The LeBow Institute for Myeloma Therapeutics and Jerome Lipper Myeloma Center, Department of Medical Oncology, Dana Farber Cancer Institute, Harvard Medical School, Boston, MA, USA

Aldo Roccaro

Research Scientist/Research Associate in Medicine, Harvard Medical School, Dana-Farber Cancer Institute, Boston, MA, USA

Giuseppe Rossi

Director of Hematology, Spedali Civili di Brescia, Brescia, Italy

Domenico Ribatti

Professor of Medicine, Department of Human Anatomy and Histology, Bari, Italy

David P. Steensma

Lecturer on Medicine, Department of Medicine, Harvard Medical School, Oncology, Brigham And Women's Hospital, Boston, MA, USA

Catherine A. Suppan

Research Assistant, Channing Laboratory, Department of Medicine, Brigham and Women's Hospital, Boston, MA, USA

Pierosandro Tagliaferri

Professor of Medicine, Medical Oncology Unit, University of Magna Græcia and T. Campanella Cancer Center, Catanzaro, Italy

Pierfrancesco Tassone

Professor of Medicine, Medical Oncology Unit, University of Magna Græcia and T. Campanella Cancer Center, Catanzaro, Italy

Giovanni Tonon

Head, Functional Genomics of Cancer Unit, Division of Molecular Oncology, Scientific Coordinator, Multiple Myeloma Unit, Department of Oncology, San Raffaele del Monte Tabor Scientific Foundation, Milan, Italy

Angelo Vacca

Professor of Medicine, Department of Internal Medicine and Clinical Oncology, Bari, Italy

Sonia Vallet

Postdoctoral Fellow, Division of Hematology-Oncology, Massachusetts General Hospital Cancer Center, Harvard Medical School, MA, USA

CHAPTER 1

A Short History of Multiple Myeloma

Robert A. Kyle[1*] and David P. Steensma[2]

[1]Division of Hematology, Mayo Clinic, Rochester, MN and [2]Department of Hematologic Malignancies Harvard Medical School, Dana-Farber Cancer Institute, Brigham & Women's Hospital, Boston, MA

Abstract: Although multiple myeloma has probably been present for centuries, the first well-documented case was published less than 160 years ago. The famous patient, Thomas Alexander McBean excreted large amounts of a peculiar protein that was studied by Henry Bence Jones. Jones was a well-recognized physician as well as chemist. Less than a half-century ago, Bence Jones protein was found to consist of monoclonal light chains. Otto Kahler described a patient with autopsy-proven multiple myeloma; this patient survived eight years after the onset of symptoms despite the absence of effective therapy. The discovery of Roentgen's rays facilitated the diagnosis of multiple myeloma. Serum electrophoresis followed by immunofixation allowed physicians to readily make the diagnosis. Melphalan was introduced for therapy half a century ago but little progress was made until autologous stem cell transplantation became available almost 20 years ago. This was followed by the introduction of the "novel" agents thalidomide, bortezomib and lenalidomide in the last decade.

Keywords: Bence Jones protein, Kahler's disease, plasma cell, multiple myeloma, immuno/electrophoresis, immunofixation, angiogenesis, urethane, Melphalan, prednisone, stem cell transplantation, thalidomide, lenalidomide.

Although multiple myeloma has very likely been present for centuries, the first well-documented case was published in a series of cases of "mollities ossium" published 1844 by Samuel Solly[1]. There is suggestive but not definitive evidence of earlier cases. For instance, the Wellcome Museum in London featured an exhibit on skeletons which included a skeleton with myeloma-like lesions in the bones of a 45-year-old Roman soldier. The skeleton of George Grenville, the Whig Prime Minister of Great Britain in the 1760s, also reveals lytic lesions resembling those of multiple myeloma.

Solly's patient, Sarah Newbury, was a 39-year-old housewife who had developed severe back pain while stooping 4 years before her death. She ultimately developed bilateral fractures of her femurs when her husband lifted her (Fig. **1**).

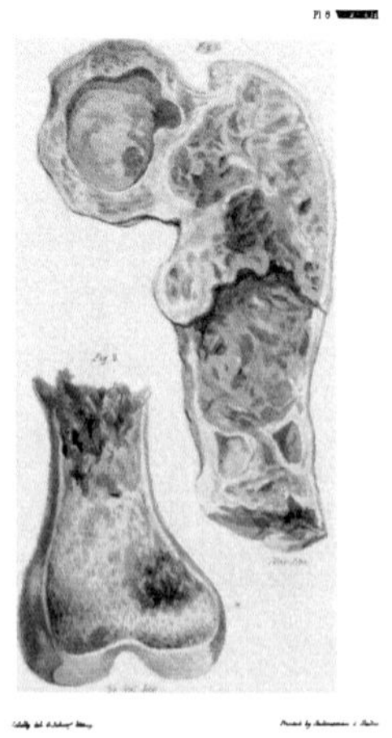

Fig. (1). Sarah Newbury. Fractures of femurs and right humerus [1].

***Address correspondence to Robert A. Kyle:** Division of Hematology, Mayo Clinic 200 First Street, SW, Rochester, MN 55905, Tel: 507-284-3039, E-mail: kyle.robert@mayo.edu

Klaus Podar and Kenneth C. Anderson

She subsequently had fractures of the clavicles, right humerus, and right radius and ulna (Fig. **1**). She was hospitalized at St. Thomas'Hospital in London and treated with an infusion of orange peel and a rhubarb pill as well as opiates for her pain. She was also given wine, arrowroot, a mutton chop and a pint of porter daily. Despite this treatment, she died four days later and, at autopsy, a peculiar "red matter" replaced the cancellous portion of her sternum (Fig. **2**).

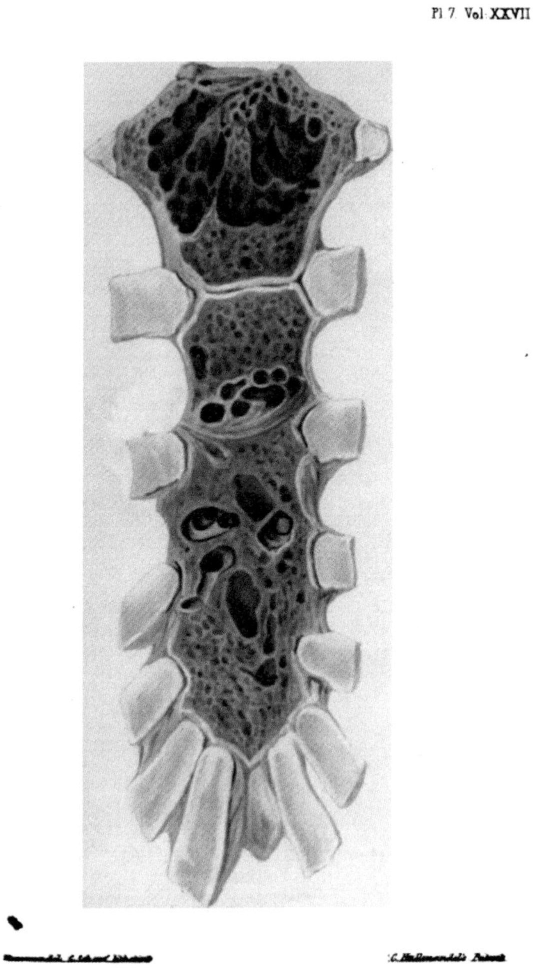

Fig. (2). Sternum of Sarah Newbury showing destruction of bone [1].

The cells were "very clear, their edge being remarkedly distinct and the clear oval outline enclosed one bright central nucleolus, rarely two, never more." Solly thought that the disease began with a "morbid action" of the blood vessels in which the "earthy matter of the bone is absorbed and thrown out by the kidneys in the urine." One-hundred and fifty years later, anti-angiogenesis drugs such as thalidomide were used for the treatment of multiple myeloma [2]. Is it possible that Solly anticipated the role of angiogenesis in the pathophysiology of multiple myeloma?

The best-described early case of multiple myeloma is that of Thomas Alexander McBean, a 45-year-old "highly-respectable tradesman" from London. He had developed fatigue and noted that his "body linen was stiffened by his urine". In September of 1844, he vaulted out of an underground cavern while on holiday and suddenly "felt as if something had snapped or given way within the chest." For some minutes, he lay unable to move because of the severe pain. A "strengthening plaster" was applied to the chest with temporary relief but symptoms recurred a few weeks later. Then, "a pound of blood" was removed and leeches were applied for "maintenance therapy". This resulted in resolution of his skeletal pain, but he complained of weakness for two or three months. Six months later, his chest pain recurred but cupping and therapeutic phlebotomy were not helpful. Steel and quinine were prescribed and this produced a rapid symptomatic improvement. Quinine was recommended for many illnesses and the combination of quinine and iron was considered appropriate for severely debilitated patients. During the summer of 1845, he travelled to Scotland for holiday where "he bounded over hills as nimbly as any of his companions" [3]. Lumbar and sciatic pain recurred after returning to London, so he was seen by a Harley Street consultant, Dr. William Macintyre on October 30, 1845. Macintyre personally examined the urine because edema had been observed and he found that it "abounded in animal matter." A sample of urine and the following note were sent to Henry Bence Jones, a chemist at St. George's Hospital.

Saturday, November 1, 1845

> *"Dear Dr. Jones,*
>
> *The tube contains urine of very high specific gravity. When boiled, it becomes slightly opaque. On the addition of nitric acid, it effervesces, assumes a reddish hue, and becomes quite clear; but as it cools, assumes the consistence and appearance which you see. Heat reliquifies it. What is it?"*

Dr. Jones confirmed the finding of Macintyre and calculated that the patient was excreting 60 grams of protein per day. He felt that the strange new protein was an oxide of albumin, specifically "hydrated deutoxide of albumen" [4]. Richard Bright had reported 20 years earlier that the presence of edema and kidney disease was frequently associated with proteinuria [5]. Despite a variety of therapies, McBean died January 1, 1846. His bones were soft, brittle and readily fractured at autopsy and contained a "gelatiniform substance of a blood-red colour and unctuous feel". The bone marrow contained round and oval-shaped cells that were one-half to twice as large as an average blood cell and each contained one or two nuclei and a bright-colored nucleolus (Fig. **3**).

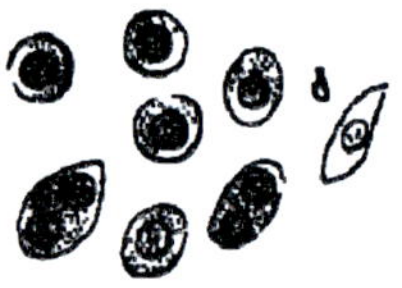

Fig. (3). Plasma cells (wood engravings made from drawings by Mr. Dalrymple) [73].

HENRY BENCE JONES

Henry Bence Jones was born on December 31, 1813, at Thorington Hall near Yoxford in Suffolk, England [6]. His maternal grandfather, Reverend Mr. Bence Sparrow, had loaned the home to his daughter, Matilda, and her husband, Lieutenant Colonel William Jones of the Dragoon Guards. Reverend Mr. Bence Sparrow was the parish priest of Beccles and was known as Reverend Bence Bence because he adopted the surname Bence in 1804 when he inherited Thorington Hall from his cousin, Anne Bence Golding. Henry attended boarding school in Putney in southwest London and then entered Harrow, a famous English public school. He was an accomplished cricketer and football and racket player but was not an outstanding student. In 1831, he entered Trinity College, Cambridge, where he rowed and took a second-class degree in 1836. He attended the Divinity lectures and received a certificate for ordination but decided not to pursue a career in the church.

He considered emigrating to New Zealand, but his father suggested that he study medicine. He began working in the apothecary shop of John Hammerton where he prepared medicines for six months. Many years later, he said that this experience "was of the utmost use to me all my life" [7]. He began medical school at St. George's Hospital on October 1, 1838. During medical school, he attended lectures of the physicist, Michael Faraday, on electricity at the Royal Institution. He also was taught to use the stethoscope by Dr. James Hope at St. George's Hospital.

St. George's Hospital had been established as a public infirmary and teaching facility in 1733 in what was then considered the open countryside outside the village of Knightsbridge. The site was noted for its clean air in contrast to the overcrowded and filthy conditions in the city of London. Faculty members at the hospital included Henry Gray (anatomist), Edward Jenner, John Hunter and Thomas Young. The Lanesborough Hotel is presently on the original site at Hyde Park Corner, but the Classical neo-Grecian structure was retained.

Jones developed rheumatic fever in the spring of 1839 and returned home for 6 weeks, but he "recovered without complications of disease of the heart" [7]. He returned to London and enrolled as a private pupil to Professor Thomas Graham who was considered to be "the father of colloid chemistry" and discoverer of the principle of dialysis. George Fownes, Graham's assistant, did most of the teaching. Fownes had studied with Justice von Liebig in Giessen, Germany; von Liebig was a strong advocate of applying chemistry to the study of animal physiology. Thus, Jones learned the principles of organic chemical analysis from Fownes and Graham and subsequently analyzed the sulfur in a cystine oxide calculus which represented his first medical publication [8]. Jones left for Giessen, Germany, on Easter Sunday in 1841, where he studied in von Liebig's laboratory for six months. He learned advanced analytical methods and remained in contact with von Liebig throughout his life. It is of interest to note that von Liebig and Bence Jones died two days apart in April of 1873, and their obituaries appeared in the same issue of *Lancet*. In 1842, Jones married a cousin, Lady Millicent Acheson, and settled at 30 Grosvenor Square, London. Jones analyzed the calculi in the Museum of University College Hospital and published his second paper in 1845 [9]. He obtained an assistant physician position and then became a full physician at St. George's Hospital. He subsequently was involved with the Royal Institution when he gave a series of lectures in 1851 and then served as Secretary for more than 20 years.

Jones stated that he would "let no year pass without doing something original in natural science as applied to medicine," despite his rapidly growing clinical practice [7] (Fig. **4**). He believed that medicine would be much better served if students spent more time studying chemistry and physics rather than memorizing Latin and Greek vocabulary and declensions. He claimed to believe in nothing that he could not separate, test and measure. He published a series of articles on the sediment, uric acid, calcium oxalate and phosphates of urine. It is interesting to note that his obituary in the *Medical Times and Gazette* listed 34 papers and 6 additional articles, but his papers on Bence Jones protein were not mentioned.

Jones began his laboratory work at 6 a.m. and then arrived at the hospital at approximately 1 p.m. for ward rounds. He was not popular with medical students because of his lack of punctuality. In addition, he frequently chided students with the phrase, "Oh! Medical facts! Medical facts!" His chief effort in the wards was to make therapeutics more scientific. In contrast to the majority of physicians, he did not mix several medications together but instead used simple, precise prescriptions. He was very skeptical of most of the therapeutic drugs.

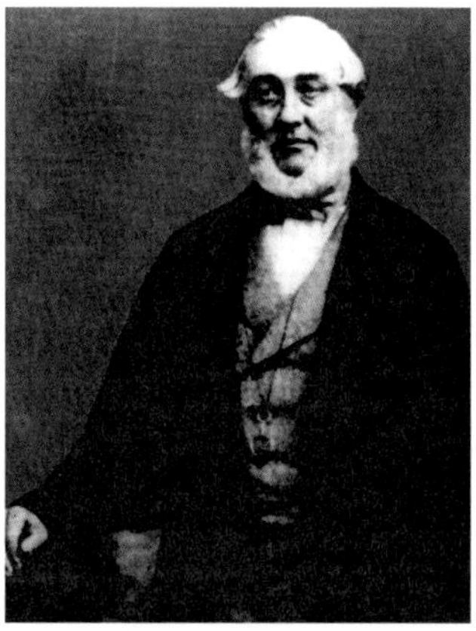

Fig. (4). Portrait of Henry Bence Jones. (From Snapper, I., and Kahn, A.[1971]. Myelomatosis: Fundamentals and Clinical Features. Baltimore: University Park Press [74]).

In fact, he made the statement that "there is scarcely a drug which may not, under different conditions, produce opposite effects..." [10].

His medical practice became large and lucrative. His profits from one year of practice were 7,400 pounds, a very large income. He bought a house at 84 Brook Street in the posh Mayfair neighborhood in West London where he lived for the remainder of his life. Nursing pioneer, Florence Nightingale, once stated that Bence Jones was "the best chemical doctor in London" [11]. Charles Darwin, the naturalist, was one of his patients. Jones had prescribed a "severe diet" for Darwin's indigestion which "half-starved him to death" [10]. Michael Faraday and the biologist, Thomas Huxley, were also his patients.

He noted palpitations in 1861, and made a diagnosis of rheumatic heart disease in himself after hearing a mitral systolic murmur with his stethoscope. He realized that his bout of rheumatic fever more than 20 years before had "done permanent damage to one of the valves" [7]. Congestive heart failure developed in 1866. In a letter to physicist John Tyndall, Jones stated, "I am very lazy and feel unfit for any work and as neither eating, drinking, or sleeping come pleasantly to me, I am a useless mortal and had better be helping the worms and the grass to grow faster than they otherwise would do..." [11]. He was forced to give up his clinical practice and resign as Secretary of the Royal Institution in 1873 because of congestive hepatomegaly, ascites, and anasarca. He died at his home at 84 Brook Street in London of congestive heart failure on April 20, 1873, and was buried at Kensall Green Cemetery.

His obituary in the *Medical Times and Gazette* described his work on renal stones, diabetes mellitus, malignant and tuberculous involvement of the kidney as well as the clinical value of microscopic analysis of the urine. There was no mention of the unique urinary protein that bears his name.

It should be emphasized that Henry Bence Jones did not hyphenate his name and no hyphen is used in any of his papers or books published during his lifetime. He may not have liked his given name "Henry", because he signed his correspondence as "H. Bence Jones". He descendants added a hyphen more than a half-century after his death [12].

OTHER CONTRIBUTIONS TO BENCE JONES PROTEINURIA

Johann Heller, an Austrian clinical chemist, described a protein in the urine that precipitated when warmed above 50° C and then dissolved on further heating, but he did not recognize the reprecipitation of the protein when the urine was cooled. The term "Bence Jones protein" was first used by Fleischer in 1880 [13]. W. Kuhne isolated a urinary protein, which precipitated upon warming to 50° C and cleared at 100° C. He called the protein "albumosurie" and stated that carbon, hydrogen and nitrogen levels were similar to those described by Bence Jones.

In 1922, Stanhope Bayne-Jones and D. W. Wilson at Johns Hopkins University reported two distinct groups of Bence Jones proteins [14]. Leonhard Korngold and Rose Lipari at Memorial Cancer Institute in New York demonstrated a close relationship between Bence Jones protein and the serum proteins of multiple myeloma in 1956 [15]. These two major classes have been designated as kappa and lambda in honor of Korngold and Lipari. One-hundred and seventeen years after the description of the unique properties of Bence Jones protein, Edelman and Gally proved that the light chains prepared from an IgG myeloma serum protein and the Bence Jones protein from the same patient's urine had an identical amino acid sequence as well as other physical chemical characteristics [16].

SOME FURTHER EARLY CASES OF MULTIPLE MYELOMA

Herman Weber described a 40-year-old man with bone pain, tenderness and deformity of the sternum in 1867. At autopsy, the sternum was almost entirely replaced by a grayish-red substance. There were several round defects in the skull, vertebrae and pelvis. Amyloid was found in the kidneys and spleen [17]. William Adams described a patient with bone pain and fractures as well as "lardaceous changes" in the liver and kidney [18]. The term, "multiple myeloma" was introduced by J. von Rustizky, a Russian pathologist working in the laboratory of von Recklinghausen in Strassburg in 1873. A patient had eight separate tumors of the bone marrow which von Rustizky called "multiple myelomas". He also noted that the nucleus of the tumor cells was located in the periphery of the cytoplasm of the cell.

The term "Kahler's disease" was often used to describe multiple myeloma. This eponym resulted from a case report by Professor Otto Kahler of Prague who described his patient, Dr. Loos. Loos was a 46-year-old physician who developed severe thoracic pain in July 1879. The pain was intermittent but aggravated by exercise. Two years later, pallor was noted and, in 1885, Dr. Loos was seen by Professor Kahler. Anemia, severe kyphosis, tenderness of many bones and albumosuria were found. The kyphosis was so severe that the patient's chin pressed against his sternum and produced a pressure ulcer. Dr. Loos died eight years after the onset of symptoms. At autopsy, many masses were noted in the ribs and microscopic examination revealed large, round cells consistent with myeloma. He maintained a high fluid intake and took sodium bicarbonate on a regular basis which may have helped prevent renal failure.

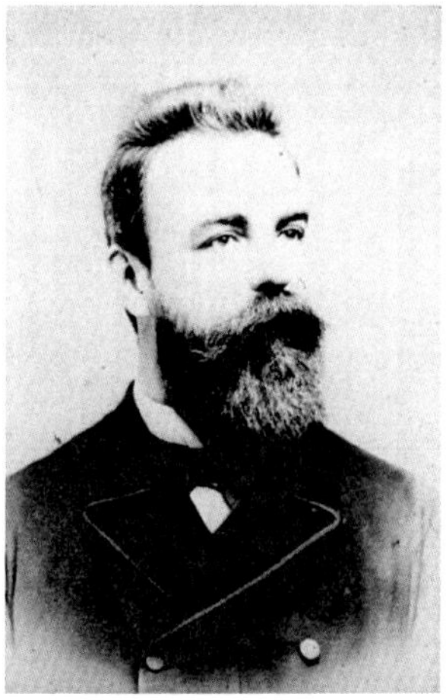

Fig. (5). Otto Kahler (Courtesy of Dr. Heinz Ludwig, Vienna) [74].

Otto Kahler, born in 1849, was the son of a well-known physician in Prague (Fig. **5**). Kahler studied in Paris after receiving his MD degree from the University of Prague in 1871. He became interested in neurology and worked with Jean Martin Charcot and Guillaume-Benjamin-Amand Duchenne. Kahler made contributions to the pathological anatomy of tabes dorsalis and the symptoms of gradual compression of the spinal cord. He returned to Prague and he became head of the second medical clinic at the German University of Prague. Kahler succeeded the Austrian internist, Heinrich von Bamberger as Professor at the University of Vienna in 1889. Unfortunately, Kahler developed a carcinoma of the tongue and died in 1893. It is of interest to note that his obituaries and eulogies made no mention of his famous case report of Dr. Loos [19]. Thus, the contributions of both Henry Bence Jones and Otto Kahler to multiple myeloma were not recognized during their lifetimes.

James Herrick and Ludvig Hektoen at Rush Medical College in Chicago in 1894 reported the first case of multiple myeloma in the United States. Frederick Parkes Weber reported a case of multiple myeloma in 1898 and stated that the diagnosis might be "greatly facilitated by the employment of Röntgen's rays" [20]. He also stated that the bone marrow was the site of production of the Bence Jones protein and that it "nearly always, if not always" indicated that the patient was suffering from "multiple myeloma" [21].

In 1928, Geschickter and Copeland analyzed all 425 cases of multiple myeloma reported since 1848 [22]. The six major features consisted of multiple involvement of the skeleton by tumors, pathologic fractures, Bence Jones proteinuria, back pain, anemia and renal insufficiency. Blood protein abnormalities were not recognized. Bone marrow examination was described in 1929 by Arinkin in Leningrad. This led to the increased recognition of multiple myeloma [23]. In fact, Rosenthal and Vogel reported that only 3 cases of multiple myeloma had been recognized in Mt. Sinai Hospital in New York from 1916 to 1935, but that 13 cases were found from 1935 to 1937 [24]. Bayrd and Heck described 83 patients with histologic proof of multiple myeloma from the Mayo Clinic through 1945. Survival ranged from 1 month to 84 months (median 15 months) [25].

PLASMA CELLS

Although the term "plasma cell" was first used in 1875 by Waldeyer, it is likely that he was observing tissue mast cells rather than plasma cells [26]. Santiago Ramón y Cajal accurately described plasma cells in 1890 [27]. He felt that the unstained perinuclear area ("hof") contained the Golgi apparatus and that the plasma cells were likely normal constituents of connective tissue. It was T. von Marschalkó, a Hungarian pathologist, who described the characteristics of plasma cells in 1895. He noted the blocked chromatin, eccentric position of the nucleus and the "hof" [28]. Wright believed that the tumor cells of myeloma consisted of plasma cells or their immediate descendants [29].

ANTIBODIES

Although Bence Jones protein had been detected in the serum by Jacobsen in 1917, it was not until 1928 that Perlzweig recognized hyperproteinemia in a patient with multiple myeloma [30]. Wintrobe and Buell recognized cryoglobulinemia in 1933, but the term "cryoglobulin" was introduced by Lerner and Watson 14 years later [31].

ELECTROPHORESIS

Arne Tiselius described the separation of serum proteins by electrophoresis in his doctoral dissertation in 1930 while working in the laboratory of Theodore Svedberg [32]. His description of the moving boundary method of electrophoresis was published in 1937, but it is of interest to note that this manuscript was rejected by the Biochemical Journal [11]. Later that year, Tiselius described the separation of serum globulins into three major components which he named alpha, beta and gamma, according to their electrophoretic mobility. He and his American postdoctoral fellow, Elvin Kabat, localized antibody activity to the gamma globulin region [33]. He noted that some antibodies sedimented in the ultracentrifuge as 7S and others as 19S molecules while some migrated in the fast gamma region and others in the slow gamma region. Before 1960, the term, "gamma globulin" was used for any protein that migrated in the gamma mobility region of the electrophoretic pattern. These gamma globulins are now recognized as IgG, IgA, IgM, IgD and IgE. The tall, narrow-based "church spire peak" was demonstrated in 1939 by Longsworth and his colleagues at the Rockefeller Institute when they studied multiple myeloma [34]. The original commercial models of the electrophoresis apparatus were 20 feet long and 5 feet high and often occupied a separate laboratory room. A single electrophoretic run required a full day and results could only be interpreted by an experienced operator [11]. The use of filter paper as a support media permitted the separation of protein into distinct zones that could be stained with various dyes [35]. Subsequently, cellulose acetate was introduced as the supporting media and now most laboratories use agarose gel electrophoresis or capillary zone electrophoresis.

Grabar and Williams described immunoelectrophoresis in 1953 [36], but it was not available as a routine laboratory procedure for more than a decade because of the difficulty in developing monospecific antisera. Immunofixation was introduced as "direct immunoelectrophoresis" 11 years later by Wilson when he applied antisera on the surface of the agarose immediately after completion of electrophoresis. IgD monoclonal protein was discovered by Rowe and Fahey in 1965 [37] and a year later, Ishizaka *et al.* isolated IgE [38].

MONOCLONAL VERSUS POLYCLONAL GAMMOPATHIES

Jan Waldenstrom introduced the concept of monoclonal versus polyclonal gammopathies in the Harvey Lecture Series in 1961 [39]. He described a monoclonal protein as having a narrow band of hyperglobulinemia in the electrophoretic pattern while those with hypergammaglobulinemia producing a broad band as having a polyclonal increase in protein. Patients with monoclonal proteins usually have multiple myeloma or macroglobulinemia, while those with polyclonal hypergammaglobulinemia have an inflammatory or infectious process. Those patients with a monoclonal pattern, but no evidence of multiple myeloma or macroglobulinemia, were considered to have "essential hypergammaglobulinemia" or a "benign monoclonal protein." Today, the preferred term is monoclonal gammopathy of undetermined significance (MGUS) because some of these proteins will remain stable for many years and not cause a problem while in others, multiple myeloma, macroglobulinemia, light chain (AL) amyloidosis or a related disorder may develop [40].

THERAPY OF MULTIPLE MYELOMA

Treatment of multiple myeloma has improved markedly since the days of Sara Newbury's treatment with rhubarb pills and infusion of orange peel, or the phlebotomy, leeches, steel, quinine and other agents given to Thomas McBean. Although many advances have occurred, multiple myeloma is still an incurable disease.

Urethane

Alwall described a patient with multiple myeloma in 1947 who was treated with urethane (ethyl carbamate) and had an increase in hemoglobin from 60% to 87%, decrease in serum globulin concentration from 5.9 g/dL to 2.2 g/dL, disappearance of proteinuria and a reduction in bone marrow plasma cells from 33% to 0% [41]. The standard of therapy for multiple myeloma was urethane until Holland *et al.* randomized 83 patients with treated or untreated multiple myeloma to receive urethane or a placebo consisting of cherry- and cola-flavored syrup [42]. The objective response and survival were not significantly different between the two treatment groups.

Melphalan

Blokhin and colleagues from Moscow reported in 1958 that 3 of 6 patients with multiple myeloma obtained benefit from sacrolysin (L-phenylalanine mustard, Melphalan) [43]. Bergsagel and his colleagues at MD Anderson reported that 8 of 24 patients with multiple myeloma had significant improvement from Melphalan while 6 others obtained more modest benefit [44].

Subsequently, Melphalan given as a loading dose for one week followed by a low dose produced some response in 78% of 64 patients with newly diagnosed or previously treated multiple myeloma [45].

Prednisone

Prednisone as a single agent produced significant decreases in serum globulin levels and increases in hematocrit in a placebo-controlled double-blind trial in 1962 [46]. There was no improvement in survival when compared with placebo. Prednisone in a single dose of 200 mg every other morning produced benefit in 8 of 10 patients with poor-risk myeloma [47]. In an analysis of two Cancer and Leukemia Group B (CALGB) myeloma treatment studies, prednisone as a single agent produced a 44% objective response [48]. Survival was 6 months longer in a randomized trial comparing Melphalan and prednisone with Melphalan alone in a trial of 183 myeloma patients published by Alexanian *et al.* in 1969 [49].

Alkylator Combinations

The first reported combination of alkylating agents included Melphalan, cyclophosphamide and carmustine (BCNU) in 1972 by Harley *et al.* [50]. The M-2 protocol consisting of a combination of carmustine, cyclophosphamide, Melphalan, vincristine and prednisone produced excellent subjective and objective responses in 60% of 36 myeloma patients [51].

The combination of carmustine, Melphalan, cyclophosphamide and prednisone (BCMP) compared to MP in 252 patients, revealed no survival benefit from the BCMP regimen [52]. The Myeloma Trialists Collaboratorive Group reported a large meta-analysis of individual data from 4,930 persons in 20 randomized trials comparing MP with various combinations of alkylating agents. The response rates were higher with combinations of chemotherapy (60% vs. 53% for MP, $p < 0.0001$). There was no significant difference in response duration or overall survival. Consequently, Melphalan remained the mainstay of myeloma treatment for decades [53].

Stem Cell Transplantation

The first report of stem cell transplantation was published in 1957 when Thomas *et al.* treated six patients (one had multiple myeloma) with total body irradiation or chemotherapy followed by an intravenous infusion of bone marrow cells [54]. Thomas moved to Seattle in 1963 and continued his research on stem cell transplantation, which finally led to his Nobel prize in 1990. Syngeneic bone marrow transplantation was reported in 1982, when two physician brothers were the patients [55]. Four years later, Fefer *et al.* described five myeloma patients who received a syngeneic bone marrow transplant [56]. Ten of 14 patients with multiple myeloma received an allogeneic bone marrow transplant from an HLA-compatible sibling donor and survived for a median of 12 months [57].

The first autologous bone marrow transplantation was reported by McElwain and Powles in 1983 [58]. Four years later, Barlogie *et al.* used Melphalan 140 mg/m^2 and total body irradiation (150 cGy) followed by autologous allogeneic bone marrow transplantation in multiple myeloma patients refractory to chemotherapy [59]. Subsequently, Barlogie developed intense treatment programs using tandem autologous transplantation which he called "total therapy" - a term and concept pioneered for childhood leukemia at St. Jude Children's Research Hospital in Memphis. Clinical trials of transplantation regimens played a major role in establishing high-dose therapy and stem cell rescue as standard therapy for multiple myeloma.

Novel Agents

In the past decade, thalidomide [60], bortezomib [61], and lenalidomide [62] have been introduced and have revolutionized the treatment of multiple myeloma.

Thalidomide

Thalidomide was introduced as a sedative and as a treatment for morning sickness of pregnancy in 1957. Four years later, it was found that severe teratogenic malformations were associated with drug exposure during the first trimester of pregnancy. Fortunately, the drug was not approved in the United States. Two separate clinical trials for patients with advanced cancer reported no benefit when treated with thalidomide [63, 64]. However, only a few myeloma patients were included in these trials. Thalidomide was used for leprosy, Behcet syndrome, graft-versus-host disease and HIV-associated oral ulcers and wasting. Thalidomide was approved for the treatment of erythema nodosum leprosum with a safety system termed "The System for Thalidomide Education and Prescribing Safety program (STEPS)." D'Amato and Folkman recognized the antiangiogenic properties of thalidomide [65]. Singhal and Barlogie published a landmark trial that enrolled 84 myeloma patients for whom Melphalan and prednisone had failed [60]. Almost one-third of the patients responded to thalidomide.

Bortezomib

The 20S proteasome cylinder hydrolyzes ubiquitin-tagged proteins into small polypeptides. Inhibition of the proteasome leads to apoptosis with malignant and proliferating cells being particularly susceptible [66, 67]. Orlowski *et al.* reported antimyeloma activity in a phase I study [68]. Bortezomib showed activity against myeloma cells in several clinical models [69]. It produced response in one-third of 202 patients with relapsed, refractory myeloma [61].

Lenalidomide

Lenalidomide is a 4-aminosubstituted analog of thalidomide and belongs to a group of "immunomodulatory drugs." Phase I trials in relapsed/refractory myeloma were reported by Richardson *et al.* in 2002 [70]. Rajkumar *et al.* reported a phase II trial conducted at Mayo Clinic which showed that 31 of 34 patients (91%) with newly diagnosed myeloma obtained an objective response with thalidomide plus dexamethasone [62]. Two large phase III trials have shown a significantly superior time to progression with lenalidomide plus dexamethasone compared with placebo plus dexamethasone in patients with relapsed myeloma [71, 72].

REFERENCES

[1] Solly S. Remarks on the pathology of mollities ossium with cases. Med Chir Trans 1844;27:435-61.

[2] Kyle RA. Multiple myeloma: anodyssey of discovery. Br J Haematol 2000; 111(4): 1035-44.

[3] Macintyre W. Case of mollities and fragilitas ossium, accompanied with urine strongly charged with animal matter. Med Chir Trans 1850; 33: 211-32.

[4] Bence Jones H. On the new substance occurring in the urine of a patient with mollities ossium. Philos Trans R Soc Lond 1848; 138: 55-62.

[5] Steensma DP, Kyle RA. A history of the kidney in plasma cell disorders. Contrib Nephrol 2007; 153: 5-24.

[6] Kyle RA. Henry Bence Jones--physician, chemist, scientist and biographer: a man for all seasons. Br J Haematol 2001; 115(1): 13-8.

[7] Bence Jones H. An autobiography (with elucidations at later dates by his son, A. B. Bence Jones). London: Crusha & Sons Limited (privately printed) 1929.

[8] Bence Jones H. On gravel, calculus and gout; chiefly an application of Professor Liebig's physiology to the prevention and cure of these diseases. London: Taylor and Walton 1842.

[9] Bence Jones H. On the state in which the uric acid exists in the urine. London: R. Kinder 1845.

[10] Rosenbloom J. An appreciation of Henry Bence Jones, M.D., F.R.S. (1814-1873). Ann Med Hist 1919; 2: 262-4.

[11] Putnam FW. Henry Bence Jones: the best chemical doctor in London. Perspect Biol Med 1993; 36(4): 565-79.

[12] Rosenfeld L. Henry Bence Jones (1813-1873): the best "chemical doctor" in London. Clin Chem 1987; 33(9): 1687-92.

[13] Fleischer R. Ueber das Vorkommen des sogenannten Bence Jones'schen Eiweisskoerpers im normalen Knochenmark. Arch Pathol Anatom Physiol Klin Med 1880; 80: 842-49.

[14] Bayne-Jones S, Wilson DW. Immunological reactions of Bence Jones proteins. II. Differences between Bence Jones proteins from various sources. Bull Johns Hopkins Hospit 1922; 33: 119-25.

[15] Korngold L, Lipari R. Multiple myeloma proteins. III. The antigenic relationship of Bence Jones proteins to normal gammaglobulin and multiple myeloma serum proteins. Cancer 1956; 9: 262-72.

[16] Edelman GM, Gally JA. The nature of Bence-Jones proteins. Chemical similarities to polypetide chains of myeloma globulins and normal gamma-globulins. J Exp Med 1962; 116: 207-27.

[17] Weber H. Molities ossium, doubtful whether carcinomatous or syphilitic. Trans Pathol Soc Lond 1867; 23: 186-7.

[18] Adams W. Mollities ossium. Trans Pathol Soc Lond 1872; 23: 186-7.

[19] Kahler O. Zur symptomatologie des multiplen myeloms: Beobachtung von Albumosurie. Prager Med Wochenschr (Prague) 1889; 14(33): 45.

[20] Weber FP. General lymphadenomatosis of bones, one form of'multiple myeloma'. J Pathol 1898; 5: 59-64.

[21] Weber FP, Hutchinson R, Macleod JJR. Multiple myeloma (myelomatosis), with Bence-Jones protein in the urine (myelopathic albumosuria of Bradhaw, Kahler's disease). Am J Med Sci 1903; 126: 644-65.

[22] Geschickter CF, Copeland MM. Multiple myeloma. Arch Surg 1928; 16: 807-63.

[23] Arinkin MI. Die intravitale Untersuchungsmethodik des Knochenmarks. Folia Haematologie 1929; 38: 233-40.

[24] Rosenthal N, Vogel P. Value of the sternal puncture in the diagnosis of multiple myeloma. J Mount Sinai Hospital 1938; 4: 1001-19.

[25] Bayrd ED, Heck FJ. Multiple myeloma: a review of eighty-three proved cases. J Am Med Assoc 1947; 133: 147-57.

[26] Waldeyer W. Ueber Bindegewebszellen. Archiv fuer Microbiol Anat 1875; 11: 176-94.

[27] Cajal SR. Estudios histologicos sobre los tumores epiteliales. Rev Trimest Microgr 1896; 1: 83-111.

[28] Marschalko T. Ueber die sogenannten Plasmazellen, ein Beitrag zur Kenntniss der Herkunft der entzuendlichen Infiltrationszellen. Arch Derm Syphilo 1895; 30: 241.

[29] Wright JH. A case of multiple myeloma. Trans Assoc Am Phys 1900; 15: 137-47.

[30] Perlzweig WA, Delrue G, Geschicter C. Hyperproteinemia associated with multiple myelomas: report of an unusual case. J Am Med Assoc 1928; 90: 755-57.

[31] Lerner AB, Watson CJ. Studies of cryoglobulins. I. Unusual purpura associated with the presence of a high concentration of cryoglobulin (cold precipitable serum globulin). Am J Med Sci 1947; 214: 410-5.

[32] Tiselius A. A new apparatus for electrophoretic analysis of colloidal mixtures. Trans Faraday Soc 1937; 33: 524.

[33] Tiselius A, Kabat EA. Electrophoretic study of immune sera and purified antibody preparation. J Exp Med 1939; 69: 119-31.

[34] Longsworth AB, Shedlovsky T, MacInnes DA. Electrophoretic patterns of normal and pathological human blood serum and plasma. J Exp Med 1939; 70: 399-413.

[35] Kunkel HG, Tiselius A. Electrophoresis of proteins on filter paper. J Gen Physiol 1951; 35(1): 89-118.

[36] Grabar P, Williams CA.[Method permitting the combined study of the electrophoretic and the immunochemical properties of protein mixtures; application to blood serum.]. Biochim Biophys Acta 1953; 10(1): 193-4.

[37] Rowe DS, Fahey JL. A New Class of Human Immunoglobulins. I. a Unique Myeloma Protein. J Exp Med 1965; 121: 171-84.

[38] Ishizaka K, Ishizaka T, Hornbrook MM. Physicochemical properties of reaginic antibody. V. correlation of reaginic activity with gamma-E-globulin antibody. J Immunol 1966; 97: 840-53.

[39] Waldenstrom J. Studies on conditions associated with disturbed gamma globulin formation (gammopathies). Harvey Lectures 1960-1961; 56: 211-31.

[40] Kyle RA. Monoclonal gammopathy of undetermined significance. Natural history in 241 cases. Am J Med 1978; 64(5): 814-26.

[41] Alwall N. Urethane and stilbamidine in multiple myeloma: report on two cases. Lancet 1947; 2: 388-9.

[42] Holland JR, Hosley H, Scharlau C, *et al.* A controlled trial of urethane treatment in multiple myeloma. Blood 1966; 27(3): 328-42.

[43] Blokhin N, Larionov L, Perevodchikova N, Chebotareva L, Merkulova N.[Clinical experiences with sarcolysin in neoplastic diseases.]. Ann N Y Acad Sci 1958; 68(3): 1128-32.

[44] Bergsagel DE, Sprague CC, Austin C, Griffith KM. Evaluation of new chemotherapeutic agents in the treatment of multiple myeloma. IV. L-Phenylalanine mustard (NSC-8806). Cancer Chemother Rep 1962; 21: 87-99.

[45] Hoogstraten B, Sheehe PR, Cuttner J, *et al.* Melphalan in multiple myeloma. Blood 1967; 30(1): 74-83.

[46] Mass RE. A comparison of the effect of prednisone and a placebo in the treatment of multiple myeloma. Cancer Chemother Rep 1962; 16: 257-9.

[47] Salmon SE, Shadduck RK, Schilling A. Intermittent high-dose prednisone (NSC-10023) therapy for multiple myeloma. Cancer Chemother Rep 1967; 51(3): 179-87.

[48] McIntyre OR, Pajak TF, Kyle RA, Cornwell GG, 3rd, Leone L. Response rate and survival in myeloma patients receiving prednisone alone. Med Pediatr Oncol 1985; 13(5): 239-43.

[49] Alexanian R, Haut A, Khan AU, *et al.* Treatment for multiple myeloma. Combination chemotherapy with different Melphalan dose regimens. JAMA 1969; 208(9): 1680-5.

[50] Harley JB, Ramanan SV, Kim I, *et al.* The cyclic use of multiple alkylating agents in multiple myeloma. W V Med J 1972; 68(1): 1-3.

[51] Lee BJ, Sahakian G, Clarkson BD, Krakoff IH. Proceedings: Combination chemotherapy of multiple myeloma with alkeran, cytoxan, vincristine, prednisone, and BCNU. Cancer 1974; 33(2): 533-8.

[52] Harley JB, Pajak TF, McIntyre OR, *et al.* Improved survival of increased-risk myeloma patients on combined triple-alkylating-agent therapy: a study of the CALGB. Blood 1979; 54(1): 13-22.

[53] Combination chemotherapy versus Melphalan plus prednisone as treatment for multiple myeloma: an overview of 6,633 patients from 27 randomized trials. Myeloma Trialists'Collaborative Group. J Clin Oncol 1998; 16(12): 3832-42.

[54] Thomas ED, Lochte HL, Jr., Lu WC, Ferrebee JW. Intravenous infusion of bone marrow in patients receiving radiation and chemotherapy. New Engl J Med 1957; 257(11): 491-6.

[55] Osserman EF, DiRe LB, DiRe J, Sherman WH, Hersman JA, Storb R. Identical twin marrow transplantation in multiple myeloma. Acta Haematol 1982; 68(3): 215-23.

[56] Fefer A, Cheever MA, Greenberg PD. Identical-twin (syngeneic) marrow transplantation for hematologic cancers. J Natl Cancer Inst 1986; 76(6): 1269-73.

[57] Gahrton G, Tura S, Flesch M, *et al.* Bone marrow transplantation in multiple myeloma: report from the European Cooperative Group for Bone Marrow Transplantation. Blood 1987; 69(4): 1262-4.

[58] McElwain TJ, Powles RL. High-dose intravenous Melphalan for plasma-cell leukaemia and myeloma. Lancet 1983; 2(8354): 822-4.

[59] Barlogie B, Alexanian R, Dicke KA, *et al.* High-dose chemoradiotherapy and autologous bone marrow transplantation for resistant multiple myeloma. Blood 1987; 70(3): 869-72.

[60] Singhal S, Mehta J, Desikan R, *et al.* Antitumor activity of thalidomide in refractory multiple myeloma.[see comment][erratum appears in N Engl J Med 2000; 342(5): 364]. New Engl J Med 1999; 341(21): 1565-71.

[61] Richardson PG, Barlogie B, Berenson J, *et al.* A phase 2 study of bortezomib in relapsed, refractory myeloma[see comment]. New Engl J Med 2003; 348(26): 2609-17.

[62] Rajkumar SV, Hayman SR, Lacy MQ, *et al.* Combination therapy with lenalidomide plus dexamethasone (Rev/Dex) for newly diagnosed myeloma. Blood 2005; 106(13): 4050-3.

[63] Grabstald H, Golbey R. Clinical experiences with thalidomide in patients with cancer. Clin Pharmacol Ther 1965; 6: 298-302.

[64] Olson KB, Hall TC, Horton J, Khung CL, Hosley HF. Thalidomide (N-Phthaloylglutamimide) in the treatment of advanced cancer. Clin Pharmacol Ther 1965; 6: 292-7.

[65] D'Amato RJ, Loughnan MS, Flynn E, Folkman J. Thalidomide is an inhibitor of angiogenesis. Proc Natl Acad Sci USA 1994;91(9):4082-5.

[66] Orlowski RZ, Eswara JR, Lafond-Walker A, Grever MR, Orlowski M, Dang CV. Tumor growth inhibition induced in a murine model of human Burkitt's lymphoma by a proteasome inhibitor. Cancer Res 1998; 58(19): 4342-8.

[67] Adams J, Palombella VJ, Sausville EA, *et al.* Proteasome inhibitors: a novel class of potent and effective antitumor agents. Cancer Res 1999; 59(11): 2615-22.

[68] Orlowski RZ, Stinchcombe TE, Mitchell BS, *et al.* Phase I trial of the proteasome inhibitor PS-341 in patients with refractory hematologic malignancies. J Clin Oncol 2002; 20(22): 4420-7.

[69] Hideshima T, Richardson P, Chauhan D, *et al.* The proteasome inhibitor PS-341 inhibits growth, induces apoptosis, and overcomes drug resistance in human multiple myeloma cells. Cancer Res 2001; 61(7): 3071-6.

[70] Richardson PG, Schlossman RL, Weller E, *et al.* Immunomodulatory drug CC-5013 overcomes drug resistance and is well tolerated in patients with relapsed multiple myeloma. Blood 2002; 100(9): 3063-7.

[71] Dimopoulos M, Spencer A, Attal M, *et al.* Lenalidomide plus dexamethasone for relapsed or refractory multiple myeloma. N Engl J Med 2007; 357(21): 2123-32.

[72] Weber DM, Chen C, Niesvizky R, *et al.* Lenalidomide plus dexamethasone for relapsed multiple myeloma in North America. N Engl J Med 2007; 357(21): 2133-42.

CHAPTER 2

Epidemiology and Etiology of Multiple Myeloma

Brenda M. Birmann[1*], Brian C.-H. Chiu[2], Kristin Muench[3], Catherine A. Suppan[1] and Wendy Cozen[3]

[1]Channing Laboratory, Department of Medicine, Brigham and Women's Hospital and Harvard Medical School, Boston, MA; [2]Department of Health Studies, University of Chicago, Chicago, IL and [3]Department of Preventive Medicine Norris Comprehensive Cancer Center, Keck School of Medicine, University of Southern California, Los Angeles, CA

Abstract: Multiple myeloma (MM) is a yet incurable malignancy of mature B lymphocytes that account for approximately 1% of all cancers in Whites and 2% of all cancers in Blacks in the United States (US). Demographic patterns of MM incidence and mortality are well described, but more precise characterization of individuals at the greatest risk for MM to have proven elusive. A vast body of literature on the etiology of MM identifies a few likely risk factors—including family history of MM or MGUS and the potentially modifiable risk factor, obesity—but also illustrates the inconsistencies that arise in the epidemiologic study of rare and lethal malignancies due to inherent methodologic and practical challenges. The study of risk factors for the benign precursor condition called monoclonal gammopathy of undetermined significance (MGUS) lags behind that of MM. However, recent studies on MGUS have provided intriguing new insights on the natural history of monoclonal gammopathy, including demonstration of the occurrence of MGUS prior to essentially all diagnoses of MM and the suggestion that MGUS and MM share several etiologic factors. Improved characterization of risk factors for MM, MGUS, and MGUS progression is necessary to inform the development of MM prevention strategies. In the following review, we offer a summary of the current understanding of the descriptive epidemiology and etiology of MM and MGUS and suggest areas of focus for future research.

Keywords: MGUS, incidence, mortality, socioeconomic status, survival, familial risk, genetic risk factors, autoimmune conditions, environmental and occupational exposures, lifestyle factors.

1. INTRODUCTION

Multiple myeloma (MM), also called plasma cell myeloma, is a malignancy of mature B lymphocytes, or plasma cells [1]. MM is characterized by monoclonal proliferation of plasma cells in the bone marrow, which is accompanied by the secretion of abnormally high levels of paraproteins such as monoclonal immunoglobulin (Ig) or Ig light chains (*i.e.*, "M-protein") into the blood and/or urine [2]. Osteolytic lesions, bone pain, anemia, hypercalcemia, and renal insufficiency are among the clinical signs and symptoms that also contribute to the diagnosis. A related tumor, plasmacytoma, is characterized by the same clinical signs as MM but occurs as a single lesion. Patients with abnormal secretions of paraproteins (<30.0 g/*L*) who lack malignant invasion of the bone marrow and the clinical syndromes typical of MM are labeled with "monoclonal gammopathy of undetermined significance (MGUS)," a premalignant lesion [3]. In addition, a proportion of patients have "smoldering multiple myeloma," a clinical intermediate between MGUS and true MM that is characterized by the presence of high paraprotein levels and/or bone marrow plasmacytosis in the absence of the clinical symptoms of organ damage [2].

MM is the second most common hematologic malignancy and is expected to account for 20,180 new cancer diagnoses and 10,650 cancer deaths in the United States (US) in 2010 [4]. As detailed in other chapters of this book, tremendous breakthroughs in clinical translational research have paved the way for novel targeted therapies and effective combinations of drugs, therefore improving the prognosis and quality of life of persons diagnosed with MM. However, research on the etiology of MM and MGUS, and in

*Address correspondence to Brenda M. Birmann: Channing Laboratory, Department of Medicine, Brigham and Women's Hospital and Harvard Medical School, 181 Longwood Avenue, Boston, MA 02115. Ph. 617-525-2251; Fax: 617-525-2008; E-mail: nhbmb@channing.harvard.edu

Klaus Podar and Kenneth C. Anderson (Eds)

particular the identification of modifiable risk factors that could be incorporated into prevention strategies, has advanced less rapidly due to numerous methodological and practical challenges. For example, the relatively low incidence and poor survival of this malignancy tend to limit the number of MM patients who can be included in any given study, especially those of prospective design. Due to the smaller sample sizes of many studies and to differing approaches to collecting data, the published data are inconsistent with regard to many putative risk factors. Nonetheless, in spite of such challenges, epidemiology studies have contributed important insights on the etiology of MM and MGUS, which have been recently reviewed in considerable detail [5]. The following review is intended to present a narrative synthesis of the published data rather than a technical discussion, with commentary on study design or data quality where relevant, and to propose areas of focus for future study.

2. DESCRIPTIVE EPIDEMIOLOGY AND DEMOGRAPHIC RISK FACTORS FOR MM INCIDENCE AND MORTALITY

MM comprises 10% of all new blood cancers and 1% of all cancer deaths. In 2009, an estimated 11,680 US men and 8,900 US women developed MM and 5,640 US men and 4,940 US women died from MM [6]. Each year in the US, there are on average 7 new diagnoses of MM in men and 4 new diagnoses in women per 100,000 persons at risk. Plasmacytoma occurs much less frequently with less than 1 newly diagnosed case per year expected per 100,000 persons at risk (men and women combined). The discussion below pertains only to MM unless otherwise specified.

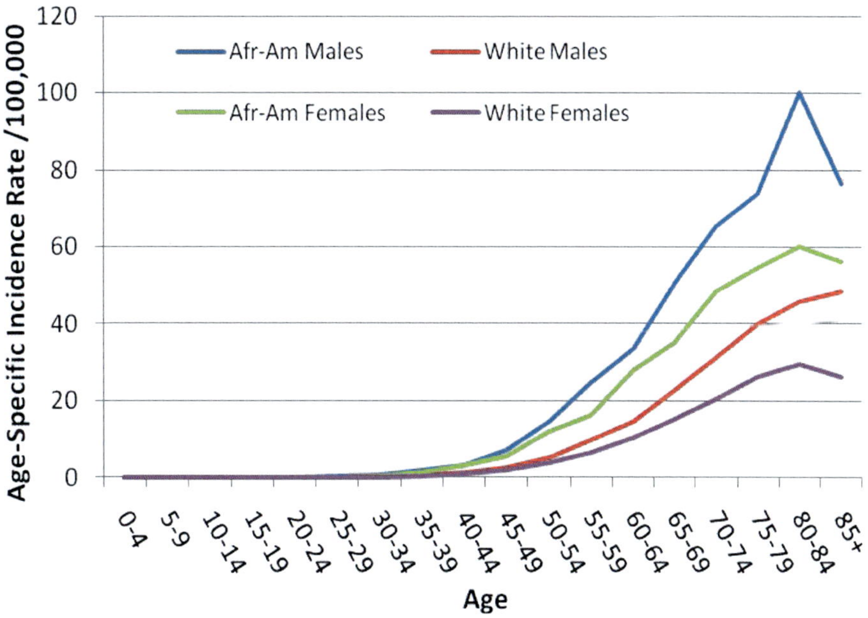

Fig. (1). Average annual age-specific incidence rates of multiple myeloma, 1973-2006, Surveillance, Epidemiology and End-Results Program.[a]

MM rarely develops before age 35 (Fig. **1**). The occurrence rises sharply between the ages of 35 and 60. Incidence rates continue to rise, though not as drastically, after age 65 and begin to decline a decade later. Men experience about 50% higher incidence rates than women, and African-Americans have much higher incidence rates than Whites (about 2.5 times higher). In fact, African-Americans have long experienced the highest incidence rates in the world (Fig. **2**) for yet unknown reasons.

---

[a]Surveillance Research Program, National Cancer Institute SEER*Stat software (www.seer.cancer.gov/seerstat), Version 6.5.2. Surveillance, Epidemiology, and End Results (SEER) Program (www.seer.cancer.gov) SEER*Stat Database: Incidence-SEER 9 Registries Limited-Use, Nov. 2008 Submission (1973-2006).

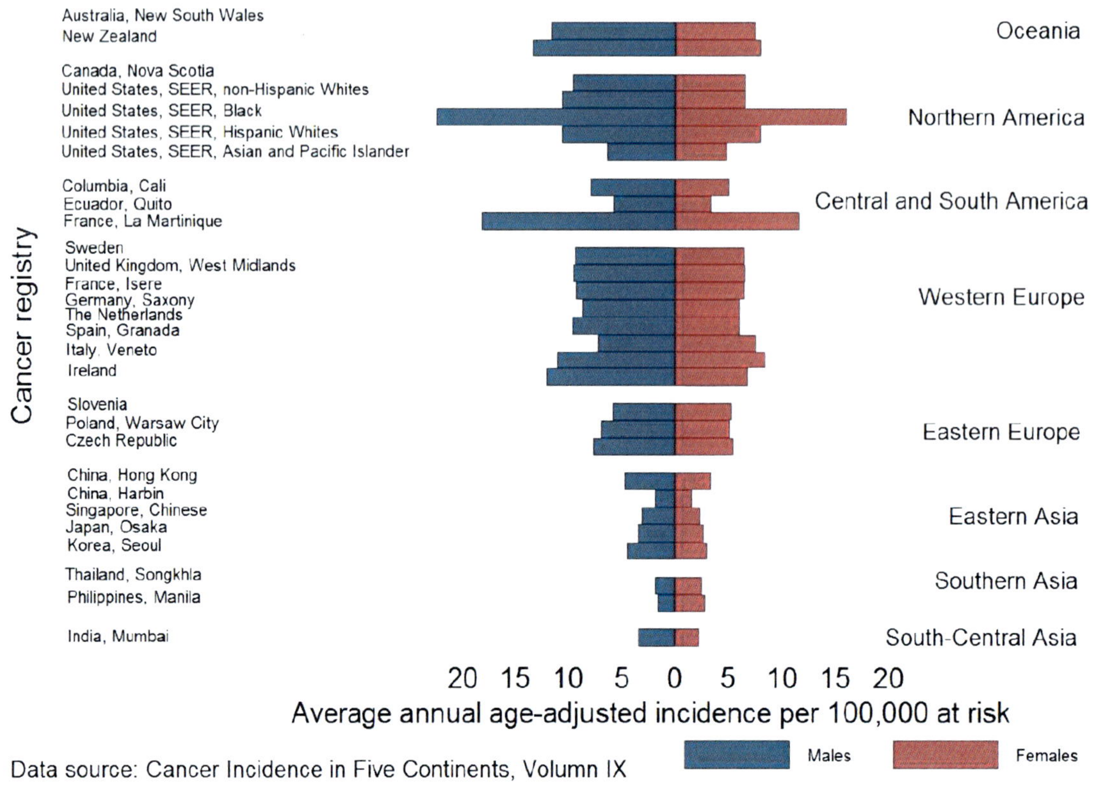

Fig. (2). International incidence rates of multiple myeloma in persons 35 years of age and older (Cancer in Five Continents, Volume IX).

The occurrence of MM shows marked geographic variation (Fig. **2**). Incidence rates tend to be higher in countries with populations of European origin and lower in countries with populations of Asian origin. Ireland has the highest incidence rate among European countries, and Filipinos have incidence rates that are intermediate between Europeans and Asians. Cancer registry data from sub-Saharan Africa are presently too limited to document what are assumed to be higher MM incidence rates in Africans; however, the population of Martinique, most of which is of African origin, has incidence rates similar to those of African-Americans (Fig. **2**). Several hospital-based studies in South Africa showed higher MM incidence rates among populations of African origin compared to those of European origin in South Africa [7,8] and Zimbabwe [9]. Higher incidence rates have been reported among the mostly African populations of Martinique [10], Jamaica [11,12], and Curacao [13]. Grulich and colleagues reported a 2- to 3-fold increased rate of death from MM among African and Caribbean migrants to England and Wales compared to the native British White population. Landgren and colleagues noted that Ghanaian men have a 2-fold increased age-adjusted prevalence of the MM precursor MGUS relative to White men from Rochester County, Minnesota [14], and thus the risk of MM may be similarly elevated. Overall, there is strong and consistent evidence of a higher risk of MM and its precursor in populations of African origin compared to those of European origin. There are no known explanations for these racial risk differences.

The incidence of MM and plasmacytoma (combined) was examined in Los Angeles, California using data from the population-based cancer registry that collects information on over 99% of cancer patients diagnosed in the region since 1972 [15]. A 2.2- to 2.4-fold higher risk among African-Americans compared to Whites was observed, consistent with other reports [16-21]. In the Los Angeles study the sharp age-related increase in MM incidence was evident at an earlier age in African-Americans than in Whites by approximately 10 years [15]; a similar earlier rise in age-incidence rates in African-Americans is also evident in the broader US population (Fig. **2**). In Los Angeles, Hispanics had the second highest risk, only slightly (about 20%), but significantly, higher than Whites. Furthermore, Hispanics who had been born in the US were 16% less likely to develop plasma cell tumors than Hispanics born elsewhere [15].

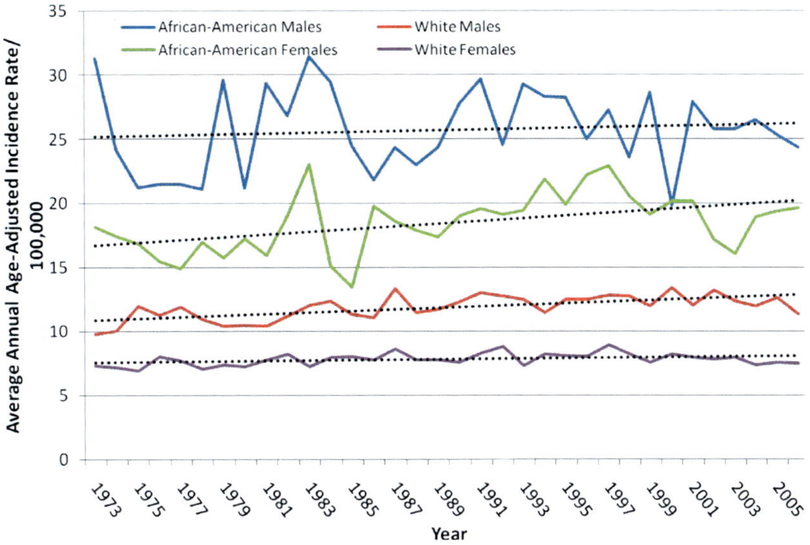

Fig. (3). Time trends of plasma cell myeloma incidence rates in the United States, 1973-2006, Surveillance, Epidemiology and End-Results Program.[b]

In the US, incidence rates of MM appear to be increasing fastest among African-American women and White men, each at a statistically significant rate of approximately 0.5% per year as observed from 1973-2006 [22] (Fig. **3**), while African-American men and White women did not experience significant increases in incidence rates over the same time period. Incidence rates did not vary notably from 1973-1997 in regions covered by 11 cancer registries in two East Asian and five European countries [23].

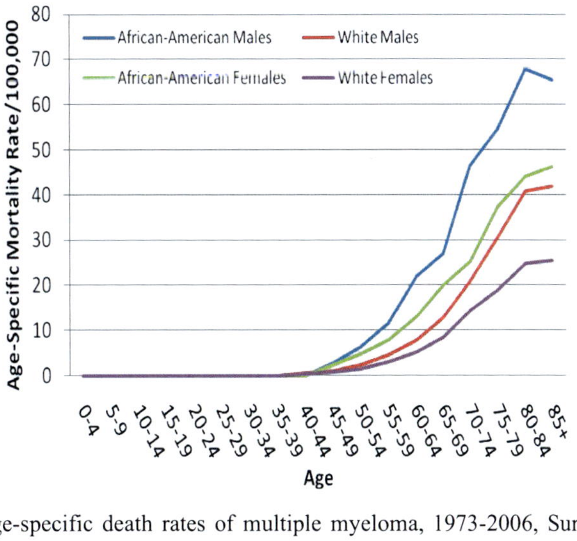

Fig. (4). Average annual age-specific death rates of multiple myeloma, 1973-2006, Surveillance, Epidemiology and End-Results Program.[c]

---

[b]Surveillance Research Program, National Cancer Institute SEER*Stat software (www.seer.cancer.gov/seerstat), Version 6.5.2. Surveillance, Epidemiology, and End Results (SEER) Program (www.seer.cancer.gov) SEER*Stat Database: Incidence-SEER 9 Registries Limited-Use, Nov. 2008 Submission (1973-2006).

[c]Surveillance Research Program, National Cancer Institute SEER*Stat software (www.seer.cancer.gov/seerstat), Version 6.5.2. Surveillance, Epidemiology, and End Results (SEER) Program (www.seer.cancer.gov) SEER*Stat Database: Incidence-SEER 9 Registries Limited-Use, Nov. 2008 Submission (1973-2006).

MM mortality rates follow very similar demographic trends to incidence rates (Fig. **4**). Starting around the age of 40 *i.e.*, shortly after incidence rates begin to rise—mortality rates begin to rise sharply in African-Americans and Whites, and in both men and women, and rise steadily until around age 80. Mortality rates tend to be 2-fold higher in men than women at any given age; race- and age-combined mortality rates are approximately 4.4 and 2.9 deaths per 100,000 for men and women, respectively [24]. Of note, this gender discrepancy in mortality rates is greater than the 1.5-fold male excess that is typically observed for incidence rates, suggesting an influence of gender on disease progression as well as on susceptibility. The mechanisms for these gender differences are not known. In the US, African-Americans have an approximately 2-fold higher MM mortality rate than Whites; the rates are highest in African-American men, at 8.2 per 100,000, and second-highest in African-American women at 5.4 per 100,000. Asian and Pacific Islanders have some of the lowest MM mortality rates at 1.7 per 100,000, age and gender combined, followed by American Indian and Alaska Natives at 2.4, and Hispanics at 2.8 [24]. Over the past few decades, MM mortality rates in the US have remained steady with few fluctuations (Fig. **5**) [25], in contrast to notable increases in MM mortality rates that were observed during the middle of the 20th century in the US and in England and Wales [26,27].

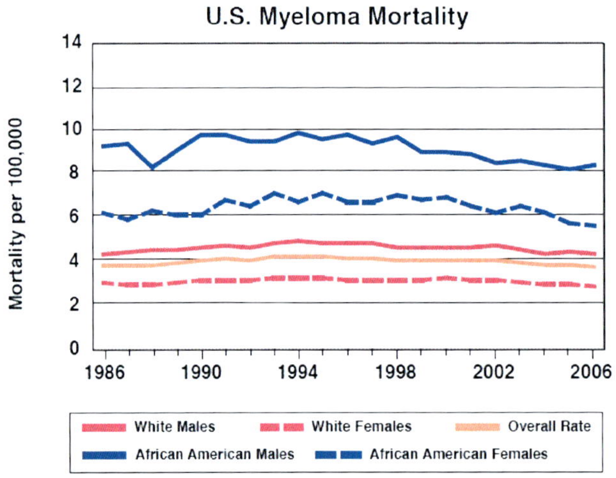

Fig. (5). Time trends of multiple myeloma mortality rates in the United States, 1986-2006.[d]

Socioeconomic Status

Two descriptive studies using data from population-based registries covering the entire populations of Sweden, the US, and Los Angeles County reported a positive relationship between indices of increasing socioeconomic status (SES) and MM risk [15,28]. In the latter study [15], SES was classified at the individual level according to census tract residence at the time of diagnosis, with each census tract assigned a ranking from 1 to 5 based on average income and education [29]. A trend toward higher incidence rates with increasing SES was observed among men and women of each racial group except Asians and was especially apparent among African-Americans. Two case-control studies used occupational indicators for SES [30,31] but found opposing results. A nested case-control study using the American Cancer Society cohort found an inverse relationship between educational level and MM risk [32], and another found no association [33].

SES was also evaluated in relation to MGUS in two studies conducted by Landgren and colleagues [14,34]. In a sample of Ghanaian men recruited from the general population in Accra there was no relationship between MGUS and educational status [14], whereas the study conducted in a cohort of southern US

[d]National Cancer Institute. 2009. A Snapshot of Myeloma. Available: http://www.cancer.gov/aboutnci/servingpeople/cancer-snapshots.

Whites and African-Americans found a non-significant inverse association of MGUS with education that appeared to be modified by obesity [34].

It is important to note that both SES and education are linked to participation in studies; in particular, persons of lower SES and extremely high SES are less likely to participate [35], therefore studies that rely on recruitment of participants are more subject to bias when examining the relationship between SES and disease. On the other hand, descriptive studies using cancer registry data for an entire population usually lack accurate data on individuals'SES, so studies evaluating SES and cancer with those data could be affected by misclassification of SES. Because occupation and obesity are MM risk factors and both are linked to SES, careful studies controlling for these factors are necessary to clarify the relationship of SES with MM and MGUS. Based on the current studies, there is no consistent evidence for a link between SES and MM risk independent of obesity and occupation.

Collectively, the descriptive epidemiologic data indicate that age, gender, and race are important demographic predictors of MM incidence and mortality, whereas the influence of SES is less clear. The mechanisms underlying these demographic associations are not known but likely involve a complex interrelationship of genetic, physiologic, lifestyle, and other environmental components.

Survival

Historically, patients with MM have had poor survival rates. Overall 5-year survival rates were 28.5% for White males, 32.1% for African-American males, 27.0% for White females and 31.3% for African-American females and were shown to decrease substantially with age in each race-gender subgroup during the years 1973-2003 [36]. African-Americans had marginally better survival than Whites during this period; however, by 10 years post-diagnosis, the majority of patients in any demographic group were deceased. With the development and introduction of several new treatment modalities in the late 1990s and early 2000s, including autologous stem cell transplantation and agents such as thalidomide and bortezomib, the survival pattern began to change [37]. Survival for patients younger than 60 years at diagnosis has improved among White men and women in the US (Fig. **6A**), with 10-year relative survival increasing from 18.5% of patients diagnosed before 1996 to 34.8% of person diagnosed after 1996. In comparison, 10-year survival for younger African-Americans, and for patients older than 60 in both ethnic groups, did not significantly improve (Fig. **6A** and **B**).

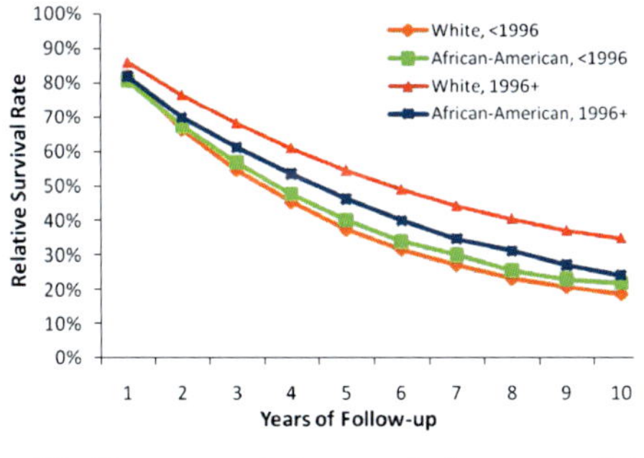

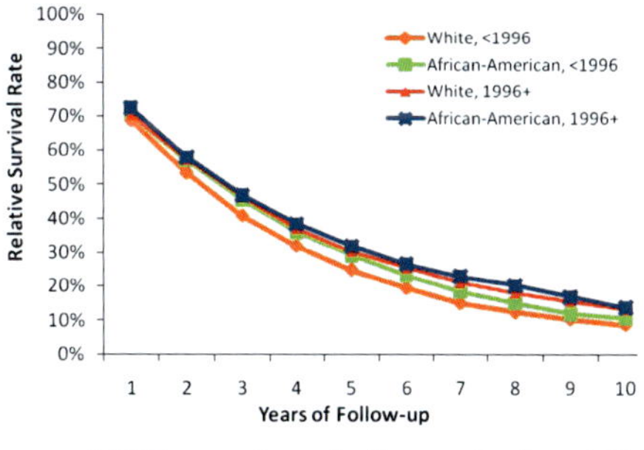

Fig. (6). Ten year relative survival curves of African-American and White patients before and after 1996, using survival data from SEER 17 registries, 1973-2006. **A** Multiple myeloma relative survival rates in patients diagnosed at < 60 years of age. **B** Multiple myeloma relative survival rates in patients diagnosed at 60+ years of age.

A study in the Netherlands also found an increase in survival for younger, White MM patients since the mid-1990s, with 5-year survival rates increasing from 34% of patients diagnosed between 1989-1992 to 56% of those diagnosed between 2001-2005 [38]. The improved survival of younger patients appeared to coincide with increasing trial participation and increasing use of high-dose chemotherapy and autologous stem-cell transplantation. Similarly, a population-based study of 773 patients diagnosed with MM in Malmö, Sweden from January 1, 1950 through December 31, 2005 reported a significant increase in the median overall survival of patients age ≤65 years at diagnosis, but not in those >65 years, across the five calendar periods examined [39]. The median overall survival of the younger patients more than doubled during the study period, with the most marked improvement observed for patients diagnosed in 2000-2005. As in the Netherlands study, the improvement in survival among younger patients appeared to coincide with an increase in the use of high-dose chemotherapy and autologous stem cell transplantation as a first-line treatment in this group [39]. The Malmö study corroborated an earlier registry-based analysis conducted in Sweden [40] on MM patients diagnosed from 1973 to 2003. In that study, Kristinsson and colleagues observed improved 1-year survival in all age groups, and significantly improved 5- and 10-year survival in patients younger than age 70 or 60 at diagnosis, respectively. In addition to the aforementioned increased use of high-dose therapy and autologous stem cell transplantation, these authors also credited improvements in supportive care measures as an important factor in the increased survival of the younger patients. In a study that followed patients from time of relapse or from time of diagnosis, the patients who had relapsed or were diagnosed with MM from January 1, 1997 through December 31, 2006 had a marked improvement in overall survival time compared to those who had relapsed or were diagnosed earlier (23.9 vs 11.8 months, $p = <0.001$ and 44.8 vs 29.9 months, $p<0.001$ respectively) [41]. They also found that patients treated with newer drugs (*i.e.* thalidomide, lenalidomide, and bortezomib) had longer survival from relapse (30.9 vs 14.8 months, $p<0.001$) confirming the important contribution of these novel therapies to recent improvements in survival.

The reported improvements in the survival of younger MM patients are encouraging, and continuing progress in the development of targeted therapies is likely to further extend survival. The recent survival data also urge several important priorities for ongoing clinical and translational research, including the improvement of therapeutic options for older patients and of access to novel modalities and clinical trials for underrepresented populations. A better understanding of the etiology and natural history of MGUS and MM through epidemiologic research is also critically important, to make possible the development of prevention strategies that will complement the clinical therapeutic approaches to diminishing the population burden, suffering, and costs from this still incurable malignancy.

3. HOST FACTORS

Monoclonal Gammopathy of Undetermined Significance (MGUS)

MGUS is itself an asymptomatic condition, but persons with MGUS are predisposed to developing MM. In the following paragraphs, we briefly summarize the current understanding of the prevalence and etiology of MGUS and predictors of progression to MM. Additional information on MGUS is incorporated, when available, into the appropriate discussions of the descriptive epidemiology and etiology of MM.

Demographic patterns of MGUS occurrence appear to closely resemble those described earlier for MM. The population prevalence of MGUS has been estimated at approximately 0.5%-1.0% of White adults of any age [42-45] and increases steadily with age; in White populations MGUS occurs in 2%-3.5% of persons age 50 years or older, in 3-5% of those age 70 years or older, and in nearly 9% of men older than 85 years [42-47]. MGUS has an approximately 3-fold higher prevalence in Blacks than in Whites in the US [48,49]. Similarly, a study of 917 African male blood donors in Accra, Ghana reported an age-adjusted prevalence of MGUS that was 2-fold higher than that observed in White men in Minnesota [14]. In a cohort of adult Japanese atomic bomb survivors in Nagasaki City, Japan [50], the overall prevalence of MGUS was 2.1% (2.4% among those 50 years of age or older). The prevalence of MGUS is higher in men than women [47,50].

At present, little is known about the etiology of MGUS. Several studies that examined familial risk of MGUS and MM support an approximate 2- to 3-fold increase in the risk of MGUS among first-degree relatives of MGUS and/or MM patients [51-53] as well as a 5-fold increase in MGUS risk among first-degree relatives of patients with Waldenström macroglobulinemia/lymphoplasmacytic lymphoma [54]. Evidence from genetic susceptibility studies supports an association with MGUS for polymorphisms in genes related to cytokine signaling [55-61]. In addition, several autoimmune, infectious, or inflammatory disorders were associated with risk of MGUS in a retrospective cohort study of US male veterans [62]. Many of the conditions that were associated with MGUS also demonstrated an association with MM in the same study population. In the Agricultural Health Study, an increased risk of MGUS was observed among male pesticide applicators, and in relation to exposure to specific pesticides [63]. Lastly, an analysis of obesity and risk of MGUS in the Southern Community Cohort Study suggested that obesity was independently associated with MGUS and predicted an 80% increase in risk of MGUS after adjustment for age and race [34]. These etiologic data are discussed in greater detail in conjunction with the corresponding discussions on MM. The findings observed to date are often based on sparse data and require confirmation in additional studies but collectively suggest that MGUS and MM share many common etiologic factors.

An important unresolved question is that of predicting risk of progression from MGUS to malignancy. MGUS patients have an average annual risk of progression of 1.5% that was shown to persist for at least 25-35 years among 241 MGUS patients in Minnesota [64,65]. Of interest, although the prevalence of MGUS is higher in Blacks than in Whites, the risk of progression to MM appeared to be similar across racial groups [49]. The concentration of the M-protein spike at time of MGUS diagnosis is a consistent predictor of risk of progression, and IgA isotype also frequently predicts persons at a higher risk of MM; other features are less consistently predictive (reviewed in [5,66]). Careful evaluation of the clinical data on MGUS progression has led to a consensus definition of progression risk profiles and recommendations for the optimal clinical monitoring of patients in the various risk categories [66]. However, many questions remain unanswered regarding predictors of progression, including the contribution of non-clinical factors such as patient lifestyle. Potential interventions are not yet available to diminish the risk of malignant transformation [67], although the natural agent curcumin has demonstrated potential in a small chemoprevention study and warrants further investigation [68]. Candidate chemopreventive agents and other preventive strategies are best examined in persons at greatest risk for progression [69]. Therefore, studies to characterize risk factors for progression remain an important priority.

Two important questions were recently addressed in large prospective US cohorts with extensive serum repositories [52,70]: First, does MGUS precede all diagnoses of MM, and second, do patterns of serum M-protein and free light chains in MGUS patients predict risk of progression to malignancy? M-protein and related tests were performed on up to 6 samples per person that had been collected 2 to 10 years before cancer diagnosis in 71 MM patients from the Prostate, Lung, Colorectal, and Ovarian Cancer Screening Trial (PLCO) [52]. All (100%) of the samples from 2 years prior to diagnosis, and 82% of the samples collected 8+ years prior to MM diagnosis, had MGUS; the prevalence of MGUS observed among samples collected in years 3-7 pre-diagnosis ranged from 93% to 100%. The second study, conducted in repeat sera collected 2 to 15 years prior to diagnosis from 30 MM patients in the Department of Defense Serum Repository (DoDSR), reported comparable results [70]. Among the DoDSR patients, 90% (27 of 30) had detectable MGUS prior to MM diagnosis, and in a majority of the patients (23 of 30), all the sera collected up to 15 years pre-diagnosis had detectable MGUS. In both studies, many of the patients—close to half in the PLCO study [52]–showed stable patterns of M-protein and serum free light chains until diagnosis or shortly before. In the remaining PLCO patients, M-protein and serum free light chains showed patterns of increasing levels with decreasing time to diagnosis [52]. In 7 DoDSR patients whose temporal patterns could be fully evaluated pre-diagnosis, there was considerable inter-individual variability in the patterns, but all demonstrated a sharp rise in the kappa-lambda serum free light chain ratio 2 or more years pre-diagnosis [70].

The latter prospective studies demonstrated that virtually all MM diagnoses are preceded by MGUS, which in some patients may develop as early as 15 years prior to MM diagnosis and remain stable for many years. Those studies also illustrate the value to etiologic research of establishing and maintaining large cohorts with prospectively acquired, well-annotated, serial biospecimens. Further studies with larger populations of MM patients are needed to confirm these novel findings, and to explore the mechanisms by which stable MGUS is influenced toward malignant disease and the contribution from the putative genetic, environmental, and lifestyle-related risk factors for MM.

Familial Risk

Most studies to explore the familial aggregation of MM and/or MGUS were performed in families of European descent [71-80], although aggregation has also been observed in African-American families [81].

Four families were identified in which cases of MM occurred in more than one generation and demonstrated "anticipation," or the occurrence of MM diagnoses at progressively earlier ages with successive generations, a phenomenon known to occur in some heritable conditions [72,76,82,83]. Anticipation was not apparent in a study in a national population-based cancer registry in Sweden [84]. Collectively, however, the data from these families support a role for heritability in MM.

There are numerous methodological challenges to determining whether multiple-case families of MM or MGUS occur by chance or due to inherited susceptibility or other aspects of a family's shared lifestyle and environment, since it is not possible to identify suitable comparison families. Insights into the role of family history are therefore typically derived from studies that examine the risk of MM or MGUS in relation to whether or not first-degree relatives also had a history of MGUS, MM, another hematologic cancer, or other type of cancer, preferably with analytic control for other risk factors. In the following paragraphs, we summarize the research that has addressed these focal questions of familial risk of MM and MGUS.

Twin concordance studies can provide some of the most convincing evidence of disease heritability but are difficult to conduct because the frequency of MM is low and twins are uncommon. From a Scandinavian twin registry [85], 64 and 95 pairs of identical and fraternal twins were identified, respectively, in which one twin was diagnosed with MM. During the follow-up period one originally unaffected identical twin of a case also developed MM but the sample size is too small for definitive conclusions [85].

Familial risk of MM has been evaluated in population-based studies with varying designs, eight of which have reported an increased risk of MM given a family history of MM [51,86-92]. In four of these studies, the risk of MM was about 2-fold greater than the expected risk estimated from the corresponding general population rates of MM [51,86,87,90]. In an earlier registry-based Swedish study, the risk of MM was more than 5-fold higher among individuals who had a first-degree relative with MM than in persons who did not [89]. In a similar US based study, White MM patients had a non-significant 1.5-fold greater probability and African-American patients had a significant 17-fold greater probability of having a relative with the same disease compared to control subjects without MM [88], however both studies were based on fewer than 10 MM patients with affected relatives [88,89]. The association of family history with MM risk appears to be stronger in women than in men [86,90].

Four population-based studies have evaluated the relationship between family history of MGUS and MM and risk of these conditions [51,53,90,93]. A 2- to 3-fold increased risk of MGUS was observed among first-degree relatives of MGUS or MM patients in Minnesota [53]. Studies in Sweden have reported 2- to 3-fold higher risks of both MGUS and MM among first-degree relatives of persons with MGUS [51,93] compared to first-degree relatives of persons without MGUS. Of interest, when the associations were further examined by characteristics of the patients or their M-protein, the increased risk of MGUS was higher for females and older relatives (> 65 years) of MGUS patients [53], and the risk of MGUS and MM was increased most notably in relatives of patients with IgA or IgG MGUS compared to IgM [93]. The study in Iceland did not observe an increased risk of MGUS among first-degree relatives of MM patients but was limited by the small numbers of MM families [90].

The risk of MM and MGUS in persons with a family history of another malignancy has also been examined. In one study, a 5-fold risk of MGUS, but not MM, was observed among first-degree relatives of Waldenström macroglobulinemia/lymphoplasmacytic lymphoma patients [54]. In another study utilizing the Swedish Family Cancer Database, offspring of chronic lymphocytic leukemia patients had a 1.8-fold increased risk of MM, and relatives over 65 years of age had a 2-fold increased risk of MGUS [94]. In contrast, the risk of MM did not appear to be increased among relatives of non-Hodgkin lymphoma patients in the same Swedish database [86,95] nor among relatives of patients with Hodgkin lymphoma, chronic lymphocytic leukemia or other leukemias [86]. Relatives of Hodgkin lymphoma patients in Sweden and Denmark also had no excess risk of MM [96]. A family history of prostate cancer was marginally associated with an increased risk of MM among Whites, but not among African-Americans; in the same study there was no association of MM with a family history of other common cancers [88]. A family history of any cancer was associated with an approximate 1.4-fold increase in risk of MM in two case-control studies [87,97].

Taken together, the studies discussed above consistently support an approximate 2- to 3-fold greater risk of MGUS and MM among first-degree relatives of patients with these conditions. The evidence for a link between MGUS and MM and family history of other malignancies, including other hematologic cancers, remains inconsistent. Familial risks appear to be somewhat stronger in women and more prevalent in White families, although fewer studies of non-White families have been conducted to date. Further study is needed to clarify the basis of the familial associations and to characterize possible hereditary factors.

Genetic Risk Factors

The data on familial aggregation of MGUS and MM strongly suggest a role for genetic susceptibility in the etiology of these conditions. Because numerous biologic pathways are known to contribute to the natural history and pathogenesis of MGUS and MM, it is plausible that variation in genes that encode signaling molecules in those pathways also influence inherited susceptibility. Studies to examine putative genetic risk factors comprise a growing segment of the literature on MM etiology, although no genetic factors have been clearly confirmed to date. After a brief review of methodological issues that are important to consider when evaluating studies on the association of genetic variants with cancer (or other chronic disease), we summarize the epidemiologic literature on genetic risk factors for MGUS and MM. The data are organized by corresponding biologic pathway, and each section begins with a brief explanation of the presumed role for the given pathway in MM etiology. Throughout this summary, the gene symbols are written in *italics*, to distinguish between the gene and its encoded protein in keeping with current conventions.

Most epidemiologic studies of genetic susceptibility examine single nucleotide polymorphisms (SNP), nucleotide repeat polymorphisms, or insertion/deletion polymorphisms and, when possible, focus on variants for which a functional effect on the encoded protein can be postulated. The distribution of these variants can vary widely across different populations, so that an allele that is considered "wild type" due to its frequency in one population may be the "variant" or less common allele in another population. This fact can create spurious genetic associations when the MM cases and control subjects that are analyzed in a given study are obtained from different source populations. We have excluded case-control studies with fewer than 100 participants because these studies have inadequate sample size to detect potential small associations of a common variant with MGUS or MM. The smaller studies are also more vulnerable to the effects of chance on the sampling of participants (and thus genotypes) into the study population. Cohort and population-based case-control study designs are considered superior to hospital-based studies because the genetic factors of interest may be related to other diseases present in hospital controls, making results difficult to interpret. Nevertheless, we included data from hospital-based studies in the following discussion and noted the study design. As with any epidemiologic finding, the replication and validation of an association with MGUS or MM risk in subsequent studies is necessary before the association can be accepted as definitive. Such replication or validation has not been performed for the studies we summarize, and therefore we recommend that the findings be viewed as preliminary and interpreted with caution.

Xenobiotic Metabolism Pathway. Personal or occupational exposure to some xenobiotics (substances that do not naturally occur in the body, such as pesticides or solvents) is associated with risk of MM (discussed below in the section entitled "Occupational and Environmental Exposures"). Thus, variation in the genes that encode xenobiotic metabolizing enzymes has been the focus of several studies of genetic susceptibility to MM. Metabolism of xenobiotics occurs in two enzyme-mediated phases that ultimately detoxify the substance in preparation for excretion from the body, but which can also lead to the creation of potentially cytotoxic reactive intermediates. Phase I (activation) features activity by enzymes such as the cytochrome P450 oxidases (including CYP2E1, CYP1B1, CYP2C9), microsomal epoxide hydrolase (mEH), and myeloperoxidase (MPO). Phase II (conjugation) involves reactions catalyzed by enzymes such as the glutathione S-transferases (GSTM1, GSTT1, or GSTP1) and NAD(P)H:quinone oxidoreductase (NQO1). Variation in the genes that encode these enzymes (*i.e., CYP2E1, CYP1B1, CYP2C9, mEH, MPO, GSTM1, GSTT1, and NQO1)* may affect their function and therefore the degree of carcinogenic effect of exposure to the corresponding xenobiotic.

Evidence for an association of phase I enzyme gene variants with MM risk includes the finding of a positive association between a functional SNP in *CYP1B1* and risk of MM among both African-Americans and Whites [98]. The higher-risk (G) allele of this SNP is associated with increased activity of the CYP1B1 enzyme on several carcinogenic compounds, including compounds that have been associated with risk of MM in other studies [98]. Two SNPs in *CYP1A1* (*i.e.*, CYP1A1*1/*2A and CYP1A1*1/*2B) were inversely associated with MM risk in a Korean study [99]. In addition, a variant genotype for a polymorphism in *mEH* that is linked to higher enzyme activity predicted an increased risk of MM in an Australian hospital-based case-control study with healthy bone marrow donor controls [100]. With regard to variants in genes that encode phase II enzymes, SNPs in *GSTM1* and *GSTT1* were not associated with MM risk in Korea [99]. In the Australian study [100], an increased risk was suggested among persons with a low-activity genotype at a SNP in *NQO1*. The latter study also supported a significant trend of increasing MM risk with increasing numbers of higher-risk genotypes at SNPs in genes coding for *GSTT1, mEH*, and *NQO1* (p for trend =.001) [100]. In contrast, Maggini *et al.* found no association between *NQO1* or *GSTP1* polymorphisms and risk of MM in Italy [101]. Similarly, variants in *GSTM1, GSTT1* or *P53* were unassociated with risk in a hospital-based study with blood donor controls, although a variant genotype in codon 72 of *P53* seemed to be associated with disease progression [102].

In summary, the few studies that examined common variants in genes important to xenobiotic metabolism have reported some biologically plausible but also some contradictory findings. In addition, most studies included only a few loci per gene, so that a lack of association with the variants examined cannot be interpreted as a lack of association of the gene itself with susceptibility to MM. The contribution of genetic variation in these pathways to inherited susceptibility to MM requires further study.

One-Carbon Metabolism Pathway. To date, only three case-control studies have examined polymorphisms in genes that encode enzymes in the one-carbon metabolism pathway in relation to MM risk [103-105]. This pathway plays an essential role in DNA synthesis and methylation, and errors in these processes due to altered enzyme activity, including the aberrant activity that has been observed in association with certain polymorphisms in genes that encode one-carbon metabolizing enzymes [106], could affect the activation status of oncogenes that influence cell proliferation or survival. Selected polymorphisms in one-carbon metabolizing enzymes have been linked to several hematologic cancers [107-109] and have been postulated to influence the risk of MGUS or MM. A functional SNP (A2756G) in the gene coding for methionine synthase (referenced as *MTR* or *MS*) is believed to reduce enzyme activity and was positively associated with risk of MM in a hospital-based case-control study in Brazil [104]. In contrast, the same variant was inversely associated with MM in a Korean case-control study [103]. Of note, the frequency of the variant (G) allele was somewhat different in the respective study populations. This factor, along with the differences in study design and other unmeasured genetic and population characteristics likely contributed to the discrepant findings. SNPs in the gene that codes for another enzyme in this pathway,5,10- methylenetetrahydrofolate reductase (*MTHFR*), have also been evaluated but were not associated with risk of MM in any study to date [103-105]. Collectively, these preliminary data do not support an important role for variation in one-carbon metabolizing genes in the etiology of MM; however, the available data are clearly insufficient for conclusive inferences.

B Cell Activation and Survival. The complex sequence of processes involved in the normal differentiation and maturation of plasma cells is replete with opportunities for DNA rearrangement errors that can inadvertently lead to carcinogenic translocations such as those that activate an oncogene. Aberrations in one such process called class switch recombination (CSR), which generates different classes of antibody, is believed to be involved in the pathogenesis of MM [110]. Thus, variation in the genes that encode enzymes important to the rejoining of DNA strands that are broken during CSR, including DNA repair genes *XRCC3*, *XRCC4, XRCC5,* and the gene that encodes the enzyme DNA ligase IV (*LIG4*) could be associated with MM risk. A hospital-based study in Ireland reported a statistically significant association of a regulatory SNP in *XRCC5* and a suggestive association for a variant in *XRCC4* with MM risk, but no association for any variant examined in

XRCC3 [110]. In a United Kingdom (UK)-based study of two polymorphisms in *LIG4* that are in linkage disequilibrium, persons who carried variant alleles at one or both loci had a diminished risk of MM, with evidence of a dose-response [111]. These findings have not been validated by other groups.

Polymorphisms in genes involved in other aspects of normal B cell growth and differentiation, some of which are also potent growth factors for malignant plasma cells, are also thought to contribute to MM susceptibility. Consistent with this hypothesis, a variable nucleotide tandem repeat (VNTR) polymorphism in the gene that encodes one important MM growth factor, interleukin-6 (*IL6*) [112-114] was associated with a 60-70% lower risk of MM, and a rare SNP in *IL6* predicted a nearly 2-fold increased risk, in a multi-ethnic case-control study in Los Angeles [115]. The latter association was not confirmed in the Nurses'Health Study and Health Professionals Follow-up Study cohorts [116]. In those cohorts, suggestive associations with MM were observed for variants in the genes coding for the IL6 receptor (*IL6R*) and for insulin receptor substrate-1 (*IRS1*), a molecule important for proper signaling by insulin-like growth factor (IGF)-I, another potent growth factor for MM. In secondary analyses with additional controls, variants in several other genes related to IGF-I or IL6 signaling also had suggestive associations [116]. A common and presumed functional variant in *IL6* (rs1800795, commonly referenced as -174 G/C or -236 C/G) has been studied in several populations without demonstrating a link to MM [61,115-117].

Genes that encode other B cell stimulatory molecules have been examined in relation to MM risk as well. A polymorphism in the gene that encodes the interleukin-4 (IL4) receptor (*IL4R*) and a variant in the Fcγ receptor IIa gene (*FCGR2A*), which encodes an antibody receptor that is important in plasma cell interactions, were both positively associated with risk in a population-based case-control study of Connecticut women [117]. In a hospital-based study with blood donor controls, risk of both MM and MGUS was associated with specific VNTR polymorphisms in the gene that codes for IL-10 (*IL10*), another potent B cell stimulatory cytokine, and in the gene coding for the IL-10 receptor (*IL10R*) [60]. A microsatellite polymorphism in the gene that codes for cytotoxic T-lymphocyte-antigen-4 *(CTLA4)*, an important mediator of B cell-T cell interactions, was also associated with MM and MGUS risk [59]. There was no association with MGUS or MM for a functional SNP in *IL10* [60], nor with variation in genes that encode other cytokines, including IL-1β (*IL1β*) and IL-1 receptor-α (*IL1Rα*) [61].

Several studies have examined MM risk in relation to variation in genes involved inflammation and innate immunity. Four studies examined common variants in the gene that encodes tumor necrosis factor (TNF)- *α* (*TNFα*) or haplotypes in a haplotype block that covers the *TNFα* and lymphotoxin-*α* (*LTA*) genes (*i.e.*, *LTA*TNF*) [55-57,117]. Two studies observed an increased risk of MM and MGUS among persons who carried *LTA*TNF* haplotypes associated with higher cytokine production [55,56,117], and a third observed an association of the same variants just with MM [117]. In contrast, Zheng and colleagues did not observe an association of individual SNPs in *TNFα* with MM or MGUS [61], whereas Morgan and colleagues found a decreased risk of MM in carriers of the high producing *TNFα* allele and no additional gain from *LTA*TNF* haplotype analysis [57]. Genes important to innate immunity were investigated in relation to risk of MM in a population-based case-control study including 103 female cases [118]. Variants in the genes that encode plasminogen activator inhibitor type 1 (referenced as *SERPINE1*), hepatocyte growth factor (*HGF*), and C-C chemokine receptor type 7 (*CCR7*) were associated with MM; the observed associations were inverse for the SNPs in *SERPINE1* (rs2227667) and *CCR7* (rs3136685) and positive for the one in *HGF* (rs17501108) [118]. These findings have yet to be replicated.

With regard to gene variation in other pathways that may also contribute MM pathogenesis, two studies examined susceptibility to MM in relation to polymorphisms in the gene coding for the inhibitor of nuclear factor (NF)-kappa B (NF-κB), known as IκBα [58,119]. The NF-κB family of proteins function as transcription factors of anti-apoptotic genes that are usually blocked due to binding to inhibitors like IκBα in the cytoplasm [119] but which have demonstrated increased activity in MM cell lines [58]. In a small population of 18 MM cases and 24 healthy controls, three of eight SNPs in the gene encoding IκBα

(*NFKBIA*) were found to be positively associated with risk of MM [58]. A larger study of 157 MM patients enrolled in a clinical trial and 196 population-based controls enrolled in an adult leukemia study in the UK examined eight SNPs in *NFKBIA* [119] and reported apparent associations for two individual SNPs and one haplotype. The risk-associated variants were not consistent across the two studies, and neither study utilized an ideal design. Nonetheless, it is plausible that constitutive differences in regulation of this pathway may predict MM risk, and further investigation is warranted.

Functional variants in genes that encode molecules in cell cycle control or apoptosis pathways, such as caspase enzymes [120] may also influence cell survival and tumor growth by interfering with signals that normally lead to programmed cell death (apoptosis). To date, only two publications have reported on the association of variants in apoptosis-related genes and risk of MM. In the aforementioned study of Connecticut women [120], SNPs in the genes coding for caspase-3 (*CASP3* rs13113) and caspase-9 (*CASP9* rs1072576) were inversely associated with risk. In a separate analysis of the same study population that was restricted to non-Hispanic Whites, women who carried certain SNPs in the pro-apoptosis genes bcl-2–associated X protein (*BAX*) and receptor-interacting serine/threonine-protein kinase 1 (*RIPK1*) had a decreased risk of MM, whereas women with the variant (G) allele at rs751643 in *CASP9* had an increased risk [121]. Table **1** summarizes the published data on genetic susceptibility to MM at these loci and at others discussed above.

Table 1. Genes with one or more statistically significant risk loci for MM.

Author	Source of Controls	Number of Cases	Gene	Association*
Xenobiotic Metabolism Genes				
Lincz *et al.*, 2007†[a]	Blood donors	102	*mEH*	Positive
Kang *et al.*, 2008‡[b]	Blood donors	116	*CYP1A1*	Inverse
One-Carbon Metabolism Pathway				
Lima *et al.*, 2008†[c]	Blood donors	123	*MTR*	Positive
B Cell Differentiation and Plasma Cell Growth				
Birmann *et al.*, 2009§[d]	Cohort risk set	82	*IGF1*	Positive, inverse
			IGFBP3	Positive
			IRS1	Positive
			IL6R	Positive
Hayden *et al.*, 2007†[e]	Epilymph and hospital-based	306	*XRCC4*	Positive, inverse
			XRCC5	Positive
Spink *et al.*, 2007‡[f]	Leukemia Research Fund (pop-based)	157	*NFKB1A*	Positive
Brown *et al.*, 2007‡[g]	Population-based	127	*LTA*TNF*	Positive
			IL4R	Positive
			FCGR2A	Positive
Cozen *et al.*, 2006‡[h]	Relative and population-based	148	*IL-6*	Positive, inverse
Roddam *et al.*, 2002‡[i]	Leukemia Research Fund (pop-based)	270	*Ligase IV*	Inverse
Morgan *et al.*, 2005‡[j]	Leukemia Research Fund (pop-based)	181	*TNFα*	Inverse
			LTA	Inverse
Davies *et al.*, 2000‡[k]	Pop-based from a previous study	63MGUS / 198MM	*TNF/LT*	Positive
Zheng *et al.*, 2000[l] and 2001‡[m]	Pop-based from Stockholm area	27MGUS / 73MM	*CTLA-4*	Inverse
			IL-10	Positive
Purdue *et al.*, 2010‡[n]	Participants from another population-based case-control study	108	*SERPINE1*	Inverse

Table 1. cont....

			HGF	Positive
			CCR7	Inverse
Cell Proliferation, Differentiation, and Apoptosis Pathways				
Hosgood *et al.*, 2008‡ [o]	Population-based	128	*CASP3*	Inverse
			CASP9	Inverse
Hosgood *et al.*, 2009‡ [p]	Population-Based	108	*BAX*	Inverse
			CASP9	Inverse
			RIPK1	Inverse

[a] reference 102.
[b] reference 101.
[c] reference 106.
[d] reference 118.
[e] reference 112.
[f] reference 121.
[g] reference 119.
[h] reference 117.
[i] reference 113.
[j] reference 58.
[k] reference 56.
[l] reference 62
[m] reference 61
[n] reference 120.
[o] reference 122.
[p] reference 123.
* Genes with both positive and inverse associations noted had SNPs demonstrating each type of effect.
† Hospital-based case-control study.
‡ Population-cased case-control study.
§ Nested case-control study.

Collectively, the evidence from these studies of genetic mutations in pathways potentially involved in the development of MM indicates a plausible role for genetic susceptibility, consistent with the findings from the familial risk studies. Due to the limited coverage of most genes investigated in the studies summarized above, the null findings do not necessarily preclude a role for the corresponding gene. Likewise, a variant observed to predict risk of MM or MGUS may be an indirect marker of a "causal" locus rather than itself the causal SNP. Hence, the rapidly expanding literature on genetic susceptibility to MM and MGUS has only begun to scratch the surface of this complex but important area of study and cannot yet offer conclusive evidence for or against a role for any biologic pathway.

Prior Medical Conditions and Treatment

Although MM is a malignancy of plasma cells, malignant transformation is believed to occur at the stem cell or pre-B cell stage, *i.e.*, prior to a B cell's first exposure to antigen [122]. Chronic antigenic stimulation is therefore unlikely to contribute to malignant transformation but may promote the progression of MM by creating an immune milieu conducive to B cell proliferation. Conditions or therapeutic regimens that result in immune suppression or B cell activation may also increase the risk of MM by diminishing anti-tumor immune responses or promoting dysregulated cell growth. This hypothesis has motivated numerous studies on the association of a history of a different primary malignancy or of medical conditions characterized by chronic antigenic stimulation with risk of MM. The results have been inconsistent due largely to limitations of the study designs. For example, many studies were not able to verify that a medical condition was diagnosed prior to the onset of preclinical disease in persons who were subsequently diagnosed with MM. In addition, the methods used to characterize personal medical history differ across studies, as do the individual conditions assessed. In the following section, we summarize the published evidence for an association of MM with a history of certain medical conditions and related treatments, with discussion of relevant methodological limitations.

Multiple Myeloma as a Second Malignancy. A previous diagnosis of cancer is a potential risk factor for developing MM, which has been identified as one of the most frequent hematologic neoplasms to occur as a multiple primary cancer [123]. The mechanisms behind the association between a first and a subsequent primary cancer have yet to be fully established. Possible explanations include unmeasured or unknown shared exposures or susceptibilities [124], increased surveillance after diagnosis of a first primary cancer [125], initial staging of individuals with a first cancer for metastatic disease or a genetic predisposition for disease [125], treatment related damage [126-129], or possible cancer related immunosuppression [124,130-133]. Studies examining risk of MM in persons with a history of a different cancer diagnosis frequently base risk estimations on standardized incidence and mortality ratios (SIR and SMR respectively), which compare observed MM incidence or death rates with the corresponding expected rates estimated from an appropriate reference population. Some of the studies published to date suggest a link between history of other first primary cancers and MM, but the data are often sparse and contradictory. Table **2** summarizes the Surveillance, Epidemiology, and End Results (SEER) data on risk of MM as a second malignancy, much of which is discussed in the following paragraphs.

A few studies have examined personal history of skin cancer as a risk factor for MM. In a prospective mortality study, women with a history of non-melanoma skin cancer had a significant 50% greater risk of dying from MM in the years following first cancer diagnosis compared to women without a history of this cancer [124]. This study observed no risk for men. In contrast, a study based in a Canadian cancer registry found a significantly increased SIR for MM among men with a previous diagnosis of non-melanoma skin cancer, including a 36% increase in MM risk following basal cell (BCC) and a 65% increased risk following squamous cell carcinoma (SCC) [134].

The associations were evident across all follow-up intervals after skin cancer diagnosis, although the highest risk was found during the first 4 years. In the same study, women were found to have a significantly decreased risk of developing MM following both BCC and SCC diagnoses across all follow-up intervals with the exception of the first 4 years after diagnosis of BCC, when the risk of MM increased significantly.

Table 2. Risk of multiple myeloma as a second cancer following a previous cancer diagnosis, by site of first primary malignancy, from SEER Cancer Registries, 1973-2000.[a]

Site of First Primary Cancer*	#Subjects	Age at 1st Cancer Diagnosis (AAD)	Follow-up Interval (years)	Sex	O/E	Overall Excess Absolute Risk
Buccal Cavity and Pharynx						
Lip	1	Across all ages	1-4	Both	0.16	-0.28
Oral Cavity/Pharynx	14	Across all ages	Overall	Males	0.56	-0.99
Bone, Soft Tissue, and Kaposi's Sarcoma						
Kaposi's Sarcoma	3	Across all ages	Overall	Both	4.53†	10.71
Cancer of Soft Tissues¶	10	Across all ages§	1-4	Both ‡	2.76	0.52
Digestive Tract						
Liver/Intrahepatic Bile Duct	5	Across all ages	Overall	Males	3.77	5.28
Rectum	8	<50	Overall	Both	3.26	1.3
Colon	243	Across all ages	Overall	Both	0.92†	-0.23
Stomach	21	Across all ages§	Overall	Both	0.87†	-0.33
Pancreas	1	Across all ages	Overall	Both	0.15	-1.87
	1	>50	Overall	Both	0.15	-2.14
Gallbladder	0	Across all ages	Overall	Males	0†	-3.08

Table 2. cont....

Melanoma and Eye						
Ocular Melanoma	5	Across all ages§	1-4	Both ‡	3.34	1.35
	6	Across all ages	Overall	Female	3.15	3.35
	5	>50	1-4	Both	3.45	2.10
Lymphoma and Myeloma						
Hodgkin Lymphoma¶	5	40-59	Overall	Both	2.03†	1.02
Multiple Myeloma	3	Across all ages§	Overall	Both ‡	0.17	-2.09
	0	>70	Overall	Both	0	-3.76
NHL¶	35	Across all ages§	Overall	Both ‡	0.56	-0.8
Urinary Tract						
Renal Cell Carcinoma	11	>18	<1	Both	2.6	0.59
Kidney Parenchyma	12	>18	<1	Both	2.53	0.58
Thyroid and other Endocrine						
Thyroid	13	Across all ages	1-4	Both ‡	2.27	0.35
	3	40-49	1-4	Both	5.6	0.08
Male Genital Tract						
Prostate¶	11	Across all ages	>20	Males	3.24	0.01
	118	>70	5-9	Males	1.21	0.01
	13	>70	>10	Males	0.52	0.01
	4	Across all ages, with radiotherapy	>20	Males	4.11	0.04
Respiratory Tract						
Non-small Cell Lung¶	6	Across all ages, no radiotherapy	>10	Both	0.45	-0.34
Lung	91	Across all ages	Overall	Both	0.82†	-0.41
	5	50-69	>10	Both	0.41	-0.46
Larynx	21	Across all ages	Overall	Males	0.61	-1.06

Curtis RE, Freedman DM, Ron E, Ries LAG, Hacker DG, Edwards BK, Tucker MA, Fraumeni JF Jr. (eds). New Malignancies Among Cancer Survivors: SEER Cancer Registries, 1973-2000. National Cancer Institute.
NIH Publ. No. 05-5302. Bethesda, MD, 2006.

*Organized by organ system, modified from Cutis, *et al.*

† Non-significant findings

‡ EAR differences between genders

§ EAR changes based on AAD

¶ EAR changes based on radiotherapy treatment history

A recent systematic review of non-melanoma skin cancer and risk of second primary cancers found a significantly increased summary relative risk for MM among 21 registry-based studies [135]. In contrast to the non-melanoma skin cancer studies, a study in a Swedish cancer registry did not observe a clear excess of MM in men or women with a history of malignant melanoma [136].

Aside from skin cancer, several other cancers have been evaluated as potential risk factors for MM. One study based on the SEER program found a significant 61% increase in MM incidence following thyroid cancer among women (SIR= 1.61, 95% confidence interval (CI)=1.04–2.37) and a non-significant increase of similar magnitude among men [137]. When the analysis was stratified by age at diagnosis of MM, the SIRs remained elevated but were no longer statistically significant. This study was consistent with an earlier study completed in a cohort of thyroid cancer patients compiled from 13 population-based cancer registries (SIR=1.26, 95% CI= 0.89–1.74) [138] as well as a meta-analysis suggesting a similar significant association [139].

A few studies have looked at breast cancer and risk of MM with results varying by gender. One found a non-significant increase in risk of MM in men previously diagnosed with breast cancer; the risk of MM was evident across all follow-up periods combined and highest during the first year of follow-up [140]. In contrast, women with breast cancer had a significant 10% decrease in risk of MM in a study conducted in cancer registries around the world (SIR = 0.90; 95% CI = 0.82-0.99) [141]. Andersson *et al.* reported similar but non-significant reductions in MM risk that were apparent across age at first diagnosis and follow-up intervals, with the exception of increased risks observed for women aged 70+ at diagnosis and during 10 to 19 years of follow-up. Of note, Andersson *et al.* also found a decreased risk of MM among women who underwent radiotherapy for breast cancer (SIR= 0.1, 95% CI= 0.0-0.4) and those treated with Tamoxifen (SIR=0.4, 95% CI=0.0-1.0) and chemotherapy (SIR=0.6, 95% CI=0.0-1.5), as opposed to an increased risk of MM among women who did not undergo radiotherapy for breast cancer (SIR=1.3, 95% CI=0.8-1.8) or were not treated with Tamoxifen (1.1, 95% CI=0.7-1.6) or chemotherapy (1.0, 0.6-1.4). The heterogeneity in the risk of MM by breast cancer treatment modality was statistically significant for radiotherapy treatment [142].

One study to date has examined the risk of MM following endometrial cancer in the SEER population. Among women with endometrial cancer, the observed incidence of MM (543 per 100,000; 95% CI: 66-1962 per 100,000) was nearly 120-fold greater than the expected incidence ($P<0.05$) [143]. A 27-fold increase in MM was observed for first- degree relatives of these patients, suggesting a possible genetic link between endometrial cancer and MM [143]. Similarly, incidence of lymphatic and hematopoietic diseases, which included MM, was significantly increased in patients with hairy cell leukemia across all follow-up periods after leukemia diagnosis (SIR=3.09, $P <.05$) [133]. The SMR for death from lymphatic and hematopoietic diseases was also significantly elevated among these patients (SIR=33.81, $P<.05$). Both risk ratios decreased with length of follow-up (see Table **2**) [22].

In conclusion, the evidence does not strongly support an association between previous other malignancy and MM for most cancer sites. A possible exception is history of non-melanoma skin cancer, for which multiple individual studies and a systematic review observed a modest increase in MM risk. Studies of the association of MM with prior primary malignancies at other sites typically included too few MM patients to be informative and/or have not been replicated, and so their findings cannot be considered conclusive. Furthermore, most studies report the strongest increases in risk of MM during the first year of follow-up, which may reflect detection bias or an effect of immunologic alterations due to preclinical MM rather than an effect of the first primary cancer or its treatment on MM risk. Well-designed future studies of MM as a second malignancy may nonetheless provide insights into biologic pathways that contribute to MM etiology or help to identify cancer patients at higher risk for subsequent cancers and who could benefit from increased clinical surveillance or cancer prevention measures.

Autoimmune Conditions. Autoimmune diseases are frequently characterized by substantial up-regulation of inflammatory and B cell-stimulatory cytokines, and persons with these conditions have been hypothesized to have an increased risk of MM. Two early studies did not observe significant associations for history of autoimmune disorders or number of autoimmune disorders but lacked the statistical power to examine individual conditions [144,145]. In a retrospective cohort of Black and White US veterans [62], a history of any autoimmune disorder and a history of autoimmune disorders with systemic involvement each predicted a modest increase in risk of MM and MGUS.

Comparatively few individual autoimmune diseases have been reported in more than one or two publications in relation to risk of MM [5]. Several cohort [146-149] and case-control studies [150-154] reported modest to strong increases in MM risk among persons with a history of rheumatoid arthritis, but the relative risk estimates varied widely (1.2-8.0) and were in most instances based on 9 or fewer exposed MM cases. Other studies reported no association [62,92,155-157] or a non-significant inverse association of rheumatoid arthritis with MM [158,159]. Patients who were hospitalized for rheumatoid arthritis, who may have more severe or more accurately reported disease than those who self-reported a diagnosis, either did not have an increased risk of MM [152,160-162] or demonstrated an increased risk that appeared to diminish steadily with increasing time since hospitalization [161,163]. Apparent increases in MM risk soon after a hospital discharge may be explained by the existence of preclinical malignancy at the time of the hospitalization for rheumatoid arthritis. There is no evidence that an increased risk of MM in rheumatoid arthritis patients is explained by any particular treatment modality [155,164-167].

Persons with a history of pernicious anemia were also found to have an increased risk of MM. Cohort studies of patients with pernicious anemia in Sweden, Denmark, and the US reported a consistent and statistically significant 2- to 3-fold increase in MM risk among Whites [62,168-170] and a non-significant 1.7-fold increased risk among Black US veterans [62]. The US study also observed a significant 2-fold increase in risk of MGUS in Blacks and Whites combined [62]. In Denmark the association of pernicious anemia with MM appeared to be restricted to the earlier years of follow-up [170] and may be biased by preclinical MM. In contrast, in the US veterans, significant or marginal associations with MM (relative risks ranging from 2.0-2.5) persisted at 5 to 9 and 10+ years after diagnosis with pernicious anemia [62]. Population-based case-control studies in Sweden [92] and the US [158,160] also reported significant or suggested increases in risk (ORs ranging from 1.5 to 3.3). In Sweden, as in the Danish cohort, when the analysis was stratified by time since diagnosis of pernicious anemia, the association of pernicious anemia with MM was most striking within the first year and was not evident in more distant time intervals following diagnosis [92].

Numerous other conditions have been examined in only one or two studies or have repeatedly shown no association with MM [5,62,92,160]. For example, persons with a history of polymyalgia rheumatica had a nearly 2-fold increase in risk of MM in Sweden [92] but not in a US population-based study [160]. In the Swedish study, the association was restricted to the first year after diagnosis with polymyalgia rheumatica [92]. Autoimmune hemolytic anemia was associated with a 2- to 3-fold increase in MM risk that was statistically significant in the cohort study of US veterans [62] and non-significant in two case-control studies [92,171]. Of interest, autoimmune hemolytic anemia was also significantly associated with MGUS risk in the US veterans study [62]. In the Swedish case-control study a family history of systemic lupus erythematosus was associated with a statistically significant 2.7-fold increase in risk of MM [92], but a personal history of lupus was not significantly associated with MM in that or other study populations [62,92,157,158,160,172]. Autoimmune thyroid diseases have demonstrated an increased risk of MM in some [158,173] but not all [92,160] studies. The positive associations were not specific to a particular autoimmune thyroid condition and were based on sparse data. The US veterans study reported significant or suggested positive associations with MGUS for two systemic autoimmune disorders that were not associated with MM in the same study population: polymyositis/dermatomyositis, which was non-significantly associated with a 2-fold increased risk of MGUS, and systemic sclerosis, which predicted a significant 4-fold increase in MGUS risk [62].

Collectively, although some studies reported strong associations between one or more autoimmune conditions and MM, the data are inconsistent and the observed associations often limited to periods soon after diagnosis of the autoimmune disease. It remains unclear whether chronic antigenic stimulation from active autoimmune disease promotes the development of MM or whether the emergence of autoimmunity is itself a manifestation of immune disruptions from the preclinical malignancy. The conditions that were associated with both MM and MGUS are particularly intriguing, such as pernicious anemia and autoimmune hemolytic anemia. These associations warrant confirmation and further investigation to explore possible shared underlying mechanisms.

Asthma, Allergy, and Inflammatory Disorders. Numerous studies have examined the relation of a history of asthma with MM and found no evidence of an association between asthma [62,150,153,154,158,171,174-179], hospitalization for asthma [180], or use of asthma medications [153] with MM. Similarly, neither a history of allergy (in general) nor number of allergies was associated with MM in most population-based studies [137,144,158,178,181]. In the First National Health and Nutrition Examination Survey (NHANES I) study, a prospective analysis with only 7 exposed cases suggested a non-significantly increasing risk of MM with increasing number of allergies [145]. In contrast, two case-control studies, one hospital-based [182] and one population-based [153], reported a modest reduction in risk of MM among persons with a history of allergy. In one small hospital-based case control study that reported an increased risk of MM in persons with a history of allergy or allergy treatments [183], the types of allergies reported differed among MM patients and controls. Cases primarily reported symptoms such as hives, rashes, or swelling, whereas controls most frequently reported breathing difficulties. Other studies did not observe an association with MM for allergy shots or other allergy treatment such as anti-histamine [153,158,184]. Among studies that examined specific allergic conditions in relation to MM risk [62,150,154,158,159,175-178,181,185], the findings are inconsistent and collectively not supportive of a link for any specific type of allergy. The question of allergy and risk of MGUS has yet to be addressed.

In contrast to the null findings for asthma and allergy and related medications, several studies have suggested an increased risk of MM in persons with a history of inflammatory conditions, although the conditions included in the respective studies varied, rendering the findings difficult to compare. The aggregated entity, "total inflammatory disorders," which comprised a diagnosis of any of 11 inflammatory conditions, was associated with an 18% increase in risk of MM in the US veterans study [62]. A stronger 60% increase in MM risk was reported in persons with a history of chronic inflammatory conditions in a hospital-based case-control study in northern Italy [182]. In the prospective NHANES I study, number of inflammatory conditions was positively associated with MM in an analysis with only 8 exposed cases [145]. When individual conditions were examined separately, no specific chronic or acute inflammatory disease demonstrated a consistent association with MM (reviewed in [5]). Glomerulonephritis, nephrotic syndrome, and osteoarthritis were positively associated with both MGUS and MM among US veterans; latencies of up to 9 years were suggested for the association of glomerulonephritis or nephrotic syndrome with MM, whereas a latency as long as 10 or more years was apparent for some MGUS or MM patients with a history of osteoarthritis [62]. The authors of this study noted that physiologic effects of undetected MM may explain the association of these inflammatory conditions with MM, although the associations of the same conditions with MGUS (in some instances with similarly long latencies) help to mitigate those concerns [62].

Infections. The literature on infectious diseases and risk of MM features many of the methodological limitations noted for studies of other medical conditions: small numbers of exposed cases, inconsistent classifications of infection histories, and an uncertainty as to the relevance of the timing of the diseases of interest with regard to the prodromal period of MM. For example, in many instances it is difficult to conclude whether an observed association of a history of an infectious condition is a contributor to, or a manifestation of immune disruptions related to preclinical MM.

There is no clear evidence of an association of acute [158,182] or chronic bacterial infections [144,158,182] with MM risk. All four studies reporting on number of bacterial infections, including one prospective and three case-control studies, used different numbers of categories and boundaries. Not surprisingly, the findings were also inconsistent, suggesting an inverse association in the prospective study based on only 2 exposed cases [145], a positive association in the hospital-based case-control study [182], and no association [184] or a non-significant and weak inverse association [158] in the population-based case-control studies. A diverse panel of individual bacterial infections, as well as history of immunization against common bacterial infections, have been examined, but few have been reported by more than one or two studies [5]. Overall, most bacterial infections and related immunization histories were not consistently or significantly associated with MM.

The most consistent findings pertain to a personal history of pneumonia, which was non-significantly associated with a higher risk of MM among Blacks [158] but not Whites [158,184] in earlier US case-control studies but which has demonstrated a statistically significant positive association with MM in both Blacks and Whites in more recent studies in the US [62] and Denmark [186]. The Danish study was the most detailed and reported similarly increased risks of MM across subgroups of participants defined by latency interval (<5, 5+ years), number of infections (1, 2, 3+), and sex; the relative risks ranged from 1.4 to 1.8 across those strata [186]. Analyses stratified by age at MM diagnosis suggested a slightly stronger association of pneumonia with MM in younger (<65 years; relative risk (RR)=2.3) than older (65+ years; RR=1.5) MM patients. In the US veterans, the association of pneumonia with MM diminished somewhat but nonetheless persisted at 10+ years post-pneumonia [62]. A history of pneumonia also predicted risk of MGUS in the US veterans cohort—most strongly 2 to 4 years prior to MGUS diagnosis but apparent at 10+ years prior to MGUS [62]. Among the less consistent findings for bacterial infections, a history of bronchitis was positively associated with MM in one study [150] but not in two larger studies [153,186]. Likewise, an imprecise positive association observed in one study for history of pyelonephritis [182] was not subsequently confirmed [137]. A history of scarlet fever appeared to predict a 2-fold increase in risk of MM in the Italian hospital-based study [182] but was associated with a statistically significant 50% decrease in risk of MM in a larger population-based case-control study of women in Connecticut [153].

Findings related to a personal history of viral infections are similarly inconsistent in the classification of exposure, due in part to the varying approaches to classify infection history—*i.e.*, based on serologic confirmation of past or chronic infection by a specific agent versus self-report of a condition typically associated with a virus infection. There is little evidence to support an important role for a history of any viral infection [182], number of viral infections [184], or any of several individual viruses [5,62,186], in the etiology of MM. Patients with AIDS have demonstrated an increased risk of MM in several studies designed to study AIDS-related malignancy [187-189]. Strong associations of MM with HIV seropositivity in the range of 2.6 to 12 have been reported [189-191]. In an Australian cohort study, an increased risk of MM was reported that was primarily restricted to persons with a prior diagnosis with AIDS, and MM risk increased with increasing time since AIDS onset [190]. As has been observed for other non-AIDS-defining hematologic cancers, in the era of highly active antiretroviral therapy the elevated risk of MM in HIV-infected persons has persisted or even increased due in part to prolonged survival with HIV [192-195]. Hepatitis C virus (HCV) has also been positively associated with MM in population-based studies of varying designs [196-198] but not in hospital-based case-control studies in Europe [199-201] or a US cohort [202]. Of interest, a marginally significant 30% increase in MGUS risk was observed among HCV-positive members of a cohort of US veterans, whereas HCV infection was not associated with MM in that population [203]. An increased risk of MM in persons with a history of hepatitis was apparent in some [137,159] but not all [158,184] studies. Lastly, an increased risk of MM was suggested in persons with a history of history of *Herpes zoster* (shingles) in several studies [137,176,182] but was restricted to Blacks in a US study [158] and not evident in others [151,184]. The association of shingles with MM was strongest in the first 10 years post-shingles diagnosis in one population [176] but was weakest in the first 4 years post-diagnosis in a US retrospective cohort [62].

In summary, the role of bacterial and viral infections in the etiology of MM remains unclear, possibly due in part to the uncertainty regarding the relative onsets of an infectious disease and preclinical MM. Prospective studies with the ability to consider latency and to serologically confirm infection status are necessary to further explore the more intriguing virus-MM associations, such as HIV and possibly HCV. At present, the literature does not support a strong association of bacterial or viral infections with risk of MM.

Other Conditions. Limited data are available on a variety of other chronic or acute diseases and risk of MM, and most conditions do not appear to be associated [5]. In contrast, one recent, large US population-based case-control study reported that a history of solid organ transplantation, and especially kidney transplantation, was approximately twice as prevalent in persons with MM as in population controls [204]. The relative risk of MM increased sharply with increasing number of years since transplantation. These findings support an etiologic role for immune suppression in MM and warrant confirmation in other populations.

4. ENVIRONMENTAL AND OCCUPATIONAL EXPOSURES

Radiation

Several studies have been conducted investigating the effects of radiation on the development and etiology of MM; however the findings are varied and often contradictory. Radiation exposure can cause DNA damage that can interfere with switch recombination machinery to increase the likelihood of IgH translocations and oncogene deregulation that may ultimately promote the development of MM [205]. Among Hiroshima and Nagasaki atomic bomb survivors, an excess of death from MM was noted [206,207]. However, a comprehensive analysis of data on the incidence of MM in those populations from 1950-1987 showed no evidence for an increased risk of MM [208]. Radiation does not appear to affect the incidence of MGUS either. Neriishi *et al.* [209] performed serum electrophoresis in the A-bomb survivor cohort and found no significant increase in the prevalence of M-proteinemia with increasing radiation dose. However, the frequency of transformation from MGUS to MM appeared to be higher in the exposed than in the non-exposed survivors (26% v. 16%, respectively) [210]. This difference was not statistically significant and the transformation rate is similar to that previously reported in the general population [65].

There is little evidence for an association of occupational exposure in the nuclear industry with the development of MM [211,212]. Compared with unexposed workers, a higher risk of death from MM was found among radiation-exposed workers at three US nuclear weapons plants [213]. However, no excess of MM mortality was reported by the British Nuclear Fuels occupational cohort [214] or a cohort of Japanese radiation workers at nuclear facilities [215]. Epidemiologic studies have also evaluated the association between radiation and risk of MM among atmospheric nuclear test participants, and the findings are generally null [216,217].

There is no strong evidence supporting an excess risk of MM among medical radiation workers. In an early study, Lewis [218] reported an excess of MM deaths among American radiologists, but no association was found in the 90,305 men and women participating in the US Radiologic Technologists Health Study [219]. Similarly, no excess of MM was found among 27,000 diagnostic X-ray workers in China during a 30-year period [220]. There was no excess risk of MM among Canadian dental workers exposed to ionizing radiation either [221].

Individuals receiving diagnostic or therapeutic radiation also do not appear to be at a higher risk of MM. Although a small, non-significant association was found between the highest cumulative number of diagnostic X-ray procedures and the risk of MM in a nested case-control study with over 200 cases of MM [222], no association has been reported in most case-control [175,223] or cohort [224] studies. Exceptions include a significantly higher risk of plasmacytoma observed in Danish women who had received alpha-emitting thorotrast for cerebral arteriography [225], and small excesses of MM deaths reported in patients who received X-ray treatment for ankylosing spondylitis [226] and metropathia hemorrhagica [227]. While the work done regarding radiation and MM is reasonably extensive, the results from this work are not yet conclusive.

Agricultural Work and Pesticides

The association between MM and farming has been extensively studied [228]. Although findings are not entirely consistent, the majority of cohort [229-231] and case-control [232-234] studies reported a positive association that was typically small to moderate in magnitude [228]. These studies included a cohort of almost 3 million Swedish workers followed for 19 years [231], which found a significantly elevated incidence of MM in the agriculture/forestry/fishing sector. Separate meta-analyses of mortality and of cancer incidence that examined studies conducted among farmers found reasonably consistent excesses for MM [235,236]. In one meta-analysis of 13 case-control studies of hematopoietic cancer occurrence in pesticide related occupations, Merhi *et al.* [235,236] found a small positive association between occupational exposure to pesticides and MM (OR=1.16; 95% CI=0.99-1.36). Another meta-analysis of 32 peer-reviewed studies of MM and farming published between 1981 and 1996 found a slightly stronger positive association between farming and MM (OR=1.23; 95% CI=1.14-1.32) [235].

Despite this evidence for an association between farming activities and risk of MM, the exposures responsible for this association are not entirely clear. Farmers may come into contact with many potentially hazardous chemicals such as pesticides, chemical fertilizers, solvents and other chemicals, engine fuels and exhausts, organic and inorganic dusts, welding fumes, and zoonotic viruses [205,228]. Pesticides may operate through a variety of mechanisms, including genotoxicity, tumor promotion, and immunotoxicity [237]. Several studies have investigated the association between pesticides and MM; some reported elevated risks and others did not [205,228,237]. Pesticides encompass a heterogeneous group of chemicals and only a handful of studies have evaluated the role of specific pesticides. The results from those studies are inconsistent [238,239]. In contrast, the Agricultural Health Study cohort recently reported an excess risk of MM associated with several specific herbicides, including alachlor, atrazine, and glyphosate [234,240,241]. Of note, the prevalence of MGUS among 678 pesticide applicators in the Agricultural Health Study was twice that observed in a comparison to population-based sample of 9469 men from Minnesota [63]. In addition, among pesticide applicators, a 5.6-fold (95% CI, 1.9-16.6), 3.9-fold (95% CI, 1.5-10.0), and 2.4-fold (95% CI, 1.1-5.3) increased prevalence of MGUS was observed among users of the chlorinated insecticide dieldrin, the fumigant mixture carbon-tetrachloride/carbon disulfide, and the fungicide chlorothalonil respectively [63]. Thus, while important questions remain regarding the specific associations of farming activities, pesticides, and herbicides with risk of MM, these studies collectively suggest that exposure to these activities and chemicals can increase the risk of MM and may influence disease pathogenesis at an early stage.

Benzene and Other Organic Solvents

Benzene, which is present in crude oil at most stages of petroleum production and distribution, is classified as a group 1 human carcinogen by the International Agency for Research on Cancer [242]. Numerous epidemiologic studies have evaluated the potential role of benzene exposure in the development of MM, and the results are generally null [243-247]. In particular, individual studies found no evidence for excess mortality or dose-response [246], or of increased MM incidence [248]. Results from meta-analyses also provide little support for an association between benzene or organic solvent exposure and MM. In a meta-analysis of 55 cohort mortality studies across different industries, Chen and Seaton [244] found a non-significant excess of death from MM. In an analysis of the published case-control studies, Bezabeh *et al.* [249] found no increase of MM from exposure to benzene or to chemical groups that included benzene. However, a recent meta-analysis of seven benzene cohort studies with 22 observed deaths from MM (13.67 expected) reported a weighted relative risk of 2.13 (95% CI = 1.31-3.46) [250]. Thus, the question of benzene and risk of MM remains somewhat controversial.

Another important source of exposure to potentially toxic organic solvents is employment in the petrochemical or petroleum distribution industry. Epidemiologic studies of workers in these industries have not reported significant excesses of MM, including a mortality study of 28,840 Texaco workers [224], a cohort of petroleum workers exposed to gasoline [251], and a meta-analysis of 22 cohort studies involving more than 250,000 petroleum workers [252]. Overall, the evidence does not support an association between exposure to petroleum products and the risk of MM [243].

Other Occupations and Exposures

Epidemiologic studies have examined the relation between MM and several other occupations and related exposures, including cosmetologists and hair dyes (discussed in section 5), engine exhaust, paint-related occupations, rubber and plastic manufacturing, wood products industries, chemical workers, asbestos, and metals [5,253]. These studies were usually based on small numbers of cases and did not consistently show positive associations.

Sunlight

An association between sunlight or ultraviolet (UV)-B exposure and cancer has been suggested for some sites (reviewed in [254]), including breast cancer [255], colon cancer [256], prostate cancer [257], and non-Hodgkin lymphoma [258], but the data for MM are contradictory. The use of several different exposure indicators across the different studies, including geographical location, duration or frequency of exposure, and physical characteristics indicative of sun sensitivity, contributes to the apparent discrepancies in the findings. The mechanisms behind a UV-B-cancer association are also still under investigation, with beneficial effects on MM risk thought to be linked to the role of UV light in vitamin D production [259-263], and harmful effects thought to reflect the capacity of UV light to mediate immune function [260,264,265]. The question of whether UV-B acts through a shared mechanism in skin cancer and MM remains somewhat more elusive because of the mixed results for history of skin cancer and MM risk (discussed above in "Prior Medical Conditions and Treatment") [260,265]. The following section addresses the few publications that have investigated the link between UV-B exposure and risk of MM, and is organized by the approach used to characterize exposure to UV-B.

Evidence supporting an inverse association between UV-B exposure and MM risk comes from studies that use latitude as an index of exposure to solar UV-B radiation. In several ecologic studies, residence in areas closer to the equator, where UV-B light is stronger, was found to be associated with a decreased risk of death due to MM [266-269]. Those findings were corroborated by an ecologic comparison of MM incidence and mortality in relation to county-level satellite-estimated annual average UV-B radiation exposure levels in the northern and southern US [259]. In non-Hispanic Whites, men and women who resided in northern areas had significantly higher rates of MM incidence and mortality than those who resided in southern states. Specifically, both incidence and mortality rates were approximately 20% greater in persons with estimated annual average UV-B exposures of 650 kJ/m^2-year, which are characteristic of northern regions, than in those with estimated annual average levels of 1540 kJ/m^2-year, which are more typical of southern states. Among Blacks, a north-south gradient in MM rates was evident in women but not in men [259]. In contrast, an ecologic study conducted in Japan found no geographic correlation between estimated ambient UV-B exposure and mortality from MM [270].

Time and frequency of exposure to UV-B radiation have also been used as measures of exposure. In a multi-center European case-control study with 242 cases, Boffetta *et al.* found a suggested increased risk of MM with increasing time spent outdoors as an adult during free days, *i.e.* days not at work or school (OR for highest vs lowest quartile 1.49, 95% CI 0.88–2.50, p_{trend} 0.10) [265]. No significant change in risk was seen based on amount of time spent outdoors during childhood, occupational exposure to natural or artificial UV light, intensity of UV light exposure, or sunlamp use [265]. Findings in a population-based case-control study with 72 MM cases were generally null for amount of UV-B exposure and risk of MM, with the exception of a suggested decrease in MM risk for time spent on vacation in sunny places and a suggested increase in risk for cumulative hours spent doing outdoor leisure activities excluding vacations [260].

The multi-center European study also considered indirect characterizations of UV-B exposure based on physical characteristics indicative of increased sensitivity to sunlight in relation to risk of MM. Risk of MM was increased in people with hazel or green eye color compared to those with blue, grey or mixed eye color (OR 1.77, 95% CI 1.24–2.52), as well as in people with red hair in comparison to those with brown hair (OR 4.14, 95% CI 1.71–10.0) [265]. Skin tone and skin reaction to sun at first or after several exposures were not associated with MM in that study. A French case-control study that examined similar physical characteristics of sun sensitivity did not replicate the multi-center study findings [271].

In summary, evidence is limited for UV exposure as a risk factor for MM. Of interest, an extensive body of evidence supports an inverse association of UV-B exposure with NHL [258,272-276], but the evidence for an inverse association of UV-B exposure with MM is primarily limited to ecologic studies that may be influenced by misclassification of individual exposure or disease status or affected by uncontrolled confounding. The observational epidemiologic studies reported contradictory results but primarily supported an increased rather than a decreased risk of MM with increasing personal sun exposure or sun sensitivity. Boffetta and colleagues considered their findings consistent with the hypothesis that UV-B affects MM *via* similar mechanisms as in skin cancer [265], in contrast to the vitamin D-mediated mechanisms hypothesized to explain the UV-B association with NHL. Improved tools for classifying personal UV-B exposure will support a better characterization of the association of UV exposure with MM. Studies of this exposure in relation to MGUS risk and progression are also necessary, as this association has not yet been examined to our knowledge. As has been stated for virtually all the putative risk factors for MM, the present data are insufficient to support firm conclusions regarding the direction or the likely strength of an association of UV-B exposure with MM.

5. LIFESTYLE FACTORS

Tobacco and Alcohol

Tobacco use and alcohol intake have been investigated as lifestyle risk factors for many cancers, and numerous epidemiologic studies have examined their association with risk of MM. The vast majority have demonstrated no significant association for tobacco use [144,175,183,238,277-288]. However, an analysis conducted in a cohort of 34,000 Seventh Day Adventists found an increased risk among smokers that was strong, but statistically imprecise (OR=6.79, 95% CI=1.37-33.61) [289]. A case-control study in Germany [290] also observed an increased risk for current smokers that was statistically significant in women (OR=2.90, 95% CI=1.14-7.40) and of borderline significance in men (OR=2.37, 95% CI=0.98-5.74). No study has reported evidence of a dose-response. Collectively, the published data do not support an association of tobacco use with risk of MM. Fewer studies have examined intake of alcohol; however, most of those reports indicate no association with MM risk [144,175,183,278,287,288,290-292]. Exceptions include two case-control studies, including a hospital-based study in Shanghai [293] and a population-based study in the US [291], that reported marginally significant positive associations for consumption of combined types of alcohol (*i.e.*, hard liquors, any alcoholic beverage). In addition, two recent analyses, one in the Japan Public Health Center-based cohort of 95,520 middle-aged and older Japanese adults [294] and one from a population-based case-control study of 11 areas in Italy [295], reported a non-significantly diminished risk among current drinkers. In the Japanese population, the number of cases reporting regular weekly alcohol intake was small and the trend was not statistically significant [294]. In the Italian study, a trend of decreasing risk of MM with increasing weekly intake was marginally significant for total alcohol consumption but not significant for specific types of alcohol [295]. The suggestive findings of an inverse association with current regular alcohol intake are consistent with two US population-based case-control studies that observed statistically significant inverse associations [175,296]. In summary, most of the published data do not support an association of alcohol intake with MM risk or provide strong evidence for a dose response. Nevertheless, several studies have reported significant or marginally significant associations in either a positive or an inverse direction, leaving lingering questions about alcohol intake and risk of MM that may be best resolved through pooled studies or a meta-analysis.

Obesity

In epidemiologic studies, overweight and obesity are often characterized by body mass index (BMI), which is computed as weight (kg) divided by height (m) squared. The World Health Organization (WHO) defines overweight individuals as those with a BMI between 25 and 29.9 kg/m^2, and persons with a BMI of 30 kg/m^2 or greater are considered obese [297]. A rapidly expanding amount of literature has examined the association of BMI with MM incidence or mortality. Most articles have reported an excess risk among persons who are overweight or obese by WHO standards. The reported increased risk was modest in overweight persons, with relative risks ranging from 1.1 to 1.6 compared to individuals with a BMI lower than 25 kg/m^2 [115,298-304]. In obese persons, the associations were somewhat stronger, with relative risks between 1.4 and 2.5 reported [115,298-305]. The Million Women Study [306] reported a 1.3-fold increase in risk of MM incidence and a 1.6-fold increase in MM mortality per 10-unit increase in BMI. Oh and colleagues [307] followed 781,283 Korean men for 10 years and observed a 1.7-fold excess of MM incidence in men with a BMI between 23.0 and 24.9 kg/m^2 compared to those with a BMI between 18.5 and 22.9 kg/m^2.

Of the studies that did not report a statistically significant association of BMI with MM risk [280,308-314], many [308-310,313,314], but not all [280,311,312], found non-significant or marginally significant associations of similar strength to the significant relative risks. In addition, an excess risk of MM was observed in persons with a clinical diagnosis of obesity compared to those without a diagnosis of obesity in two populations, including a cohort of more than 4.5 million hospitalized male US veterans and a cohort of 143,574 out-patients of a US health maintenance organization (HMO) [315,316]. However, a population-based cohort of 28,129 hospital patients in Sweden [317] did not confirm those findings, and a confirmatory study in an independent pharmacy cohort from the same US HMO (N=163,561) confirmed the result only among men [316]. Two recent meta-analyses concluded that overweight and obese persons are at a modestly increased risk of MM [318,319]. Those studies affirm the overall consistency of the data on obesity or BMI and MM risk. As noted previously (section 3), obesity predicted an approximate 80% increase in risk of MGUS after adjustment for age and race in the Southern Community Cohort Study [34].

Other Anthropometric Factors

Fewer studies have examined weight change or other anthropometric measures in relation to risk of MM [298,299,308,310-312,314,316]. Net weight change from age 35 to study enrollment and episodes of intentional weight loss over a 20-year period were not significantly associated with MM risk among the 81,219 participants in the Women's Health Initiative [310]. However, the reported episodes of weight loss appeared to reflect weight cycling and net weight gain, and likely do not capture an effect of weight loss *per se.* Weight change following a diagnosis of obesity (0.3 kg/yr or greater weight loss, 0-0.3 kg loss or gain, 0.3 kg/yr weight gain) did not predict a subsequent diagnosis of MM in the cohort of 163,561 HMO pharmacy patients from the US [315].

Findings for other anthropometric measures varied by study population, but the observed associations were usually in directions consistent with the BMI data, *i.e.*, towards a positive association. In the Iowa Women's Health Study cohort [299], tertile of weight, waist circumference, and hip circumference were positively associated with MM risk, whereas no association was evident for height or waist-to-hip ratio. Modest increases in MM risk were observed with increasing height in a cohort of more than 2 million Norwegian men and women [303] and in the California Teachers Study [311]. The observed positive association of height with MM may implicate early life exposures such as nutritional status and/or growth-related hormone levels. In a large multi-center European cohort with 371,983 participants [308], weight was positively associated with MM risk in men, and height was positively associated with risk among women, but no other anthropometric factor was associated. In other populations from the Netherlands (N=120,852, with 279 incident cases of MM) and from Australia (N=40,909, with 55 incident MM diagnoses), no anthropometric measure demonstrated an association with MM [312,314].

Physical Activity

Only two studies have examined physical activity and risk of MM [305,313]. Among 136,623 members of the Nurses'Health Study and Health Professionals Follow-up Study cohorts, which included 215 incident cases of MM, a non-significantly diminished risk of MM was observed in participants with a cumulative average of two or more hours per week of moderate or vigorous exercise [298]. Those suggestive associations were corroborated by Khan and colleagues [305], who reported a 2-fold excess of mortality from MM among 109,698 Japanese men and women who walked fewer than 30 minutes per day, compared to those who walked 1 hour or more per day. Of interest, adjustment for physical activity in the former study did not attenuate the previously noted BMI associations [298], and adjustment for BMI did not attenuate the physical activity associations in the latter population [305]. These observations offer some reassurance that BMI and physical activity may be independent risk factors for MM, although the suggested association of physical activity with MM requires confirmation and further characterization in additional large study populations.

Important unresolved questions exist regarding the association of BMI and related factors with risk of MM, such as whether childhood or early adult weight status also impacts risk [311], and whether these factors are also associated with MGUS or progression from MGUS to MM. Nonetheless, the existing data on these factors related to adiposity and energy balance are remarkably consistent across most populations reported to date. The consistency of the data corroborates the hypothesis that one or more aspects of obesity (*i.e.*, adiposity and/or a positive energy balance) may have a causal role in the etiology of MM [298]. It is plausible that dysregulation in several biologic pathways may underlie the observed effect, *i.e.* pathways known to be altered in obese individuals and important in MM pathogenesis. Candidate pathways would include IGF-1 [320-323] and IL-6 [324-327]. Altered levels of some adipose tissue cytokines ("adipokines") have been reported in newly diagnosed MM patients [328-331], but their etiologic role has not been prospectively evaluated. Further characterization of the biologic mechanisms behind the BMI/energy balance associations, and of their relation to MGUS and progression, will be critical for the translation of these findings to effective prevention strategies.

Diet

A handful of studies have evaluated the relation between dietary factors and risk of MM. Although findings are not entirely consistent, an inverse association has been observed for intake of vegetables [287], and of cruciferous vegetables in particular [301,332]. A higher consumption of fish has also been linked to a lower risk of MM in several case-control studies [301,332,333]. No clear pattern has been observed for specific nutrients and MM risk.

Use of Hair Dyes

The identification of carcinogenic compounds in hair coloring products [334] led to public concern regarding their safety [335] and the removal of several carcinogens from many of the products in the 1980s [336]. Early reports of an excess risk of MM among cosmetologists and hairdressers motivated numerous subsequent studies of both occupational and personal exposure to hair-coloring products, with contrasting data reported across cohort and case-control studies. Persons with occupational exposure to hair dyes were shown to have an excess risk of MM in several [281,284,337-340], but not all studies [238,341,342]. A recent meta-analysis of cancer risk among hairdressers and related workers reported a statistically significant 62% increase in risk of MM that was remarkably consistent across analyses stratified by study design or gender despite the observation of substantial heterogeneity across individual studies [343].

With regard to personal exposure, women in a large prospective US cohort who reported ever using permanent hair dyes did not have a significantly higher rate of mortality from MM compared to women who never used hair dyes [344,345]. However, women from this cohort who reported 20 or more years of use of black hair dyes appeared to be at more than 4-fold greater risk of mortality from MM [344]. The initial observation was based on only two exposed MM deaths. One more exposed death was observed after 5 more years of follow-up, at which time the association was somewhat attenuated and only marginally significant [345]. In another prospective analysis that included 30 MM cases, eight of whom reported ever using hair dyes, permanent hair dye use was inversely associated with MM incidence [346]. Similar contrasts are present in the data from case-control studies of personal use of hair coloring products. A study by Zahm and colleagues [347] reported non-significant positive associations in both men and women, with evidence of heterogeneity by type of product (*i.e.*, permanent versus semi- or non-permanent). Brown *et al.* [348] reported an increased risk of MM in men who used hair dyes. Other case-control studies did not observe an association in men or women [338,349-351]. In contrast to the findings among professional hairdressers, a meta-analysis of studies that examined personal use of hair dyes did not suggest an association with MM risk in all studies combined [335]. Restriction of the meta-analysis to the four published case-control studies suggested a modest 28% increase in risk among ever users that was not strengthened by restriction to more extensive exposure or exclusive use of permanent hair dye products. The relatively small effect size, the lack of evidence for a dose-response, and the null findings among the cohort studies led the authors to argue against a causal effect of personal hair dye use [335]. They postulated that the lack of association could be explained in part by the relatively low concentration of carcinogenic compounds in the products and the discontinuation of some of the more toxic formulations several years prior to the onset of many of the studies.

In summary, the present evidence does not support an important role of personal use of hair coloring products in the etiology of MM. However, it does appear that professional hairdressers and related workers may be at increased risk and may benefit from further studies to identify the most toxic exposures and potential genetic or environmental modifiers of the observed effect [352], as well as the use of measures to limit exposure to those products.

Medication Use

Data are sparse on the association of medication use with risk of MM. Most studies have focused on medications that influence biologic pathways of known or suspected importance to MM pathogenesis, such as IL-6- or NF-κB-mediated processes. Few types of medication have been examined in more than one or two studies, and thus the evidence on any agent is far from conclusive. The following summary of available evidence is organized by class of medication.

Hormone Replacement Therapy (HRT). Estrogen has been shown to block IL-6-mediated proliferation of MM cell lines [353] and therefore postmenopausal HRT may influence risk of MM in women. To date, three case-control studies have examined this association including one conducted in the US [153] and two studies from Italy that appear to include a common series of participants [354,355]. All three studies reported a reduced risk of MM among women who used HRT. Relative risk estimates suggested a 40-80% reduction in risk that was of borderline statistical significance in the US study (RR=0.4, 95% CI=0.4-0.99, based on 28 exposed cases) [153] and in one of the Italian analyses (RR=0.2, 95% CI=0.1-1.0, based on 3 exposed cases) [354]. None of these studies had sufficient numbers of MM patients with a history of HRT use to examine details such as duration or formulation. Due to the controversial nature of postmenopausal HRT, it is critical to confirm and more clearly characterize the suggested association in large studies with detailed information on HRT use. Of note, the few studies that examined other reproductive factors did not provide evidence of an important role for hormonal factors in the etiology of MM [356-358].

Analgesics and Non-Steroidal Anti-inflammatory Drugs (NSAID). A few studies have examined the use of analgesic or NSAID formulations in relation to risk of MM. Acetaminophen, in contrast to aspirin and other NSAIDs, has the effect of increasing NF-κB activation [359] and IL-6 transcription [360] and has been shown to have genotoxic properties [361]. Acetaminophen was significantly associated with a nearly 3-fold increase in risk of MM in a US hospital-based case-control study [362]. The association was independent of aspirin use and demonstrated significant trends of increasing risk with increasing frequency and duration of regular use. These findings corroborate the non-significant 2-fold increase in MM risk among users of salicylates or paracetamol that was previously observed in a population-based case-control study conducted in Sweden [151]. The US study did not observe an association with MM for regular use of aspirin or ibuprofen, consistent with a report from a population-based case-control study of women in Connecticut that did not observe an association for aspirin, analgesics, or NSAIDs [153]. Few women reported use of those agents in the Connecticut study. In contrast to the case-control studies, a recent prospective analysis in the Nurses'Health Study and Health Professionals Follow-up Study cohorts with a total of 279 incident cases of MM observed an inverse association of MM risk with quantity and duration of regular aspirin use [363]. The analysis incorporated a 4-year lag in the classification of exposure to minimize the influence of preclinical disease on patterns of aspirin use. In pooled analyses across the two cohorts, persons who reported a cumulative average of 5 or more 325 mg tablets per week had a significantly lower risk of MM compared to non-users of aspirin after adjustment for age, gender, and BMI. The trend of diminishing risk with increasing quantity of use was marginally significant among men and in combined analyses but not among women. Duration of continuous regular aspirin use was also inversely associated with MM, although the trend was not statistically significant. The intriguing differences in the association by gender may be due to chance or may reflect gender differences in the pattern of regular aspirin use [363].

The association of aspirin use with a diminished risk of MM is plausible since aspirin inhibits cyclooxygenase (COX)-1 and -2 as well as NF-κB and IL-6, pathways that contribute to MM pathogenesis. A similar protective effect for other NSAIDs could be hypothesized but has not been demonstrated in studies with sufficient information on individual agents. Collectively, the few published findings on this class of medications must be considered preliminary and confirmed in large populations with detailed information on the frequency, dose and duration of their use.

Other Medications. In the case-control study of women in Connecticut, use of anti-diabetic medication (*i.e.*, insulin) was 3 times more prevalent in women with MM than in matched controls, although the analyses included only 8 cases and 8 controls who reported insulin use [153]. The association appeared to be somewhat stronger for moderate to longer duration of insulin use, although the data were too sparse for a robust stratified analysis. Whether these findings suggest a physiologic effect of insulin or whether insulin use should be viewed as a surrogate marker for diabetes is unclear and could not be explored in the Connecticut study. A large prospective study in Europe reported a modest and non-significant increase in MM risk in persons with a history of type 2 diabetes diagnosed after age 30 [364], whereas an earlier case-control study did not observe an association of history of diabetes with MM [158]. The association of diabetes or insulin use with MM merits further examination. The Connecticut study also reported that use of medication for gout was nearly 7 times as common among cases than controls in the same study, albeit based on only 4 exposed cases and 2 exposed controls, whereas anti-lipid statin therapy was approximately 60% less common among cases than controls based on 7 exposed cases [153]. A summary of the association with MM for the environmental and occupational exposures and lifestyle factors discussed in the sections above are summarized in Table **3**.

Table 3. Risk of multiple myeloma and MGUS in relation to selected host, environmental, and lifestyle factors.*

Exposure Type	Exposure	Analytic Exposure	Risk†
Host Factors	**Familial Risk**	Family member with multiple myeloma or MGUS	Moderate increased risk‡
		Family member with another malignancy	Suggested increased risk‡

Table 3. cont….

	Autoimmune Conditions	Pernicious anemia	Moderate increased risk‡
		Autoimmune hemolytic anemia	Weak to moderate increased risk§
		Polymyositis/dermatomyositis	Weak to moderate increased risk§
		Systemic sclerosis	Weak to moderate increased risk§
	Inflammatory Disorders	General inflammatory conditions	Weak increased risk‡
	Infection	Pneumonia	Moderate increased risk‡
		Hepatitis C virus	Weak increased risk‡
		AIDS	Moderate increased risk
Environmental and Occupational Exposures	**Radiation**	Radiation from Hiroshima and Nagasaki atomic bombs	Moderate increased risk of death; Higher progression rate to MGUS‡
		Occupational exposure in the nuclear industry	Weak increased risk of death
		Therapeutic radiation	Weak increased risk
	Occupation	Farming	Significant moderate increased risk
		Pesticide related occupations	Moderate increased risk‡
		Working with herbicides	Moderate increased risk‡
	UV-B/sunlight exposure	As measured by latitudinal location	Weak suggested decreased risk
Lifestyle Factors	**Diet**	Vegetable, coniferous vegetables in particular, intake	Weak to moderate decreased risk
		Fish intake	Weak to moderate decreased risk
	Smoking	Smokers	Weak positive association, generally no consistent association
	Alcohol	Among current drinkers	Weak decreased risk
		Consumption of combined types of alcohol	Weak increased risk
	Anthropometric Characteristics	Obesity	Moderate increased risk§
		Overweight	Weak increased risk
		Tertile of weight, waist circumference, and hip circumference	Weak increased risk
		Height	Moderate increased risk
	Physical Activity	2+ hours per day	Weak decreased risk
	Use of Hair Dye	Cosmetologists and hairdressers	Moderate increased risk in some studies
	Medication Use	Acetaminophen	Moderate to strong increased risk
		Aspirin (and other NSAIDs)	Preliminary findings of a decreased risk
		Use of Hormone Replacement Therapy	Weak decreased risk
		Use of insulin	Moderate increased risk

* References for associations listed in this table can be found in the narrative in the corresponding sections. Additional information on genetic risk factors and first primary cancers as risk factors can be found in Tables 1 and 2 respectively.

† Associations are only for MM, unless otherwise specified.

‡ Associations are for both MM and MGUS.

§Associations are only for MGUS.

6. CONCLUSIONS AND FUTURE DIRECTIONS

The preceding review describes a vast body of literature of variable quality on a broad spectrum of demographic, genetic, personal/lifestyle, and other environmental risk factors for MM and its precursor, MGUS. Many of the summaries feature a series of first reports with findings that have yet to be confirmed. Inherent in the more consistent findings are several insights that could shape the direction of future research, including:

1. MGUS appears to precede essentially all MM diagnoses and to share many features of the descriptive epidemiology and etiology of MM, from familial/genetic risk factors to aspects of personal medical history and obesity.

2. Obesity likely has a causal association with MM and potentially also with MGUS, and thus represents a modifiable risk factor for these conditions that could potentially be exploited for disease prevention.

3. Several risk factors that have demonstrated associations with MM or MGUS correspond to biologic pathways known to be important in MM pathogenesis, lending credibility to the etiologic findings. To the degree that such pathogenesis pathways can be interrupted by targeted molecular therapies, opportunities for chemoprevention with those therapies may also arise. However, prevention strategies cannot be explored without improved characterization of high risk individuals who could benefit from a given intervention.

A clear message from this review is that few, if any, etiologic questions can be considered settled at this time regarding MM. Furthermore, most putative risk factors for MM have not yet been evaluated in the etiology of MGUS or in relation to MGUS progression. These lingering questions of etiology and etiopathogenesis will be most effectively addressed through collaboration—in the form of multidisciplinary exchanges of novel insights of common interest, and in the form of pooled analyses. Such collaborative efforts could ultimately identify persons at risk and provide opportunities to intervene in the natural history of monoclonal gammopathy to prevent MM, thereby alleviating substantial suffering, costs, and population burden from this as yet incurable disease.

REFERENCES

[1] Swerdlow S, Harris N, Jaffe E, *et al.* WHO Classification of Tumours of Haematopoietic and Lymphoid Tissues. International Agency for Research on Cancer, Lyon, (2008).

[2] International Myeloma Working Group. Criteria for the classification of monoclonal gammopathies, multiple myeloma and related disorders: a report of the International Myeloma Working Group. Br J Haematol 2003; 121: 749-757.

[3] Kyle R. Monoclonal gammopathy of undetermined significance: natural history in 241 cases. Am J Med 1978; 64: 814–826.

[4] American Cancer Society. Cancer Facts & Figures 2010 American Cancer Society, Inc. 2010.

[5] De Roos AJ, Baris D, Weiss NS, Herrinton LJ: Multiple myeloma. In Cancer Epidemiology and Prevention. Schottenfeld D, *et al.* (eds) Oxford, (2006): 919-945.

[6] American Cancer Society. Cancer Facts and Figures 2009 American Cancer Society, Inc. 2009.

[7] Shulman G, Jacobson RJ. Immunocytoma in black and white South Africans. Trop Geogr Med 1980; 32: 112-117.

[8] Blattner W, Jacobson R, Shulman G. Multiple myeloma in South African blacks. Lancet 1979; 1: 928-929.

[9] Levy LM. The pattern of haematological and lymphoreticular malignancy in Zimbabwe. Trop Geogr Med 1988; 40: 109-114.

[10] Besson C, Gonin C, Brebion A, *et al.* Incidence of hematological malignancies in Martinique, French West Indies, overrepresentation of multiple myeloma and adult T cell leukemia/lymphoma. Leuk 2001; 15: 828-831.

[11] McFarlane H. Multiple myeloma in Jamaica: a study of 40 cases with special reference to the incidence and laboratory diagnosis. J Clin Pathol 1966; 19: 268-271.

[12] McFarlane H, Talerman A, Steinberg AG. Immunoglobulins in Jamaicans and Nigerians with immunogenetic typing of myeloma and lymphoma in Jamaicans. J Clin Pathol 1970; 23: 124-126.

[13] Nossent JC, Winkel CN, van Leeuwen JC. Multiple myeloma in the Afro-Caribbean population of Curacao. Neth J Med 1993; 43: 210-214.

[14] Landgren O, Katzmann JA, Hsing AW, *et al.* Prevalence of monoclonal gammopathy of undetermined significance among men in Ghana. Mayo Clin Proc 2007; 82: 1468-1473.

[15] Gebregziabher M, Bernstein L, Wang Y, Cozen W. Risk patterns of multiple myeloma in Los Angeles County, 1972-1999 (United States). Cancer Causes Control 2006; 17: 931-938.

[16] Bergsagel D. The incidence and epidemiology of plasma cell neoplasms. Stem Cells 1995; Suppl 2: 1-9.
[17] Riedel D, Pottern L. The epidemiology of multiple myeloma. Hematol Oncol Clin North Am 1992; 6: 225-247.
[18] Hernández J, Land K, McKenna R. Leukemias, myeloma, and other lymphoreticular neoplasms. Cancer 1995; 75: 381-394.
[19] Walker B, Figgs L, Zahm S. Differences in cancer incidence, mortality, and survival between African Americans and whites. Environ Health Perspect 1995; 103: 275-281.
[20] Benjamin M, Reddy S, Brawlay O. Myeloma and race: a review of the literature. Cancer Metastatsis Rev 2003; 22: 87-93.
[21] Miller B, Kolonel L, Bernstein L, *et al.* (1996) Racial/Ethnic Patterns of Cancer in the United States 1988-1992 (NIH Pub. No. 96-4104) National Cancer Institute.
[22] Surveillance Research Program, National Cancer Institute SEER*Stat software (www.seer.cancer.gov/ seerstat), Version 6.5.2. Surveillance, Epidemiology, and End Results (SEER) Program (www.seer.cancer.gov) SEER* Stat Database: Incidence-SEER 9 Registries Limited-Use, Nov. 2008 Submission (1973-2006).
[23] Hirabayashi Y, Katanoda K. Comparison of time trends in multiple myeloma incidence (1973-1997) in East Asia, Europe and United States, from Cancer Incidence in Five Continents, Vols IV-VIII. Jpn J Clin Oncol 2008; 38: 720-721.
[24] United States Cancer Statistics Working Group. (2010) United States cancer Statistics: 1999-2006 Incidence and Mortality Web-based Report. U.S. Department of Health and Human Services, Centers for Disease Control and Prevention National Cancer Institute.
[25] National Cancer Institute. A snapshot of myeloma. 2009.
[26] Devesa SS, Silverman DT, Young JL, Jr., *et al.* Cancer incidence and mortality trends among whites in the United States, 1947-84. J Natl Cancer Inst 1987; 79: 701-770.
[27] Velez R, Beral V, Cuzick J. Increasing trends of multiple myeloma mortality in England and Wales; 1950-79: are the changes real? J Natl Cancer Inst 1982; 69: 387-392.
[28] Blattner W, Blair A, Mason T. Multiple myeloma in the United States, 1950-1975. Cancer 1981; 48: 2547-2554.
[29] Liu L, Cozen W, Bernstein L, Ross R, Deapen D. The changing relationship between socioeconomic status and prostate cancer incidence. JNCI 2001; 93: 705-709.
[30] Nandakumar A, Armstrong B, De Klerk N. Multiple myeloma in Western Australia: A case-control study in relation to occupation, father's occupation, socioeconomic status and country of birth. Int J Cancer 1986; 37: 223-226.
[31] Baris D, Brown L, Silverman D, *et al.* Socioeconomic status and multiple myeloma among US blacks and whites. Am J Pub Health 2000; 90: 1277-1281.
[32] Boffetta P, Stellman S, Garfinkel L. A case-control study of multiple myeloma nested in the American Cancer Society prospective study. Int J Cancer 1989; 43: 554-559.
[33] Cuzick J, De Stavola B. Multiple myeloma- a case-control study. Br J Cancer 1998; 57: 516-520.
[34] Landgren O, Katzmann J, Hsing A, *et al.* Prevalence of monoclonal gammopathy of undetermined significance among men in Ghana. Mayo Clin Proc 2007; 82: 1468-1473.
[35] Landgren O, Rajkumar V, Pfeiffer R, *et al.* Obesity is associated with an increased risk of monoclonal gammopathy of undetermined significance among black and white women. Blood 2010; 116: 1056-1059.
[36] Shen M, Cozen W, Huang L, *et al.* Census and geographic differences between respondents and nonrespondents in a case-control study of non-Hodgkin lymphoma. Am J Epidemiol 2008; 167: 350-361.
[37] Han X, Kilfoy B, Zheng T, *et al.* Lymphoma survival patterns by WHO subtype in the United States, 1973-2003. Cancer Causes Control 2008; 19: 841-858.
[38] Brenner H, Gondos A, Pulte D. Expected long-term survival of patients diagnosed with multiple myeloma in 2006-2010. Haematologica 2009; 94: 270-275.
[39] Schaapveld M, Visser O, Siesling S, *et al.* Improved survival among younger but not among older patients with Multiple Myeloma in the Netherlands, a population-based study since 1989. Eur J Cancer 2010; 46: 160-169.
[40] Turesson I, Velez R, Kristinsson SY, Landgren O. Patterns of improved survival in patients with multiple myeloma in the twenty-first century: a population-based study. J Clin Oncol 2010; 28: 830-834.
[41] Kristinsson SY, Landgren O, Dickman PW, Derolf AR, Bjorkholm M. Patterns of survival in multiple myeloma: a population-based study of patients diagnosed in Sweden from 1973 to 2003. J Clin Oncol 2007; 25: 1993-1999.
[42] Kumar S, Rajkumar S, Dispenzieri A, *et al.* Improved survival in multiple myeloma and the impact of novel therapies. Blood 2008; 111: 2516-2520.

[43] Axelsson U, Bachmann R, Hällén J. Frequency of pathological proteins (M-components) in 6,995 sera from an adult population. Acta Med Scand 1966; 179: 235-247.

[44] Colls B. Monoclonal gammopathy of undetermined significance (MGUS)-31 year follow up of a community study. Aust N Z J Med 1999; 29: 500-504.

[45] Kyle R, Finkelstein S, Elveback L, Kurland L. Incidence of monoclonal proteins in a Minnesota community with a cluster of multiple myeloma. Blood 1972; 40: 719-724.

[46] Saleun J, Vicariot M, Deroff P, Morin J. Monoclonal gammopathies in the adult population of Finistère, France. J Clin Pathol 1982; 35: 63-68.

[47] Hallen J. Frequency of "abnormal" serum globulins (M-components) in the aged. Acta Med Scand 1963; 173: 737-744.

[48] Kyle R, Therneau T, Rajkumar S, *et al.* Prevalence of monoclonal gammopathy of undetermined significance. N Engl J Med 2006; 354: 1362-1369.

[49] Schechter G, Shoff N, Chan C, McManus C, Hawley H: The frequency of monoclonal gammopathy of unknown significance in Black and Caucasian veterans in a hospital population. In: Epidemiology and Biology of Multiple Myeloma. Obrams G, *et al.* (eds) Springer, New York, NY (1991): 83-85.

[50] Landgren O, Gridley G, Turesson I, *et al.* Risk of monoclonal gammopathy of undetermined significance (MGUS) and subsequent multiple myeloma among African American and white veterans in the United States. Blood 2006; 107: 904-906.

[51] Iwanaga M, Tagawa M, Tsukasaki K, Kamihira S, Tomonaga M. Prevalence of monoclonal gammopathy of undetermined significance: study of 52,802 persons in Nagasaki City, Japan. Mayo Clin Proc 2007; 82: 1474-1479.

[52] Kristinsson SY, Bjorkholm M, Goldin LR, *et al.* Patterns of hematologic malignancies and solid tumors among 37,838 first-degree relatives of 13,896 patients with multiple myeloma in Sweden. Int J Cancer 2009; 125: 2147-2150.

[53] Landgren O, Kyle RA, Pfeiffer RM, *et al.* Monoclonal gammopathy of undetermined significance (MGUS) consistently precedes multiple myeloma: a prospective study. Blood 2009; 113: 5412-5417.

[54] Vachon C, Kyle R, Therneau T, *et al.* Increased risk of monoloconal gammopathy in first-degree relatives of patients with multiple myeloma or monoclonal gammopathy of undertermined significance. Blood 2009; 114: 785-790.

[55] Kristinsson S, Bjorkholm M, Goldin L, *et al.* Risk of lymphoproliferative disorders among first-degree relatives of lymphoplasmacytic lymphoma/Waldenstrom macroglobulinemia patients: a population-based study in Sweden. Blood 2008; 112: 3052-3056.

[56] Davies FE, Rollinson SJ, Rawstron AC, *et al.* High-producer haplotypes of tumor necrosis factor alpha and lymphotoxin alpha are associated with an increased risk of myeloma and have an improved progression-free survival after treatment. J Clin Oncol 2000; 18: 2843-2851.

[57] Dring AM, Davies FE, Rollinson SJ, *et al.* Interleukin 6, tumour necrosis factor alpha and lymphotoxin alpha polymorphisms in monoclonal gammopathy of uncertain significance and multiple myeloma. Br J Haematol 2001; 112: 249-251.

[58] Morgan GJ, Adamson PJ, Mensah FK, *et al.* Haplotypes in the tumour necrosis factor region and myeloma. Br J Haematol 2005; 129: 358-365.

[59] Parker KM, Ma MH, Manyak S, *et al.* Identification of polymorphisms of the IkappaBalpha gene associated with an increased risk of multiple myeloma. Cancer Genet Cytogenet 2002; 137: 43-48.

[60] Zheng C, Huang D, Liu L, *et al.* Cytotoxic T-lymphocyte antigen-4 microsatellite polymorphism is associated with multiple myeloma. Br J Haematol 2001; 112: 216-218.

[61] Zheng C, Huang D, Liu L, *et al.* Interleukin-10 gene promoter polymorphisms in multiple myeloma. Int J Cancer 2001; 95: 184-188.

[62] Zheng C, Huang DR, Bergenbrant S, *et al.* Interleukin 6, tumour necrosis factor alpha, interleukin 1beta and interleukin 1 receptor antagonist promoter or coding gene polymorphisms in multiple myeloma. Br J Haematol 2000; 109: 39-45.

[63] Brown LM, Gridley G, Check D, Landgren O. Risk of multiple myeloma and monoclonal gammopathy of undetermined significance among white and black male United States veterans with prior autoimmune, infectious, inflammatory, and allergic disorders. Blood 2008; 111: 3388-3394.

[64] Landgren O, Kyle RA, Hoppin JA, *et al.* Pesticide exposure and risk of monoclonal gammopathy of undetermined significance in the Agricultural Health Study. Blood 2009; 113: 6386-6391.

[65] Kyle R, Therneau T, Rajkumar S, *et al.* Long-term follow-up of 241 patients with monoclonal gammopathy of undetermined significance: the original Mayo Clinic series 25 years later. Mayo Clinic Proc 2004; 79: 859–866.

[66] Kyle RA, Therneau TM, Rajkumar SV, *et al.* A long-term study of prognosis in monoclonal gammopathy of undetermined significance. N Engl J Med 2002; 346: 564-569.

[67] Kyle R, Rajkumar S. Monoclonal gammopathy of undetermined significance and smoldering multiple myeloma. Curr Hematol Malig Rep 2010; 5: 62-69.

[68] Bladé J, Rosiñol L, Cibeira M. Are all myelomas preceded by MGUS? Blood 2009; 113: 5370.

[69] Golombick T, Diamond T, Badmaev V, Manoharan A, Ramakrishna R. The potential role of curcumin in patients with monoclonal gammopathy of undefined significance--its effect on paraproteinemia and the urinary N-telopeptide of type I collagen bone turnover marker. Clin Cancer Res 2009; 15: 5917-5922.

[70] Rajkumar S. Prevention of progression in monoclonal gammopathy of undetermined significance. Clin Cancer Res 2009; 15: 5606-5608.

[71] Weiss B, Abadie J, Verma P, Howard R, Kuehl W. A monoclonal gammopathy precedes multiple myeloma in most patients. Blood 2009; 113: 5418-5422.

[72] Lynch H, Sanger W, Pirruccello S, Quinn-Laquer B, Weisenburger D. Familial multiple myeloma: a family study and review of the literature. JNCI 2001; 93: 1479-1483.

[73] Lynch H, Watson, Tarantolo S, *et al.* Phenotypic heterogeneity in multiple myeloma families. J Clin Oncol 2005; 23: 685-693.

[74] Lynch HT, Ferrara K, Barlogie B, *et al.* Familial myeloma. N Engl J Med 2008; 359: 152-157.

[75] Lynch H, Thome S. Familial multiple myeloma. Blood 2009; 114: 749-750.

[76] Sobol H, Vey N, Sauvan R, *et al.* Familial multiple myeloma: A family study and review of the literature. JNCI 2002; 94: 461-462.

[77] Groisbois B, Jego P, Attal M, *et al.* Familial multiple myeloma: report of fifteen families. Br J Haematol 1999; 150: 768-770.

[78] Gerkes E, de Jong M, Sijmons R, Vellengo E. Familial multiple myeloma: Report on two families and discussion of screening options. Hered Cancer Clin Practice 2007; 5: 72-78.

[79] Roddie P, Dang R, Parker A. Multiple myeloma in three siblings. Clin Lab Haematol 1998; 20: 191-193.

[80] Horowitz L, Levy R, Rosner F. Multiple myeloma in three siblings. Arch Int Med 1985; 145: 1449-1450.

[81] Crozes-Bony P, Palazzo E, Meyer O, De Bandt M, Kahn M. Familial multiple myeloma. Report of a case in a father and daughter. Review of the literature. Rev Rhum Engl Ed 1995; 62: 439-445.

[82] Jain M, Ascensao J, Schechter GP. Familial myeloma and monoclonal gammopathy: a report of eight African American families. Am J Hematol 2009; 84: 34-38.

[83] Deshpandc II, Hu X-P, Marno P, Jan N, Wiernik P. Anticipation in familial plasma cell dyscrasias Br J Haematol 1988; 103: 696-703.

[84] Molee P, Taylor K, Durrant S, Wright S. Familial myeloma. Blood 1999; 94 (Part 2 Suppl 1): 4574.

[85] Daugherty S, Pfeiffer R, Mellemkjaer L, Hemminki K, LR G. No evidence for anticipation in lymphoproliferative tumors in population-based samples. Cancer Epideimol Biomark Preven 2005; 14: 1245-1250.

[86] Lichenstein P, Holm N, Verkasalo P, *et al.* Environmental and heritable factors in the causation of cancer. New Eng J Med 2000; 343: 78-85.

[87] Mack T, Cozen W, Shibata D, *et al.* Concordance for Hodgkin's disease in identical twins suggesting genetic susceptibility to the young-adult form of the disease. N Eng J Med 1995; 332: 413-418.

[88] Altieri A, Chen B, Bermejo JL, Castro F, Hemminki K. Familial risks and temporal incidence trends of multiple myeloma. Eur J Cancer 2006; 42: 1661-1670.

[89] Bourguet CC, Grufferman S, Delzell E, DeLong ER, Cohen HJ. Multiple myeloma and family history of cancer. A case-control study. Cancer 1985; 56: 2133-2139.

[90] Brown LM, Linet MS, Greenberg RS, *et al.* Multiple myeloma and family history of cancer among blacks and whites in the U.S. Cancer 1999; 85: 2385-2390.

[91] Eriksson M, Hallberg B. Familial occurrence of hematologic malignancies and other diseases in multiple myeloma: a case-control study. Cancer Causes Control 1992; 3: 63-67.

[92] Ogmundsdottir HM, Haraldsdottirm V, Johannesson GM, *et al.* Familiality of benign and malignant paraproteinemias. A population-based cancer-registry study of multiple myeloma families. Haematologica 2005; 90: 66-71.

[93] Altieri A, Bermejo J, Hemminki K. Familial risk for non-Hodgkin lymphoma and other lymphoproliferative malignancies by histopathologic subtype: the Swedish Family-Cancer Database. Blood 2005; 106: 668-672.

[94] Landgren O, Linet MS, McMaster ML, *et al.* Familial characteristics of autoimmune and hematologic disorders in 8,406 multiple myeloma patients: a population-based case-control study. Int J Cancer 2006; 118: 3095-3098.
[95] Landgren O, Kristinsson S, Goldin L, *et al.* Risk of plasma-cell and lymphoproliferative disorders among 14,621 first-degree relatives of 4,458 patients with monoclonal gammopathy of undetermined significance (MGUS) in Sweden. Blood 2009; 114: 791-795.
[96] Goldin L, Bjorkholm M, Kristinsson S, Turesson I, Landgren O. Elevated risk of chronic lymphocytic leukemia and other indolent non-Hodgkin's lymphomas among relatives of patients with chronic lymphocytic leukemia. Haematologica 2009; 94: 647-653.
[97] Goldin L. Familial aggregation and heterogeneity of non-Hodgkin lymphoma in population-based samples. Cancer Epideimol Biomark Preven 2005; 14: 2402-2406.
[98] Goldin L, Pfeiffer R, Gridley G, *et al.* Familial aggregation of Hodgkin lymphoma and related tumors. Cancer 2004; 100: 109-114.
[99] McDuffie H, Pahwa P, Karunanayake C, Spinelli J, Dosman J. Clustering of cancer among families of cases with Hodgkin lymphoma (HL), multiple myeloma (MM), non-Hodgkin's lymphoma (NHL), soft tissue sarcoma (STS) and control subjects. BMC Cancer 2009; 9: 1-9.
[100] Gold LS, De Roos AJ, Brown EE, *et al.* Associations of common variants in genes involved in metabolism and response to exogenous chemicals with risk of multiple myeloma. Cancer Epidemiol 2009; 33: 276-280.
[101] Kang SH, Kim TY, Kim HY, *et al.* Protective role of CYP1A1*2A in the development of multiple myeloma. Acta Haematol 2008; 119: 60-64.
[102] Lincz LF, Scorgie FE, Robertson R, Enno A. Genetic variations in benzene metabolism and susceptibility to multiple myeloma. Leuk Res 2007; 31: 759-763.
[103] Maggini V, Buda G, Galimberti S, *et al.* Lack of association of NQO1 and GSTP1 polymorphisms with multiple myeloma risk. Leuk Res 2008; 32: 988-990.
[104] Ortega MM, Honma HN, Zambon L, *et al.* GSTM1 and codon 72 P53 polymorphism in multiple myeloma. Ann Hematol 2007; 86: 815-819.
[105] Kim HN, Kim YK, Lee IK, *et al.* Polymorphisms involved in the folate metabolizing pathway and risk of multiple myeloma. Am J Hematol 2007; 82: 798-801.
[106] Lima CS, Ortega MM, Ozelo MC, *et al.* Polymorphisms of methylenetetrahydrofolate reductase (MTHFR), methionine synthase (MTR), methionine synthase reductase (MTRR), and thymidylate synthase (TYMS) in multiple myeloma risk. Leuk Res 2008; 32: 401-405.
[107] Gonzalez-Fraile MI, Garcia-Sanz R, Mateos MV, *et al.* Methylenetetrahydrofolate reductase genotype does not play a role in multiple myeloma pathogenesis. Br J Haematol 2002; 117: 890-892.
[108] Bolufer P, Barragan E, Collado M, *et al.* Influence of genetic polymorphisms on the risk of developing leukemia and on disease progression. Leuk Res 2006; 30: 1471-1491.
[109] Skibola CF, Smith MT, Hubbard A, *et al.* Polymorphisms in the thymidylate synthase and serine hydroxymethyltransferase genes and risk of adult acute lymphocytic leukemia. Blood 2002; 99: 3786-3791.
[110] Niclot S, Pruvot Q, Besson C, *et al.* Implication of the folate-methionine metabolism pathways in susceptibility to follicular lymphomas. Blood 2006; 108: 278-285.
[111] Skibola CF, Forrest MS, Coppede F, *et al.* Polymorphisms and haplotypes in folate-metabolizing genes and risk of non-Hodgkin lymphoma. Blood 2004; 104: 2155-2162.
[112] Hayden PJ, Tewari P, Morris DW, *et al.* Variation in DNA repair genes XRCC3, XRCC4, XRCC5 and susceptibility to myeloma. Hum Mol Genet 2007; 16: 3117-3127.
[113] Roddam PL, Rollinson S, O'Driscoll M, *et al.* Genetic variants of NHEJ DNA ligase IV can affect the risk of developing multiple myeloma, a tumour characterised by aberrant class switch recombination. J Med Genet 2002; 39: 900-905.
[114] Hwang WY, Gullo CA, Shen J, *et al.* Decoupling of normal CD40/interleukin-4 immunoglobulin heavy chain switch signal leads to genomic instability in SGH-MM5 and RPMI 8226 multiple myeloma cell lines. Leukemia 2006; 20: 715-723.
[115] Arpin C, Dechanet J, Van Kooten C, *et al.* Generation of memory B cells and plasma cells *in vitro*. Science 1995; 268: 720-722.
[116] Jelinek DF. Mechanisms of myeloma cell growth control. Hematol Oncol Clin North Am 1999; 13: 1145-1157.
[117] Cozen W, Gebregziabher M, Conti DV, *et al.* Interleukin-6-related genotypes, body mass index, and risk of multiple myeloma and plasmacytoma. Cancer Epidemiol Biomarkers Prev 2006; 15: 2285-2291.

[118] Birmann B. Insulin-like Growth Factor-1- and Interleukin-6-related Gene Variation and Risk of Multiple Myeloma. Cancer Epidemiol Biomarkers Prev 2009; 18: 282-288.

[119] Brown EE, Lan Q, Zheng T, *et al.* Common variants in genes that mediate immunity and risk of multiple myeloma. Int J Cancer 2007; 120: 2715-2722.

[120] Purdue MP, Lan Q, Menashe I, *et al.* Variation in innate immunity genes and risk of multiple myeloma. Hematol Oncol 2011; 29(1): 42-6.

[121] Spink CF, Gray LC, Davies FE, Morgan GJ, Bidwell JL. Haplotypic structure across the I kappa B alpha gene (NFKBIA) and association with multiple myeloma. Cancer Lett 2007; 246: 92-99.

[122] Hosgood HD, 3rd, Baris D, Zhang Y, *et al.* Caspase polymorphisms and genetic susceptibility to multiple myeloma. Hematol Oncol 2008; 26: 148-151.

[123] Hosgood HD, 3rd, Baris D, Zhang Y, *et al.* Genetic variation in cell cycle and apoptosis related genes and multiple myeloma risk. Leuk Res 2009; 33: 1609-1614.

[124] Wolvekamp MC, Marquet RL. Interleukin-6: historical background, genetics and biological significance. Immunol Lett 1990; 24: 1-9.

[125] Maddali L, Maddali S. Multiple primary cancers involving nonbreast sites. J Clini Oncol 2010; 28: May 20 Supplement.

[126] Kahn HS, Tatham LM, Patel AV, Thun MJ, Heath CW, Jr. Increased cancer mortality following a history of non-melanoma skin cancer. JAMA 1998; 280: 910-912.

[127] Bradford PT, Freedman DM, Goldstein AM, Tucker MA. Increased risk of second primary cancers after a diagnosis of melanoma. Arch Dermatol 2010; 146: 265-272.

[128] Dong C, Hemminki K. Second primary neoplasms in 633,964 cancer patients in Sweden, 1958-1996. Int J Cancer 2001; 93: 155-161.

[129] Boice JD, Jr., Day NE, Andersen A, *et al.* Second cancers following radiation treatment for cervical cancer. An international collaboration among cancer registries. J Natl Cancer Inst 1985; 74: 955-975.

[130] Wright JD, St Clair CM, Deutsch I, *et al.* Pelvic radiotherapy and the risk of secondary leukemia and multiple myeloma. Cancer 2010; 116: 2486-2492.

[131] Little MP, Muirhead CR, Haylock RG, Thomas JM. Relative risks of radiation-associated cancer: comparison of second cancer in therapeutically irradiated populations with the Japanese atomic bomb survivors. Radiat Environ Biophys 1999; 38: 267-283.

[132] Dong C, Hemminki K. Second primary neoplasms among 53 159 haematolymphoproliferative malignancy patients in Sweden, 1958-1996: a search for common mechanisms. Br J Cancer 2001; 85: 997-1005.

[133] Howard RA, Dores GM, Curtis RE, Anderson WF, Travis LB. Merkel cell carcinoma and multiple primary cancers. Cancer Epidemiol Biomarkers Prev 2006; 15: 1545-1549.

[134] Hemminki K, Jiang Y, Steineck G. Skin cancer and non-Hodgkin's lymphoma as second malignancies. markers of impaired immune function? Eur J Cancer 2003; 39: 223-229.

[135] Hisada M, Chen BE, Jaffe ES, Travis LB. Second cancer incidence and cause-specific mortality among 3104 patients with hairy cell leukemia: a population-based study. J Natl Cancer Inst 2007; 99: 215-222.

[136] Nugent Z, Demers AA, Wiseman MC, Mihalcioiu C, Kliewer EV. Risk of second primary cancer and death following a diagnosis of non-melanoma skin cancer. Cancer Epidemiol Biomarkers Prev 2005; 14: 2584-2590.

[137] Wheless L, Black J, Alberg AJ. Nonmelanoma skin cancer and the risk of second primary cancers: a systematic review. Cancer Epidemiol Biomarkers Prev 2010; 19(7): 1686-95.

[138] Wassberg C, Thorn M, Yuen J, Ringborg U, Hakulinen T. Second primary cancers in patients with cutaneous malignant melanoma: a population-based study in Sweden. Br J Cancer 1996; 73: 255-259.

[139] Brown AP, Chen J, Hitchcock YJ, *et al.* The risk of second primary malignancies up to three decades after the treatment of differentiated thyroid cancer. J Clin Endocrinol Metab 2008; 93: 504-515.

[140] Sandeep TC, Strachan MW, Reynolds RM, *et al.* Second primary cancers in thyroid cancer patients: a multinational record linkage study. J Clin Endocrinol Metab 2006; 91: 1819-1825.

[141] Subramanian S, Goldstein DP, Parlea L, *et al.* Second primary malignancy risk in thyroid cancer survivors: a systematic review and meta-analysis. Thyroid 2007; 17: 1277-1288.

[142] Hemminki K, Scelo G, Boffetta P, *et al.* Second primary malignancies in patients with male breast cancer. Br J Cancer 2005; 92: 1288-1292.

[143] Mellemkjaer L, Friis S, Olsen JH, *et al.* Risk of second cancer among women with breast cancer. Int J Cancer 2006; 118: 2285-2292.

[144] Andersson M, Jensen MB, Engholm G, Henrik Storm H. Risk of second primary cancer among patients with early operable breast cancer registered or randomised in Danish Breast Cancer cooperative Group (DBCG) protocols of the 77, 82 and 89 programmes during 1977-2001. Acta Oncol 2008; 47: 755-764.

[145] Zighelboim I, Babb S, Gao F, *et al.* Excess of early onset multiple myeloma in endometrial cancer probands and their relatives suggests common susceptibility. Gynecol Oncol 2007; 105: 390-394.

[146] Linet MS, Harlow SD, McLaughlin JK. A case-control study of multiple myeloma in whites: chronic antigenic stimulation, occupation, and drug use. Cancer Res 1987; 47: 2978-2981.

[147] Bourguet CC, Logue EE. Antigenic stimulation and multiple myeloma. A prospective study. Cancer 1993; 72: 2148-2154.

[148] Hakulinen T, Isomaki H, Knekt P. Rheumatoid arthritis and cancer studies based on linking nationwide registries in Finland. Am J Med 1985; 78: 29-32.

[149] Isomaki HA, Hakulinen T, Joutsenlahti U. Excess risk of lymphomas, leukemia and myeloma in patients with rheumatoid arthritis. J Chronic Dis 1978; 31: 691-696.

[150] Katusic S, Beard CM, Kurland LT, Weis JW, Bergstralh E. Occurrence of malignant neoplasms in the Rochester, Minnesota, rheumatoid arthritis cohort. Am J Med 1985; 78: 50-55.

[151] Kauppi M, Pukkala E, Isomäki H. Elevated incidence of hematologic malignancies in patients with Sjögren's syndrome compared with patients with rheumatoid arthritis (Finland). Cancer Causes Control 1997; 8: 201-204.

[152] Doody MM, Linet MS, Glass AG, *et al.* Leukemia, lymphoma, and multiple myeloma following selected medical conditions. Cancer Causes Control 1992; 3: 449-456.

[153] Eriksson M. Rheumatoid arthritis as a risk factor for multiple myeloma: a case-control study. Eur J Cancer 1993; 29A: 259-263.

[154] Gridley G, McLaughlin JK, Ekbom A, *et al.* Incidence of cancer among patients with rheumatoid arthritis. J Natl Cancer Inst 1993; 85: 307-311.

[155] Landgren O, Zhang Y, Zahm SH, *et al.* Risk of multiple myeloma following medication use and medical conditions: a case-control study in Connecticut women. Cancer Epidemiol Biomarkers Prev 2006; 15: 2342-2347.

[156] Pearce N, Smith A, Howard J, *et al.* Case-control study of multiple myeloma and farming. Br J Cancer 1986; 54: 493-500.

[157] Askling J, Fored C, Baecklund E, *et al.* Haematopoietic malignancies in rheumatoid arthritis: lymphoma risk and characteristics after exposure to tumour necrosis factor antagonists. Ann Rheum Dis 2005; 64: 1414-1420.

[158] Becker N, Fortuny J, Alvaro T, *et al.* Medical history and risk of lymphoma: results of a European case-control study (EPILYMPH). J Cancer Res Clin Oncol 2009; 135: 1099-1107.

[159] Cuzick J, Stavola BD. Autoimmune disorders and multiple myeloma. Int J Epidemiol 1989; 18: 283.

[160] Lewis DR, Pottern LM, Brown LM, *et al.* Multiple myeloma among blacks and whites in the United States: the role of chronic antigenic stimulation. Cancer Causes Control 1994; 5: 529-539.

[161] Vineis P, Crosignani P, Sacerdote C, *et al.* Haematopoietic cancer and medical history: a multicentre case control study. J Epidemiol Commun Health 2000; 54: 431-436.

[162] Anderson LA, Gadalla S, Morton LM, *et al.* Population-based study of autoimmune conditions and the risk of specific lymphoid malignancies. Int J Cancer 2009; 125: 398-405.

[163] Mellemkjaer L, Linet MS, Gridley G, *et al.* Rheumatoid arthritis and cancer risk. Eur J Cancer 1996; 32A: 1753-1757.

[164] Parikh-Patel A, White RH, Allen M, Cress R. Risk of cancer among rheumatoid arthritis patients in California. Cancer Causes Control 2009; 20: 1001-1010.

[165] Thomas E, Brewster D, Black R, Macfarlane G. Risk of malignancy among patients with rheumatic conditions. Int J Cancer 2000 88: 497-502.

[166] Baker G, Kahl L, Zee B, *et al.* Malignancy following treatment of rheumatoid arthritis with cyclophosphamide. Long-term case-control follow-up study. Am J Med 1987 83: 1-9.

[167] Beauparlant P, Papp K, Haraoui B. The incidence of cancer associated with the treatment of rheumatoid arthritis. Semin Arthritis Rheum 1999; 29: 148-158.

[168] MacFarlane G, Black R. Rheumatoid arthritis and lymphatic cancer. Eur J Cancer 1996; 32: 1630-1632.

[169] Setoguchi S, Solomon D, Weinblatt M, *et al.* Tumor necrosis factor alpha antagonist use and cancer in patients with rheumatoid arthritis. Arthritis Rheum 2006; 54: 2757-2764.

[170] Brinton LA, Gridley G, Hrubec Z, Hoover R, Jr JFF. Cancer risk following pernicious anaemia. Br J Cancer 1989; 59: 810–813.

[171] Hsing A, Hansson L, McLaughlin J, *et al.* Pernicious anemia and subsequent cancer. A population-based cohort study. Cancer 1993; 71: 745-750.

[172] Mellemkjaer L, Gridley G, Møller H, *et al.* Pernicious anaemia and cancer risk in Denmark. Br J Cancer 1996; 73: 998–1000.

[173] Soderberg KC, Jonsson F, Winqvist O, Hagmar L, Feychting M. Autoimmune diseases, asthma and risk of haematological malignancies: a nationwide case-control study in Sweden. Eur J Cancer 2006; 42: 3028-3033.

[174] Björnådal L, Löfström B, Yin L, Lundberg I, Ekbom A. Increased cancer incidence in a Swedish cohort of patients with systemic lupus erythematosus. Scand J Rheumatol 2002; 31: 66-71.

[175] Dalamaga M, Karmaniolas K, Papadavid E, Pelecanos N, Migdalis I. Association of thyroid disease and thyroid autoimmunity with multiple myeloma risk: a case-control study. Leuk Lymphoma 2008; 49: 1545-1552.

[176] Birmann BM, Tamimi RM, Giovannucci E, *et al.* Insulin-like growth factor-1- and interleukin-6-related gene variation and risk of multiple myeloma. Cancer Epidemiol Biomarkers Prev 2009; 18: 282-288.

[177] Boffetta P, Stellman SD, Garfinkel L. A case-control study of multiple myeloma nested in the American Cancer Society prospective study. Int J Cancer 1989; 43: 554-559.

[178] Cuzick J, Stavola BD. Multiple myeloma- a case-control study. Br J Cancer 1988; 57: 516-520.

[179] Mills P, Beeson W, Fraser G, RL RP. Allergy and cancer: organ site-specific results from the Adventist Health Study. Am J Epidemiol 1992; 136: 287-295.

[180] Turner M, Chen Y, Krewski D, *et al.* Cancer mortality among US men and women with asthma and hay fever. Am J Epidemiol 2005; 162: 212-221.

[181] Vesterinen E, Pukkala E, Timonen T, Aromaa A. Cancer incidence among 78,000 asthmatic patients. Int J Epidemiol 1993; 22: 976-982.

[182] Ji J, Shu X, Li X, *et al.* Cancer risk in hospitalized asthma patients. Br J Cancer 2009; 100: 829-833.

[183] Eriksson N, Mikoczy Z, Hagmar L. Cancer incidence in 13811 patients skin tested for allergy. J Investig Allergol Clin Immunol 2005; 15: 161-166.

[184] Gramenzi A, Buttino I, D'Avanzo B, *et al.* Medical history and the risk of multiple myeloma. Br J Cancer 1991; 63: 769–772.

[185] Gallagher RP, Spinelli JJ, Elwood JM, Skippen DH. Allergies and agricultural exposure as risk factors for multiple myeloma. Br J Cancer 1983; 48: 853-857.

[186] Koepsell T, Daling J, Weiss N, *et al.* Antigenic stimulation and the occurrence of multiple myeloma. Am J Epidemiol 1987; 126: 1051-1062.

[187] Becker N, Deeg E, Rüdiger T, Nieters A. Medical history and risk for lymphoma: results of a population-based case-control study in Germany. Eur J Cancer 2005; 41: 133-142.

[188] Landgren O, Rapkin J, Mellemkjaer L, *et al.* Respiratory tract infections in the pathway to multiple myeloma: a population-based study in Scandinavia. Haematologica 2006; 91: 1697-1700.

[189] Fordyce E, Wang Z, Kahn A, *et al.* Risk of cancer among women with AIDS in New York City. AIDS Public Policy J 2000; 15: 95-104.

[190] Goedert J, Coté T, Virgo P, *et al.* Spectrum of AIDS-associated malignant disorders. Lancet 1998; 351: 1833-1839.

[191] Grulich A, Wan X, Law M, Coates M, Kaldor J. Risk of cancer in people with AIDS. AIDS 1999; 13: 839-843.

[192] Grulich A, Li Y, McDonald A, *et al.* Rates of non-AIDS-defining cancers in people with HIV infection before and after AIDS diagnosis. AIDS 2002 16: 1155-1161.

[193] Shiels M, Cole S, Kirk G, Poole C. A meta-analysis of the incidence of non-AIDS cancers in HIV-infected individuals. J Acquir Immune Defic Syndr 2009; 52: 611-622.

[194] Rabkin C. AIDS and cancer in the era of highly active antiretroviral therapy (HAART). Eur J Cancer 2001; 37: 1316-1319.

[195] Bower M, Palmieri C, Dhillon T. AIDS-related malignancies: changing epidemiology and the impact of highly active antiretroviral therapy. Curr Opin Infect Dis 2006; 19: 14-19.

[196] Pantanowitz L, Schlecht H, Dezube B. The growing problem of non-AIDS-defining malignancies in HIV. Curr Opin Oncol 2006; 18: 469-478.

[197] Carbone A, Gloghini A, Serraino D, Spina M. HIV-associated Hodgkin lymphoma. Curr Opin HIV AIDS 2009; 4: 3-10.

[198] Montella M, Crispo A, Bellis GD, *et al.* HCV and cancer: a case-control study in a high-endemic area. Liver 2001; 21: 335-341.

[199] Montella M, Crispo A, Frigeri F, *et al.* HCV and tumors correlated with immune system: a case-control study in an area of hyperendemicity. Leuk Res 2001; 25: 775-781.

[200] Duberg A, Nordström M, Törner A, *et al.* Non-Hodgkin's lymphoma and other nonhepatic malignancies in Swedish patients with hepatitis C virus infection. Hepatology 2005; 41: 652-659.

[201] Bianco E, Marcucci F, Mele A, *et al.* Prevalence of hepatitis C virus infection in lymphoproliferative diseases other than B-cell non-Hodgkin's lymphoma, and in myeloproliferative diseases: an Italian Multi-Center case-control study. Haematologica 2004; 89: 70-76.

[202] de Sanjose S, Nieters A, Goedert J, *et al.* Role of hepatitis C virus infection in malignant lymphoma in Spain. Int J Cancer 2004; 111: 81-85.

[203] Hausfater P, Cacoub P, Sterkers Y, *et al.* Hepatitis C virus infection and lymphoproliferative diseases: prospective study on 1,576 patients in France. Am J Hematol 2001; 67: 168-171.

[204] Rabkin C, Tess B, Christianson R, *et al.* Prospective study of hepatitis C viral infection as a risk factor for subsequent B-cell neoplasia. Blood 2002; 99: 4240-4242.

[205] Giordano T, Henderson L, Landgren O, *et al.* Risk of non-Hodgkin lymphoma and lymphoproliferative precursor diseases in US veterans with hepatitis C virus. JAMA 2007; 297: 2010-2017.

[206] Quinlan S, Morton L, Pfeiffer R, *et al.* Increased risk for lymphoid and myeloid neoplasms in elderly solid-organ transplant recipients. Cancer Epidemiol Biomarkers Prev 2010; 19: 1229-1237.

[207] Morgan GJ, Davies FE, Linet M. Myeloma aetiology and epidemiology. Biomed Pharmacother 2002; 56: 223-234.

[208] Ichimaru M, Ishimaru T, Mikami M, Matsunaga M. Multiple myeloma among atomic bomb survivors in Hiroshima and Nagasaki, 1950-76: relationship to radiation dose absorbed by marrow. J Natl Cancer Inst 1982; 69: 323-328.

[209] Shimizu Y, Kato H, Schull WJ. Studies of the mortality of A-bomb survivors. 9. Mortality, 1950-1985: Part 2. Cancer mortality based on the recently revised doses (DS86). Radiat Res 1990; 121: 120-141.

[210] Preston DL, Kusumi S, Tomonaga M, *et al.* Cancer incidence in atomic bomb survivors. Part III. Leukemia, lymphoma and multiple myeloma, 1950-1987. Radiat Res 1994; 137: S68-97.

[211] Neriishi K, Yoshimoto Y, Carter RL, *et al.* Monoclonal gammopathy in atomic bomb survivors. Radiat Res 1993; 133: 351-359.

[212] Neriishi K, Nakashima E, Suzuki G. Monoclonal gammopathy of undetermined significance in atomic bomb survivors: incidence and transformation to multiple myeloma. Br J Haematol 2003; 121: 405-410.

[213] Carpenter L, Higgins C, Douglas A, *et al.* Combined analysis of mortality in three United Kingdom nuclear industry workforces, 1946-1988. Radiat Res 1994; 138: 224-238.

[214] Muirhead CR, Goodill AA, Haylock RG, *et al.* Occupational radiation exposure and mortality: second analysis of the National Registry for Radiation Workers. J Radiol Prot 1999; 19: 3-26.

[215] Gilbert ES, Fry SA, Wiggs LD, *et al.* Analyses of combined mortality data on workers at the Hanford Site, Oak Ridge National Laboratory, and Rocky Flats Nuclear Weapons Plant. Radiat Res 1989; 120: 19-35.

[216] Omar RZ, Barber JA, Smith PG. Cancer mortality and morbidity among plutonium workers at the Sellafield plant of British Nuclear Fuels. Br J Cancer 1999; 79: 1288-1301.

[217] Iwasaki T, Murata M, Ohshima S, *et al.* Second analysis of mortality of nuclear industry workers in Japan, 1986-1997. Radiat Res 2003; 159: 228-238.

[218] Muirhead CR, Bingham D, Haylock RG, *et al.* Follow up of mortality and incidence of cancer 1952-98 in men from the UK who participated in the UK's atmospheric nuclear weapon tests and experimental programmes. Occup Environ Med 2003; 60: 165-172.

[219] Pearce N, Winkelmann R, Kennedy J, *et al.* Further follow-up of New Zealand participants in United Kingdom atmospheric nuclear weapons tests in the Pacific. Cancer Causes Control 1997; 8: 139-145.

[220] Lewis EB. Leukemia, Multiple Myeloma, and Aplastic Anemia in American Radiologists. Science 1963; 142: 1492-1494.

[221] Sigurdson AJ, Doody MM, Rao RS, *et al.* Cancer incidence in the US radiologic technologists health study, 1983-1998. Cancer 2003; 97: 3080-3089.

[222] Wang JX, Boice JD, Jr., Li BX, Zhang JY, Fraumeni JF, Jr. Cancer among medical diagnostic x-ray workers in China. J Natl Cancer Inst 1988; 80: 344-350.

[223] Zielinski JM, Garner MJ, Krewski D, *et al.* Decreases in occupational exposure to ionizing radiation among Canadian dental workers. J Can Dent Assoc 2005; 71: 29-33.

[224] Boice JD, Jr., Morin MM, Glass AG, *et al.* Diagnostic x-ray procedures and risk of leukemia, lymphoma, and multiple myeloma. Jama 1991; 265: 1290-1294.

[225] Hatcher JL, Baris D, Olshan AF, *et al.* Diagnostic radiation and the risk of multiple myeloma (United States). Cancer Causes Control 2001; 12: 755-761.

[226] Davis FG, Boice JD, Jr., Hrubec Z, Monson RR. Cancer mortality in a radiation-exposed cohort of Massachusetts tuberculosis patients. Cancer Res 1989; 49: 6130-6136.

[227] Andersson M, Storm HH. Cancer incidence among Danish Thorotrast-exposed patients. J Natl Cancer Inst 1992; 84: 1318-1325.

[228] Darby SC, Doll R, Gill SK, Smith PG. Long term mortality after a single treatment course with X-rays in patients treated for ankylosing spondylitis. Br J Cancer 1987; 55: 179-190.

[229] Darby SC, Reeves G, Key T, Doll R, Stovall M. Mortality in a cohort of women given X-ray therapy for metropathia haemorrhagica. Int J Cancer 1994; 56: 793-801.

[230] Blair A, Freeman LB. Epidemiologic studies in agricultural populations: observations and future directions. J Agromedicine 2009; 14: 125-131.

[231] Kristensen P, Andersen A, Irgens LM, Laake P, Bye AS. Incidence and risk factors of cancer among men and women in Norwegian agriculture. Scand J Work Environ Health 1996; 22: 14-26.

[232] Lee E, Burnett CA, Lalich N, Cameron LL, Sestito JP. Proportionate mortality of crop and livestock farmers in the United States, 1984-1993. Am J Ind Med 2002; 42: 410-420.

[233] Lope V, Perez-Gomez B, Aragones N, *et al.* Occupation, exposure to chemicals, sensitizing agents, and risk of multiple myeloma in Sweden. Cancer Epidemiol Biomarkers Prev 2008; 17: 3123-3127.

[234] Mester B, Nieters A, Deeg E, *et al.* Occupation and malignant lymphoma: a population based case control study in Germany. Occup Environ Med 2006; 63: 17-26.

[235] Orsi L, Delabre L, Monnereau A, *et al.* Occupational exposure to pesticides and lymphoid neoplasms among men: results of a French case-control study. Occup Environ Med 2009; 66: 291-298.

[236] Pahwa P, McDuffie HH, Dosman JA, *et al.* Hodgkin lymphoma, multiple myeloma, soft tissue sarcomas, insect repellents, and phenoxyherbicides. J Occup Environ Med 2006; 48: 264-274.

[237] Khuder SA, Mutgi AB. Meta-analyses of multiple myeloma and farming. Am J Ind Med 1997; 32: 510-516.

[238] Merhi M, Raynal H, Cahuzac E, *et al.* Occupational exposure to pesticides and risk of hematopoietic cancers: meta-analysis of case-control studies. Cancer Causes Control 2007; 18: 1209-1226.

[239] Zahm S, Ward MH, Blair A: Pesticides and cancer. In Human health effects of pesticides. KEIFER MC (ed.) Hanley & Belfus, Inc., Philadelphia, PA (1997): 269-289.

[240] Eriksson M, Karlsson M. Occupational and other environmental factors and multiple myeloma: a population based case-control study. Br J Ind Med 1992; 49: 95-103.

[241] Metayer C, Johnson ES, Rice JC. Nested case-control study of tumors of the hemopoietic and lymphatic systems among workers in the meat industry. Am J Epidemiol 1998; 147: 727-738.

[242] De Roos AJ, Blair A, Rusiecki JA, *et al.* Cancer incidence among glyphosate-exposed pesticide applicators in the Agricultural Health Study. Environ Health Perspect 2005; 113: 49-54.

[243] Lee WJ, Blair A, Hoppin JA, *et al.* Cancer incidence among pesticide applicators exposed to chlorpyrifos in the Agricultural Health Study. J Natl Cancer Inst 2004; 96: 1781-1789.

[244] International Agency for Research on Cancer. Monograph on the Evaluation of the Carcinogenic Risk of Chemicals: Some Industrial Chemicals and Dyestuffs. In: International Agency for Research on Cancer, Lyon, France (1982): 93-148.

[245] Bergsagel DE, Wong O, Bergsagel PL, *et al.* Benzene and multiple myeloma: appraisal of the scientific evidence. Blood 1999; 94: 1174-1182.

[246] Chen R, Seaton A. A meta-analysis of mortality among workers exposed to organic solvents. Occup Med (Lond) 1996; 46: 337-344.

[247] Goldstein BD, Shalat SL. The casual relation between benzene exposure and multiple myeloma. Blood 2000; 95: 1512-1514.

[248] Rinsky RA, Hornung RW, Silver SR, Tseng CY. Benzene exposure and hematopoietic mortality: A long-term epidemiologic risk assessment. Am J Ind Med 2002; 42: 474-480.

[249] Sorahan T, Kinlen LJ, Doll R. Cancer risks in a historical UK cohort of benzene exposed workers. Occup Environ Med 2005; 62: 231-236.

[250] Hayes RB, Yin S, Rothman N, *et al.* Benzene and lymphohematopoietic malignancies in China. J Toxicol Environ Health A 2000; 61: 419-432.

[251] Bezabeh S, Engel A, Morris CB, Lamm SH. Does benzene cause multiple myeloma? An analysis of the published case-control literature. Environ Health Perspect 1996; 104 Suppl 6: 1393-1398.

[252] Infante PF. Benzene exposure and multiple myeloma: a detailed meta-analysis of benzene cohort studies. Ann N Y Acad Sci 2006; 1076: 90-109.

[253] Wong O, Trent L, Harris F. Nested case-control study of leukaemia, multiple myeloma, and kidney cancer in a cohort of petroleum workers exposed to gasoline. Occup Environ Med 1999; 56: 217-221.

[254] Wong O, Raabe GK. Multiple myeloma and benzene exposure in a multinational cohort of more than 250,000 petroleum workers. Regul Toxicol Pharmacol 1997; 26: 188-199.

[255] Alexander DD, Mink PJ, Adami HO, *et al.* Multiple myeloma: a review of the epidemiologic literature. Int J Cancer 2007; 120 Suppl 12: 40-61.

[256] Garland CF, Garland FC, Gorham ED, *et al.* The role of vitamin D in cancer prevention. Am J Public Health 2006; 96: 252-261.

[257] John EM, Schwartz GG, Koo J, Wang W, Ingles SA. Sun exposure, vitamin D receptor gene polymorphisms, and breast cancer risk in a multiethnic population. Am J Epidemiol 2007; 166: 1409-1419.

[258] Garland C, Garland F. Do sunlight and vitamin D reduce the likelihood of colon cancer? Int J Epidemiol 1980; 9: 227–231.

[259] Colli JL, Grant WB. Solar ultraviolet B radiation compared with prostate cancer incidence and mortality rates in United States. Urology 2008; 71: 531-535.

[260] Kricker A, Armstrong BK, Hughes AM, *et al.* Personal sun exposure and risk of non Hodgkin lymphoma: a pooled analysis from the Interlymph Consortium. Int J Cancer 2008; 122: 144-154.

[261] Boscoe FP, Schymura MJ. Solar ultraviolet-B exposure and cancer incidence and mortality in the United States, 1993-2002. BMC Cancer 2006; 6: 264.

[262] Weihkopf T, Becker N, Nieters A, *et al.* Sun exposure and malignant lymphoma: a population-based case-control study in Germany. Int J Cancer 2007; 120: 2445-2451.

[263] Polesel J, Talamini R, Montella M, *et al.* Linoleic acid, vitamin D and other nutrient intakes in the risk of non-Hodgkin lymphoma: an Italian case-control study. Ann Oncol 2006; 17: 713-718.

[264] Rhee HV, Coebergh JW, Vries ED. Sunlight, vitamin D and the prevention of cancer: a systematic review of epidemiological studies. Eur J Cancer Prev 2009: 458-475.

[265] Giovannucci E. The epidemiology of vitamin D and cancer incidence and mortality: a review (United States). Cancer Causes Control 2005; 16: 83-95.

[266] Ullrich SE. Mechanisms underlying UV-induced immune suppression. Mutat Res 2005; 571: 185-205.

[267] Boffetta P, van der Hel O, Kricker A, *et al.* Exposure to ultraviolet radiation and risk of malignant lymphoma and multiple myeloma--a multicentre European case-control study. Int J Epidemiol 2008; 37: 1080-1094.

[268] Grant WB. An ecologic study of the role of solar UV-B radiation in reducing the risk of cancer using cancer mortality data, dietary supply data and latitude for European countries. In Biologic effects of light 2001, Proceedings of the Biologic Effects of Light Symposium. HOLICK M (ed.) Boston, Massachusetts (2002): 267–276.

[269] Grant WB. Ecologic studies of solar UV-B radiation and cancer mortality rates. Recent Results Cancer Res 2003; 164: 371-377.

[270] Grant WB. An ecologic study of cancer mortality rates in Spain with respect to indices of solar UVB irradiance and smoking. Int J Cancer 2007; 120: 1123-1128.

[271] Grant WB. Lower vitamin-D production from solar ultraviolet-B irradiance may explain some differences in cancer survival rates. J Natl Med Assoc 2006; 98: 357-364.

[272] Uehara M, Takahashi K, Hoshuyama T, Pan G, Feng Y. Geographical correlation between ambient UVB level and mortality risk of leukemia in Japan. Environ Res 2003; 92: 78-84.

[273] Grandin L, Orsi L, Troussard X, *et al.* UV radiation exposure, skin type and lymphoid malignancies: results of a French case-control study. Cancer Causes Control 2008; 19: 305-315.

[274] Hu S, Ma F, Collado-Mesa F, Kirsner RS. Ultraviolet radiation and incidence of non-Hodgkin's lymphoma among Hispanics in the United States. Cancer Epidemiol Biomarkers Prev 2004; 13: 59-64.

[275] Hughes AM, Armstrong BK, Vajdic CM, *et al.* Sun exposure may protect against non-Hodgkin lymphoma: a case-control study. Int J Cancer 2004; 112: 865-871.

[276] Purdue MP, Hartge P, Davis S, *et al.* Sun exposure, vitamin D receptor gene polymorphisms and risk of non-Hodgkin lymphoma. Cancer Causes Control 2007; 18: 989-999.

[277] Smedby KE, Hjalgrim H, Melbye M, *et al.* Ultraviolet radiation exposure and risk of malignant lymphomas. J Natl Cancer Inst 2005; 97: 199-209.

[278] Grant WB. An estimate of premature cancer mortality in the U.S. due to inadequate doses of solar ultraviolet-B radiation. Cancer 2002; 94: 1867-1875.

[279] Adami J, Nyren O, Bergstrom R, *et al.* Smoking and the risk of leukemia, lymphoma, and multiple myeloma (Sweden). Cancer Causes Control 1998; 9: 49-56.
[280] Brown LM, Pottern LM, Silverman DT, *et al.* Multiple myeloma among Blacks and Whites in the United States: role of cigarettes and alcoholic beverages. Cancer Causes Control 1997; 8: 610-614.
[281] Brownson RC. Cigarette smoking and risk of myeloma. J Natl Cancer Inst 1991; 83: 1036-1037.
[282] Fernberg P, Odenbro A, Bellocco R, *et al.* Tobacco use, body mass index, and the risk of leukemia and multiple myeloma: a nationwide cohort study in Sweden. Cancer Res 2007; 67: 5983-5986.
[283] Flodin U, Fredriksson M, Persson B. Multiple myeloma and engine exhausts, fresh wood, and creosote: a case-referent study. Am J Ind Med 1987; 12: 519-529.
[284] Friedman GD. Cigarette smoking, leukemia, and multiple myeloma. Ann Epidemiol 1993; 3: 425-428.
[285] Herrinton LJ, Koepsell TD, Weiss NS. Smoking and multiple myeloma. Cancer Causes Control 1992; 3: 391-392.
[286] Miligi L, Seniori Costantini A, Crosignani P, *et al.* Occupational, environmental, and life-style factors associated with the risk of hematolymphopoietic malignancies in women. Am J Ind Med 1999; 36: 60-69.
[287] Rogot E, Murray JL. Smoking and causes of death among U.S. veterans: 16 years of observation. Public Health Rep 1980; 95: 213-222.
[288] Stagnaro E, Ramazzotti V, Crosignani P, *et al.* Smoking and hematolymphopoietic malignancies. Cancer Causes Control 2001; 12: 325-334.
[289] Vlajinac HD, Pekmezovic TD, Adanja BJ, *et al.* Case-control study of multiple myeloma with special reference to diet as risk factor. Neoplasma 2003; 50: 79-83.
[290] Williams RR, Horm JW. Association of cancer sites with tobacco and alcohol consumption and socioeconomic status of patients: interview study from the Third National Cancer Survey. J Natl Cancer Inst 1977; 58: 525-547.
[291] Mills PK, Newell GR, Beeson WL, Fraser GE, Phillips RL. History of cigarette smoking and risk of leukemia and myeloma: results from the Adventist health study. J Natl Cancer Inst 1990; 82: 1832-1836.
[292] Nieters A, Deeg E, Becker N. Tobacco and alcohol consumption and risk of lymphoma: results of a population-based case-control study in Germany. Int J Cancer 2006; 118: 422-430.
[293] Brown LM, Gibson R, Burmeister LF, *et al.* Alcohol consumption and risk of leukemia, non-Hodgkin's lymphoma, and multiple myeloma. Leuk Res 1992; 16: 979-984.
[294] Tavani A, Pregnolato A, Negri E, *et al.* Diet and risk of lymphoid neoplasms and soft tissue sarcomas. Nutr Cancer 1997; 27: 256-260.
[295] Wong O, Harris F, Wang Y, Fu H. A hospital-based case-control study of non-Hodgkin lymphoid neoplasms in Shanghai: analysis of personal characteristics, lifestyle, and environmental risk factors by subtypes of the WHO classification. J Occup Environ Med 2010; 52: 39-53.
[296] Kanda J, Matsuo K, Inoue M, *et al.* Association of alcohol intake with the risk of malignant lymphoma and plasma cell myeloma in Japanese: a population-based cohort study (Japan Public Health Center-based Prospective Study). Cancer Epidemiol Biomarkers Prev 2010; 19: 429-434.
[297] Gorini G, Stagnaro E, Fontana V, *et al.* Alcohol consumption and risk of Hodgkin's lymphoma and multiple myeloma: a multicentre case-control study. Ann Oncol 2007; 18: 143-148.
[298] Brown LM, Everett GD, Gibson R, *et al.* Smoking and risk of non-Hodgkin's lymphoma and multiple myeloma. Cancer Causes Control 1992; 3: 49-55.
[299] World Health Organization. (1995) Physical Status: The use and interpretation of anthropometry: report of a WHO expert committee. World Health Organization
[300] Birmann BM, Giovannucci E, Rosner B, Anderson KC, Colditz GA. Body mass index, physical activity, and risk of multiple myeloma. Cancer Epidemiol Biomarkers Prev 2007; 16: 1474-1478.
[301] Blair CK, Cerhan JR, Folsom AR, Ross JA. Anthropometric characteristics and risk of multiple myeloma. Epidemiology 2005; 16: 691-694.
[302] Bosetti C, Negri E, Gallus S, *et al.* Anthropometry and multiple myeloma. Epidemiology 2006; 17: 340-341.
[303] Brown LM, Gridley G, Pottern LM, *et al.* Diet and nutrition as risk factors for multiple myeloma among blacks and whites in the United States. Cancer Causes Control 2001; 12: 117-125.
[304] Calle EE, Rodriguez C, Walker-Thurmond K, Thun MJ. Overweight, obesity, and mortality from cancer in a prospectively studied cohort of U.S. adults. N Engl J Med 2003; 348: 1625-1638.
[305] Engeland A, Tretli S, Hansen S, Bjorge T. Height and body mass index and risk of lymphohematopoietic malignancies in two million Norwegian men and women. Am J Epidemiol 2007; 165: 44-52.
[306] Pan SY, Johnson KC, Ugnat AM, Wen SW, Mao Y. Association of obesity and cancer risk in Canada. Am J Epidemiol 2004; 159: 259-268.

[307] Khan MM, Mori M, Sakauchi F, *et al.* Risk factors for multiple myeloma: evidence from the Japan Collaborative Cohort (JACC) study. Asian Pac J Cancer Prev 2006; 7: 575-581.

[308] Soderberg KC, Kaprio J, Verkasalo PK, *et al.* Overweight, obesity and risk of haematological malignancies: a cohort study of Swedish and Finnish twins. Eur J Cancer 2009; 45: 1232-1238.

[309] Reeves GK, Pirie K, Beral V, *et al.* Cancer incidence and mortality in relation to body mass index in the Million Women Study: cohort study. BMJ 2007; 335: 1134.

[310] Britton JA, Khan AE, Rohrmann S, *et al.* Anthropometric characteristics and non-Hodgkin's lymphoma and multiple myeloma risk in the European Prospective Investigation into Cancer and Nutrition (EPIC). Haematologica 2008; 93: 1666-1677.

[311] Chiu BC, Gapstur SM, Greenland P, Wang R, Dyer A. Body mass index, abnormal glucose metabolism, and mortality from hematopoietic cancer. Cancer Epidemiol Biomarkers Prev 2006; 15: 2348-2354.

[312] De Roos AJ, Ulrich CM, Ray RM, *et al.* Intentional weight loss and risk of lymphohematopoietic cancers. Cancer Causes Control 2009; 21: 223-236.

[313] Lu Y, Sullivan-Halley J, Henderson KD, *et al.* Anthropometric characteristics and multiple myeloma risk. Epidemiology 2010; 21: 272-273.

[314] MacInnis RJ, English DR, Hopper JL, Giles GG. Body size and composition and the risk of lymphohematopoietic malignancies. J Natl Cancer Inst 2005; 97: 1154-1157.

[315] Oh SW, Yoon YS, Shin SA. Effects of excess weight on cancer incidences depending on cancer sites and histologic findings among men: Korea National Health Insurance Corporation Study. J Clin Oncol 2005; 23: 4742-4754.

[316] Pylypchuk RD, Schouten LJ, Goldbohm RA, Schouten HC, van den Brandt PA. Body mass index, height, and risk of lymphatic malignancies: a prospective cohort study. Am J Epidemiol 2009; 170: 297-307.

[317] Friedman GD, Herrinton LJ. Obesity and multiple myeloma. Cancer Causes Control 1994; 5: 479-483.

[318] Samanic C, Gridley G, Chow WH, *et al.* Obesity and cancer risk among white and black United States veterans. Cancer Causes Control 2004; 15: 35-43.

[319] Wolk A, Gridley G, Svensson M, *et al.* A prospective study of obesity and cancer risk (Sweden). Cancer Causes Control 2001; 12: 13-21.

[320] Larsson SC, Wolk A. Body mass index and risk of multiple myeloma: a meta-analysis. Int J Cancer 2007; 121: 2512-2516.

[321] Renehan AG, Tyson M, Egger M, Heller RF, Zwahlen M. Body-mass index and incidence of cancer: a systematic review and meta-analysis of prospective observational studies. Lancet 2008; 371: 569-578.

[322] Ge NL, Rudikoff S. Insulin-like growth factor I is a dual effector of multiple myeloma cell growth. Blood 2000; 96: 2856-2861.

[323] Kaaks R, Lukanova A. Effects of weight control and physical activity in cancer prevention: role of endogenous hormone metabolism. Ann N Y Acad Sci 2002; 963: 268-281.

[324] Mitsiades CS, Mitsiades N, Poulaki V, *et al.* Activation of NF-kappaB and upregulation of intracellular anti-apoptotic proteins *via* the IGF-1/Akt signaling in human multiple myeloma cells: therapeutic implications. Oncogene 2002; 21: 5673-5683.

[325] Sandhu MS, Gibson JM, Heald AH, Dunger DB, Wareham NJ. Association between insulin-like growth factor-I: insulin-like growth factor-binding protein-1 ratio and metabolic and anthropometric factors in men and women. Cancer Epidemiol Biomarkers Prev 2004; 13: 166-170.

[326] Greenberg AS, Obin MS. Obesity and the role of adipose tissue in inflammation and metabolism. Am J Clin Nutr 2006; 83: 461S-465S.

[327] Kawano M, Hirano T, Matsuda T, *et al.* Autocrine generation and requirement of BSF-2/IL-6 for human multiple myelomas. Nature 1988; 332: 83-85.

[328] Klein B, Zhang XG, Jourdan M, *et al.* Paracrine rather than autocrine regulation of myeloma-cell growth and differentiation by interleukin-6. Blood 1989; 73: 517-526.

[329] Mohamed-Ali V, Goodrick S, Rawesh A, *et al.* Subcutaneous adipose tissue releases interleukin-6, but not tumor necrosis factor-alpha, *in vivo*. J Clin Endocrinol Metab 1997; 82: 4196-4200.

[330] Alexandrakis MG, Passam FH, Sfiridaki A, *et al.* Serum levels of leptin in multiple myeloma patients and its relation to angiogenic and inflammatory cytokines. Int J Biol Markers 2004; 19: 52-57.

[331] Dalamaga M, Karmaniolas K, Panagiotou A, *et al.* Low circulating adiponectin and resistin, but not leptin, levels are associated with multiple myeloma risk: a case-control study. Cancer Causes Control 2009; 20: 193-199.

[332] Pamuk GE, Demir M, Harmandar F, *et al.* Leptin and resistin levels in serum of patients with hematologic malignancies: correlation with clinical characteristics. Exp Oncol 2006; 28: 241-244.

[333] Reseland JE, Reppe S, Olstad OK, *et al.* Abnormal adipokine levels and leptin-induced changes in gene expression profiles in multiple myeloma. Eur J Haematol 2009; 83: 460-470.

[334] Hosgood HD, 3rd, Baris D, Zahm SH, Zheng T, Cross AJ. Diet and risk of multiple myeloma in Connecticut women. Cancer Causes Control 2007; 18: 1065-1076.

[335] Fritschi L, Ambrosini GL, Kliewer EV, Johnson KC. Dietary fish intake and risk of leukaemia, multiple myeloma, and non-Hodgkin lymphoma. Cancer Epidemiol Biomarkers Prev 2004; 13: 532-537.

[336] Ames BN, Kammen HO, Yamasaki E. Hair dyes are mutagenic: identification of a variety of mutagenic ingredients. Proc Natl Acad Sci USA 1975; 72: 2423-2427.

[337] Takkouche B, Etminan M, Montes-Martinez A. Personal use of hair dyes and risk of cancer: a meta-analysis. JAMA 2005; 293: 2516-2525.

[338] Turesky RJ, Freeman JP, Holland RD, *et al.* Identification of aminobiphenyl derivatives in commercial hair dyes. Chem Res Toxicol 2003; 16: 1162-1173.

[339] Guidotti S, Wright WE, Peters JM. Multiple myeloma in cosmetologists. Am J Ind Med 1982; 3: 169-171.

[340] Herrinton LJ, Weiss NS, Koepsell TD, *et al.* Exposure to hair-coloring products and the risk of multiple myeloma. Am J Public Health 1994; 84: 1142-1144.

[341] Spinelli JJ, Gallagher RP, Band PR, Threlfall WJ. Multiple myeloma, leukemia, and cancer of the ovary in cosmetologists and hairdressers. Am J Ind Med 1984; 6: 97-102.

[342] Baris D, Silverman DT, Brown LM, *et al.* Occupation, pesticide exposure and risk of multiple myeloma. Scand J Work Environ Health 2004; 30: 215-222.

[343] Pottern LM, Heineman EF, Olsen JH, Raffn E, Blair A. Multiple myeloma among Danish women: employment history and workplace exposures. Cancer Causes Control 1992; 3: 427-432.

[344] Teta MJ, Walrath J, Meigs JW, Flannery JT. Cancer incidence among cosmetologists. J Natl Cancer Inst 1984; 72: 1051-1057.

[345] Takkouche B, Regueira-Mendez C, Montes-Martinez A. Risk of cancer among hairdressers and related workers: a meta-analysis. Int J Epidemiol 2009; 38: 1512-1531.

[346] Thun MJ, Altekruse SF, Namboodiri MM, *et al.* Hair dye use and risk of fatal cancers in U.S. women. J Natl Cancer Inst 1994; 86: 210-215.

[347] Altekruse SF, Henley SJ, Thun MJ. Deaths from hematopoietic and other cancers in relation to permanent hair dye use in a large prospective study (United States). Cancer Causes Control 1999; 10: 617-625.

[348] Grodstein F, Hennekens CH, Colditz GA, Hunter DJ, Stampfer MJ. A prospective study of permanent hair dye use and hematopoietic cancer. J Natl Cancer Inst 1994; 86: 1466-1470.

[349] Zahm SH, Weisenburger DD, Babbitt PA, *et al.* Use of hair coloring products and the risk of lymphoma, multiple myeloma, and chronic lymphocytic leukemia. Am J Public Health 1992; 82: 990-997.

[350] Brown LM, Everett GD, Burmeister LF, Blair A. Hair dye use and multiple myeloma in white men. Am J Public Health 1992; 82: 1673-1674.

[351] Koutros S, Baris D, Bell E, *et al.* Use of hair colouring products and risk of multiple myeloma among US women. Occup Environ Med 2009; 66: 68-70.

[352] Miligi L, Costantini AS, Benvenuti A, *et al.* Personal use of hair dyes and hematolymphopoietic malignancies. Arch Environ Occup Health 2005; 60: 249-256.

[353] Tavani A, Negri E, Franceschi S, *et al.* Hair dye use and risk of lymphoid neoplasms and soft tissue sarcomas. Int J Cancer 2005; 113: 629-631.

[354] Morton LM, Bernstein L, Wang SS, *et al.* Hair dye use, genetic variation in N-acetyltransferase 1 (NAT1) and 2 (NAT2), and risk of non-Hodgkin lymphoma. Carcinogenesis 2007; 28: 1759-1764.

[355] Wang LH, Yang XY, Mihalic K, *et al.* Activation of estrogen receptor blocks interleukin-6-inducible cell growth of human multiple myeloma involving molecular cross-talk between estrogen receptor and STAT3 mediated by co-regulator PIAS3. J Biol Chem 2001; 276: 31839-31844.

[356] Altieri A, Gallus S, Franceschi S, *et al.* Hormone replacement therapy and risk of lymphomas and myelomas. Eur J Cancer Prev 2004; 13: 349-351.

[357] Fernandez E, Gallus S, Bosetti C, *et al.* Hormone replacement therapy and cancer risk: a systematic analysis from a network of case-control studies. Int J Cancer 2003; 105: 408-412.

[358] Brinton LA, Gridley G, Persson I, Baron J, Bergqvist A. Cancer risk after a hospital discharge diagnosis of endometriosis. Am J Obstet Gynecol 1997; 176: 572-579.

[359] La Vecchia C, Negri E, Franceschi S, Parazzini F. Long-term impact of reproductive factors on cancer risk. Int J Cancer 1993; 53: 215-219.

[360] Tavani A, Pregnolato A, La Vecchia C, Franceschi S. A case-control study of reproductive factors and risk of lymphomas and myelomas. Leuk Res 1997; 21: 885-888.

[361] Gadd SL, Hobbs G, Miller MR. Acetaminophen-induced proliferation of estrogen-responsive breast cancer cells is associated with increases in c-myc RNA expression and NF-kappaB activity. Toxicol Sci 2002; 66: 233-243.

[362] Blazka ME, Wilmer JL, Holladay SD, Wilson RE, Luster MI. Role of proinflammatory cytokines in acetaminophen hepatotoxicity. Toxicol Appl Pharmacol 1995; 133: 43-52.

[363] Rannug U, Holme JA, Hongslo JK, Sram R. International Commission for Protection against Environmental Mutagens and Carcinogens. An evaluation of the genetic toxicity of paracetamol. Mutat Res 1995; 327: 179-200.

[364] Moysich KB, Bonner MR, Beehler GP, *et al.* Regular analgesic use and risk of multiple myeloma. Leuk Res 2007; 31: 547-551.

[365] Birmann B, Giovannucci E, Colditz G: Regular aspirin use and risk of multiple myeloma: A prospective analysis[abstract]. AACR. Washington, DC (Apr 17-21 2010).

[366] Khan AE, Gallo V, Linseisen J, *et al.* Diabetes and the risk of non-Hodgkin's lymphoma and multiple myeloma in the European Prospective Investigation into Cancer and Nutrition. Haematologica 2008; 93: 842-850.

CHAPTER 3

Genetic and Epigenetic Mechanisms in Multiple Myeloma

Michela Frenquelli and Giovanni Tonon*

Division of Molecular Oncology, San Raffaele del Monte Tabor Scientific Foundation, Italy

Abstract: Multiple myeloma (MM) is a malignant disorder due to clonal proliferation of plasma cells in the bone marrow in association with elevated serum or urine monoclonal paraprotein levels. MM is associated, particularly in the most advanced stages of the disease, with severe complication, like lytic bone lesion, anemia, immunodeficiency and renal failure. Despite advances in the understanding of the disease and the use of high-dose chemotherapy, MM remains an incurable disease.

From a genetic standpoint, MM development is a multistep process characterized by the presence of a series of chromosomal abnormalities and complex translocations, involving known oncogenes and tumor-suppressor genes. Genomic aberrations are present with increasing frequency as disease progresses. There is an increasing evidence that, in addition to genomic abnormalities, epigenetic dysregulation plays a pivotal role in MM development, making the picture even more complex.

Keywords: Translocations, hyperdiploidy, non-hyperdiploidy, FGFR3, MMSET, MAF, minimal common regions, myc, ras, TP53, NFκB, IRF4, epigenetics, histones, microRNAs.

1. GENETIC FEATURES

MM patients usually experience an heterogeneous clinical course that is reflected by its marked genomic instability. In addition to chromosome numerical alterations, MM is frequently associated with other cytogenetic abnormalities[1]. Particularly relevant are chromosomal translocations involving the immunoglobulin heavy chain locus (IGH) at 14q32 with the most frequent partners being 11q13, 4p16, 16q23, 20q11, and 6p21. Highly represented are also deletions of chromosome 13, gain/amplification of chromosome arm 1q, and deletion of 17p. New high throughput molecular/cytogenetic approaches such as gene expression profiling and, more recently, genome-wide copy number DNA analyses have contributed to clarify the molecular and biological features of MM subtypes, and identifying putative novel molecular targets for therapy [2, 3].

Following up on previous observations [4,5], Smadja and colleagues [6] proposed in 1998 a distinction between patients presenting a hyperdiploid karyotype (number of chromosomes from 47 to 74; hyperdiploid disease, HD) with concomitant gains of several odd chromosomes, such as 3, 5, 7, 9, 11, 15, 19, 21, in various combinations, and a second group, with hypodiploid, pseudodiploid, near-diploid, or tetraploid karyotypes (non-hyperdiploid disease, NHD). HD MM includes 50% to 60% of patients and presents a more favorable prognosis [7, 8].

Within the NHD group, it is then possible to further subdivide the patients based on the presence of primary chromosomal translocations involving the Ig locus. It should be emphasized that this distinction, useful as it is, it is nevertheless an oversimplification, because primary translocations are present also in the HD group, at a frequency of approximately 10% [7].

Hyperdiploid Multiple Myeloma

Little is known about the mechanisms driving oncogenesis in this group. Gene expression data have shown that HD presents a consistent overexpression of cyclin D1 or D2, albeit a clear pathogenetic role of these cyclins in this subgroup is lacking [9]. The pattern of odd chromosome gains suggests a gene dosage effect

***Address correspondence to Giovanni Tonon:** Division of Molecular Oncology, San Raffaele del Monte Tabor Scientific Foundation Via Olgettina 58, 20132 Milan, Italy; Ph. +39 02 2643 5624; Fax +39 02 2643 2408; E-mail: tonon.giovanni@hsr.it

Klaus Podar and Kenneth C. Anderson (Eds)

resulting in the concomitant dysregulation of several oncogenic pathways. Indeed, expression profiling comparisons between HD versus NHD have suggested increased expression of genes involved in protein synthesis and defective protein catabolism and transport in this group of patients [10, 11].

Overall, this group presents a better prognosis when compared with NHD MM [8, 12, 13]. Recent studies, however, have identified subsets of HD patients with a poorer prognosis, comparable to subset of NHD patients presenting with specific chromosomal translocations [14, 15]. These patients are characterized by loss of chromosome 13 and/or gain in 1q [15]. An additional feature of this group is the lower frequency in chromosome 11 gains. These patients showed a significantly worse event-free survival, and a trend toward shorter overall survival when compared with HD patients without 1q gains/amplifications or 13 loss. Other recent studies have corroborated these findings. In a recent report using FISH and expression arrays, unsupervised clustering has confirmed the existence of two groups within the HD, one characterized by preferential gains on chromosome 11 and the second one by losses of chromosome 13 and gains of 1q [11]. This group of patients may represent an evolution of HD toward a more aggressive, high-proliferative disease, as suggested by Zhan and colleagues [16]. Another study has identified four subgroups within HD [10]. Among these, of particular interest was cluster 1, associated with high proliferation and poor prognosis when compared with the other clusters and enriched for genes mapping to chromosome 1q. Although the prognostic relevance of 1q gains/ amplifications in this subgroup of patients seems to be relatively solid, the prognostic significance of the deletion of chromosome 13 in the context of HD remains controversial [8, 13, 14]. Other genetic lesions in HD have been linked to poor prognosis in this group, as for example IgH translocations, especially those involving unknown partners [14]. These additional translocations, along with monosomies, are likely arising later in tumor development [17].

Non-Hyperdiploid Multiple Myeloma

The NHD group of patients present with high frequency chromosomal translocations affecting the Ig locus. FISH, expression array analyses, and more recently aCGH, have been able to classify these patients into several different groups, closely matching the presence of translocations and dysregulated expression of the genes at the breakpoints. An oversimplified but nevertheless useful classification of this group of patients could therefore be inferred from the presence of chromosomal translocations.

The presence of chromosomal abnormalities in MM has been recognized for a long time, but a clear model for their pathogenetic relevance in MM was lacking. In the early 1990s, a few seminal papers identified conclusively the most recurrent translocations and elucidated their anatomy. In particular, it was shown that chromosomal translocations in mouse plasmacytomas involved the immunoglobulin heavy chain (IgH) switch regions [18]. Bergsagel and colleagues [19] demonstrated that a similar mechanism was present also in the human disease. One of the hallmark features of B-cell tumors, including MM, versus other hematologic disease is the almost exclusive pattern of translocations, which does not involve the formation of fusion chimeric proteins as seen in several leukemias and lymphomas, but leads to the dysregulated expression of oncogenes induced by the juxtaposition of the oncogenes promoters with Ig regulatory elements. Indeed, the B cell–specific mechanisms of switch recombination and somatic hypermutation have been implicated in the generation of these translocations in MM, in various degrees [20, 21]. Shortly thereafter, several oncogenes whose expression was dysregulated by chromosomal translocations were identified. It should be emphasized, however, that with the exception of FGFR3 and MAF, the oncogenic role of the genes dysregulated by the different chromosomal translocations have not been experimentally proven.

Translocations Affecting Cyclins

The t(11;14)(q13;q32) dysregulates the expression of the cyclin D1 gene [22-25], with an incidence of approximately 15% in MGUS [26, 27] and in MM [28, 29]. Another translocation, t(6;14)(p21;q32), induces the dysregulation of cyclin D3 in 2% to 3% of MM patients [30]. Interestingly, Zhan and colleagues [16] have shown how cyclin D1 and D3 tumors tend to cluster together. Among the patients who had these translocations two clusters were present, each presenting t(11;14) and t(6;14) translocations. No difference in clinical parameters or survival between the two groups was evident, and the pathogenetic and clinical implications of this distinction are still unclear. Overall, patients who have cyclin D translocations tend to present a better prognosis than NHD patients who have t(4;14), t(14;16), and t(14;20). The pathogenetic consequences of these translocations remain unclear.

t(4;14) and Fibroblast Growth Factor Receptor 3 and Multiple Myeloma Set Domain

Another translocation, t(4;14), affects approximately 15% of patients [31, 32] and presents a peculiar anatomy, as a result of an error in IgH switch recombination ([32-34] for recent and comprehensive reviews on t(4;14) in MM). As a result of the translocation, IgH enhancers are separated and dysregulate the expression of the juxtaposed genes on both derivative chromosomes, at der(4) and der(14). On der(14), the 39 Eα enhancer dysregulates the expression of the receptor tyrosine kinase FGFR3 gene. On der(4), the 59 Eμ enhancer drives the expression of the WHSC1 gene, also called MMSET, which encodes a protein with homology to histone methyltransferases. Approximately 10% of the patients who have t(4;14) also develop activating mutations on FGFR3 [33, 34]. Although MMSET is almost always up-regulated in patients presenting with t(4;14) [35], FGFR3 is not always overexpressed in MM patients (up to 25% of patients do not show overexpression [16, 31, 36, 37]) suggesting that in patients who have t(4;14) the prominent oncogenic role is exerted by MMSET. On the other hand, several preclinical studies have demonstrated the oncogenic potential of the activated form of FGFR3 (present in less than 10% of the t(4;14) patients) and gain-of-function studies have consistently demonstrated the oncogenic potential of most of the mutated forms of FGFR3. Ligand-stimulated interleukin-6 (IL-6)–dependent murine B9 cells expressing wild-type FGFR3 proliferated in the absence of IL-6, whereas the growth of B9 cells transfected with mutant FGFR3 was independent from the presence of either FGF or IL-6 [38]. Most mutated forms of FGFR3, but not the wild type, were able to induce the formation of foci and tumors in nude mice after transfection of NIH3T3 cells [33, 39]. Irradiated mice injected with bone marrow hematopoietic cells infected with mutant forms of FGFR3 developed transplantable tumors within 6 weeks, whereas WT FGFR3 induced the appearance of tumors only after 1 year [40]. Moreover specific FGFR3 inhibitors are able to reduce proliferation and increase apoptosis in t(4;14) MM cell lines with activated FGFR3[43-46] and in patients who have t(4;14). The usefulness of FGFR3 inhibitors in the treatment of t(4;14) patients in the absence of activated FGFR3 therefore remains to be established.

MMSET interacts with and is likely involved in pathways with a clear relevance in carcinogenesis. For example, the helix-loop-helix transcription factor inhibitor of differentiation 1 (ID-1) has been identified as a target of MMSET [41], and different isoforms of MMSET interact with HDAC1 and Sin3b [42]. The two homologs of MMSET have strong links to cancers. Specifically, WHSC1L1 is involved in a chromosomal translocation in acute myeloid leukemia, t(8;11)(p11.2;p15) [43], is amplified in breast cancer [44] and in lung cancer, and is endowed with oncogenic activity ([45] and Giovanni Tonon, MD, PhD, unpublished data, 2005). The other homolog, NSD1, has been implicated in acute myeloid leukemia [46].

Recent studies [47, 48] shed light on the role of MMSET in MM pathogenesis. Portions of MMSET fused to the Gal4 DNA binding domain led to repression of the transcription of a Gal4 reporter gene and this repression was associated with increased H4K20 methylation and loss of histone acetylation [47]. Consistent with this repressive activity, MMSET complexes with HDAC1 and HDAC2, mSin3a, and the histone demethylase LSD1, suggesting that it is part of corepressor complexes [47]. Moreover, coexpression of MMSET and HDAC1 and HDAC2 enhances HDAC-mediated repression. It has also been shown that MMSET-knockdown reduced the viability of a myeloma cell line [47] and the clonogenic ability [48], leads to cell-cycle arrest and reduced the ability of MM cells to adhere to extracellular matrix [48]. All these findings suggest an oncogenic role in MM context.

The t(4;14) has been clearly linked to poor prognosis in several studies [31, 49, 56-59].

MAF and MAFB Translocations

The t(14;16)(q32.3;q23) is present in approximately 5% to 10% of patients who have MM [21, 50] and induces overexpression of the oncogene c-MAF [51]. Interestingly the (14;20)(q32;q11 occurs in 2% to 5% of MM cases and affects the homolog MAFB [51, 52]. Both translocations are associated with a similar expression signature [16], suggesting a shared repository of downstream targets. Surprisingly, overexpression of c-MAF has been reported even in the absence of the translocation [53], albeit the mechanism remains unclear. The oncogenic role of c-MAF has been clearly established. Forced overexpression of c-MAF enhances myeloma proliferation, likely through one of its target genes, cyclin D2, that is consistently overexpressed in this group of patients [9]. Inhibition of c-maf blocked tumor formation in immunodeficient mice. Another target of c-maf, integrin b7, was able to increase myeloma adhesion to bone marrow stroma and increased production of VEGF. It seems, therefore, that c-MAF is able to stimulate cell cycle progression and alter bone marrow stromal interactions. An additional report has proposed ARK5, an AMP-activated protein kinase (AMPK)–related protein kinase mediating Akt signals, as a target of c-MAF and MAFB signaling [54].

Previous reports have shown a reduced incidence of bone disease in this group of patients [9, 16]. Recent publications point to two genes potentially responsible for this phenotype. The gene DKK1, whose overexpression has been implicated in MM-related bone disease [55], is significantly down-regulated in this group of patients [16]. Moreover Robbiani and colleagues [56] have recently reported that the gene osteopontin (OPN) inversely correlates with MM bone disease and is specifically overexpressed in patients who have translocations affecting the MAF genes.

Although not as clearly as in the case of t(4;14), translocations affecting MAF have also been linked to poor prognosis [16, 49].

Additional Genetic Lesions Related to Poor Prognosis

Minimal Common Regions (MCR)

aCGH analysis has identified MCRs associated with poor survival (hereafter designated as PS-MCRs). These included an amplification on chromosome 8 (including MYC), amplification in 1q, and a deletion on ch17 (including TP53) - genetic events that have been previously linked to poor prognosis in MM. Of the others amplified PS-MCRs, two resided in novel MM loci. The first novel amplified PS-MCR defined a ch8q24 region spanning 6 Mb with 37 genes (distinct from MYC) and was notable for its association with a poor clinical outcome and tumor recurrence in other human cancer types [45]. The second novel amplified PS-MCR targets a ch20q region (43 genes) that is associated with disease progression and metastases in prostate cancer [57], esophageal squamous cell carcinoma, and gastric and colorectal adenocarcinoma [58]. Among the 10 deleted PS-MCRs, four discrete regions mapped to chromosome 1p that resided within a relatively large area on 1p as defined by FISH, previously implicated in poor prognosis in patients who had MM [68-70]. The remaining deleted PS-MCRs include 3 on ch16, 2 on ch17 (one of them harboring TP53) and 2 on ch20. Among these, the 16q12 region (45 genes) includes the tumor suppressor CYLD, a gene critical for the NF-κB pathway that is proving to be increasingly important in MM. The prognostic relevance of these lesions needs to be validated in prospective studies of adequate sample size, but provides a valuable entry point for gene discovery and the identification of potentially important clinical correlates.

TP53 Deletion and Mutations

Mutations in the TP53 tumor suppressor gene have been reported in MM, with a frequency ranging from 2% to 20% [71-74]. The frequency of TP53 mutations in MGUS has been reported to be low [59] but increases with progression of the disease, approaching 80% in MM cell lines [60]. Chng and colleagues [61] have shown a strong association of mutations of TP53 with poor prognosis. Moreover, in the same study, TP53 mutations were significantly more frequent in patients who had t(4;14) and t(14;16), but no association was reported with HD. Finally, although the results should be taken cautiously because of the small number of cases with mutations, patients who have these translocations show a worse prognosis if they present in addition to mutations in TP53. Other studies have used deletions in 17p13 (mostly hemizygous) as a surrogate for the inactivation of the TP53 pathway and reported a frequency that in most cases is around 10% [49, 62-64], with a strong association with poor prognosis [15, 49, 62, 64, 65]. Chng and colleagues [61] have reported that half of patients who have MM with TP53 mutations had concomitant hemizygous losses at 17p13; and, conversely, only 16% of patients who have 17p13 hemizygous deletions have mutations in the remaining copy of TP53. It is still unclear, therefore, whether the TP53 pathway is silenced in MM cases with hemizygous 17p13 deletions when no mutations are detected in the remaining copy of TP53. Moreover, whether deletions on 17p13 are indeed a surrogate of TP53 inactivation or are associated with other, yet undetermined, tumor suppressor pathways is still unclear.

RAS Mutations

Two genes belonging to the Ras family (NRAS and KRAS) are mutated with a higher frequency in patients who have MM than in those who have MGUS[80-84]. RAS mutations have been linked to increased levels of cyclin D1 expression, but not to t(4;14) [66].

MYC Alterations

Aberrant expression of c-MYC in MM has been known for many years [67-69] and has shown a strong correlation with progression of the disease [67-70]. More recently, the anatomy of the rearrangements underlying MM presenting with overexpression of c-MYC has been delineated[90-92]. These rearrangements in 25% of cases juxtapose c-MYC with an IgH or IgL locus [71], with a pattern that is more complex than the classic reciprocal translocations present in the primary translocations [20, 71]. In other cases, amplifications, deletions, inversions, and insertions without apparent translocations[14,91-93], or translocations not involving Ig loci [72, 73], have been identified. In a large patient population, rearrangements affecting c-MYC have been reported with a frequency of 3% in MGUS and 10% to 16% in MM [71, 74]. The data available on plasma cell leukemias (PCLs) are less consistent among studies, with Fabris and colleagues [74] showing c-MYC rearrangements in 3 of 4 patients who had PCL, whereas Avet-Loiseau and colleagues [71] found only 3 MYC aberrations in 23 patients.

In contrast, MM cell lines have more frequent rearrangements of the c-MYC locus, ranging from 55% [71] to more than 90%, depending on the study [72, 74]. No significant association has been reported between primary translocations and chromosome 13 deletions, whereas a direct correlation with the levels of beta-2 microglobulin have been noted [71], suggesting a potential impact of c-MYC rearrangements on prognosis. The MCR including c-MYC was among the PS-MCR in the recent aCGH survey [15], although the link between c-MYC rearrangements and prognosis has been questioned [62].

NF-κB Pathway Alterations

Genetic lesions affecting both the classical and the alternative NF-κB pathway were recently reported [75, 76]. These two pathways are tightly interconnected: many signals activate both branches and many effector proteins or target genes are shared by the two pathways. A series of mutations that result in the constitutive activation of NF-κB have been identified in 17% of the patients and in approximately 40% of cell lines Aberrations involved both positive and negative regulators acting on classical and alternative pathway. The most common event was the inactivating mutation of TRAF3, occurring in 13% of MM patients [76]. In addition inactivating mutations found in other negative regulators like TRAF2, cIAP1/2 and CYLD result in constitutive NF-κB activation. On the other hand, chromosome translocations and amplifications resulting in activation of the NF-κB-inducing kinase (NIK) [75], CD40, LTBR, TACI, NFKB1 and NFKB2 [76] were reported and all induced constitutive activation of either canonical or noncanonical pathway. Most of the mutations affecting members of the canonical pathway like TRAF2 and TRAF3 have also a negative effect on the alternative pathway. Moreover, NIK activity is usually associated with alternative pathway activation, suggesting that the alternative pathway may be more relevant in MM pathogenesis. A very recent study confirmed the importance of mutations in NF-κB family members in MM and demonstrate that compensatory and/or cooperative effects occur in MM cell lines harboring such alterations [77]. Interestingly constitutive activation of either canonical or alternative pathway resulted in regulation of the same set of genes or at least genes involved in the same biological pathway [77].

The high prevalence of mutations in NF-κB family members in MM cell lines compared to MM patients suggest that alterations in NF-κB pathway are relative late events and mainly occurs in NHD patients compared to HD ones.

Of note the proteasomal inhibitor bortezomib, widely used in MM treatment, can exert its function by blocking the activation of NF-κB pathway.

IRF4 Overexpression

MUM1/IRF4 (herein referred to as IRF4) is a transcription factor required for B lymphocyte activation and the maturation to Ig-secreting plasma cells. IRF4 was initially characterized as an oncogene involved in t(6,14) translocation in MM [78] but mechanism other than translocation are probably responsible for overexpression in MM patients not carrying t (6,14) [79]. Its high expression is associated with poor outcome in MM patients and could represent a prognostic factor [79].

IRF4 inhibition by shRNAs in MM cell lines has a dramatic effect on cell proliferation and survival regardless of the genetic background [80, 81]. Gene expression and ChIP-ChIP experiments revealed a broad set of genes regulated by IRF4, including genes involved in growth and proliferation processes, like the oncogene Myc. As IRF4 has a wide effect, controlling a large number of genes involved in metabolic control, cell cycle progression, cell death and transcriptional regulation, its targeting represent a promising tool to interfere with MM survival.

2. EPIGENETIC MECHANISMS

Along with genetic abnormalities cancer initiation and progression involve epigenetic alterations [82]. For epigenetic is intended heritable changes in gene expression that can occur in the absence of alteration in the DNA coding region [83]. The main epigenetic mechanism can be grouped in three subclasses: DNA methylation, histone modification and miRNA regulation. It is interesting to note that genetic and epigenetic both contribute to oncogenic processes, as players of the epigenetic machinery are sometimes altered at genetic level. Little is known about the contribution of these mechanisms to myeloma development and progression, but they are assuming more relevance and the understanding of epigenetic mechanisms occurring in myeloma are a promising tool to unravel new molecular target for drug development. Particularly promising is the fact that epigenetic marks are reversible, thus making very attractive the hypothesis of new epigenetic therapies.

2.1. DNA Methylation

Methylation of DNA is the most studied epigenetic mechanism controlling gene expression. It consists in the transfer of a methyl group to the c-5 position of cytosine residues in a CpG dinucleotide and is catalyzed by DNA methyltransferase enzymes (DNMTs). Methylated CpGs associate with Methyl-Cytosine-Binding proteins (MBPs) which act to prevent the binding of transcription factors to the promoter region and recruit histone modifying and chromatin remodeling enzymes leading to chromatin condensation. The role of CpG island methylation in tumorigenesis has been widely investigated and represent the first epigenetic alteration identified in cancer [84]. In normal cells the majority of promoter-associated CpG islands are hypomethylated, thus allowing transcriptional activity, with the exception of imprinted genes and tissue specific genes. Hypermethylation of CpG islands has been linked to many cancers [85, 86]. In many cases promoter hypermethylation is linked to silencing of genes such as tumor-suppressor, DNA repair or cell cycle related, conferring a growth advantage to malignant cells. Relatively little is known about the extension of CpG methylation in MM. Most of the studies on MM patients and cell lines were based on methyl-specific PCR to identify genes silenced by methylation in MM. Although is the analysis was limited to a selected panel of genes, it allowed the discovery of a wide-range of genes dysregulated in MM. Among them, was VHL, whose methylation status of CpG islands was analyzed in 45 individuals with MM and in 10 normal individuals and found to be methylated in 33.3% of the MM cases [87]. Moreover, the presence of methylation in the VHL CpG islands was significantly associated with the development of bone disease. Aberrant methylation in the VHL CpG island, causing transcriptional silencing and downregulation of VHL transcription and hence decreased HIF-1α proteolysis, could be a possible mechanism of increased angiogenesis and altered bone marrow microenvironment that is more supportive for survival and growth of MM cells, contributing to MM bone disease.

Methylation of CpG islands in the promoter region of important cell cycle regulators occurs in MM, as methylation of CDKN2A-p16[108-110], CDKN2B [88] and TP53 [89] have been reported.

A possible role in the development of MM could be also attributed to apoptosis regulator proteins. Among them, XAF1, a protein capable of interacting and so inhibiting the activity of XIAP, has been reported to be silenced by methylation of its promoter [90].

Others genes have been found methylated in MM cells, like IRF8 [91], DAPK [92], the sFRP family [93], PF4 [94], TDG [95], PTGS2,SFN,CDH1, ESR1, HIC1, CCND2 and DCC. The methylation of DAPK is particularly relevant, as present in more than 50% of the cases and correlates with clinical course, representing a potential prognostic marker [96]. Furthermore recent studies have shown correlations between disease stage and progression and the hypermethylation of some promoter regions, such as TGFBR2 [88] that correlates with a poor prognosis, and MGMT, associated with the occurrence of extramedullary disease [97]. Another gene frequently silenced by methylation is DLC1, whose ectopic expression in MM cell lines reduces cell survival and migration capacity [98].

Most of the information about DNA methylation role in MM are based on the use of demethylating agents, such as, a compound that has proved to have anti-myeloma activity in MM cell lines. In particular, it has been demonstrated that 5-azacytidine inhibits IL-6 and NF-κB signaling, key pathways in myeloma survival [99, 100]. The action on IL-6 signaling is particularly relevant as IL-6 is involved in the induction of DNMT-1, causing the manteinance of hypermethylated status in the p53 promoter region and ultimately leading to epigenetic silencing of this key molecule in cell cycle regulation [89].

It should be noted that the anti-neoplastic effect of 5-azacytidine is only partly linked to its demethylating activity, as it has direct citotoxic activity and induces double stranded DNA breaks, with consequent p53-dependent cell cycle arrest and apoptosis induction [99, 101].

2.2 Histone Modification

Histones are alkaline proteins that represent the core subunits of nucleosomes, the structures responsible for order packaging of chromatin. Histones are composed by a globular C-terminal domain and a flexible N-terminal tail. Histone modifications represent an important level of epigenetic regulation as modification in histonic tails can alter the chromatin structure and change accessibility to transcription factors and other proteins involved in the control of gene expression. Reversible modification of histone tails includes acetylation, methylation, ubiquitynation and phosphorylation, the first two being the most widely studied. Depending on the nature of the modification and on the residue affected by it, histone modifications can lead to either activation or repression of gene expression. Specific patterns of histone modifications characterize distinct cell types and differentiation stages, so alteration of this delicate balance could lead to cellular transformation and malignant outgrowth. Indeed, several groups of proteins that modify chromatin structure, such as histone deacetylases (HDAC), histone acetyltransferase (HAT) or histone methylases and demethylases, have been implicated in various cancers.

Histone Methylation and Acetylation

Histone methylation occurs on lysine (K) and arginine (R) residues, altough the K residues modifications have been studied more extensively, in particular the tails of histones H3 and H4. Lysine residues can be mono-, di- and thri-methylated and the degree of methylation of the same residue differentially affects chromatin structure and transcription, defining a sort of "histone code". As a general rule, methylation of the residues H3K4, H3K36 and H3K79 is associated to transcriptional activation, while H3K9, H3K27 and H4K20 with repression, although this is not always true, depending on cellular context.

In the MM context, not so much is known about histone methylation and methylating-demethylating mechanisms.

One of the recurrent translocations in MM, namely (t4;14)(p16;q32), involves FGFR3 [102] and MMSET genes [51]. MMSET is a functional histone methyltransferase acting on histones H3 and H4 [42, 47], specifically on H3K9, H3K27 and H4K20, all residues being involved in repressory mechanisms. It also interacts with histone deacetylases HDAC1 and HDAC2, suggesting a coordinated action with others histone modifiers [47]. The transcriptional repression activity of the RE-IIBP MMSET family member is confirmed by a subsequent work showing activity of this protein on H3K27 methylation. RE-IIBP also represses transcription via interaction with HDAC1 and 2 [103].

Beside the action of histone methyltransferase enzymes, the "histone code" is dictated by several histone demethylases. Each demethylase preferentially targets one specific K residue and importantly the activity of the different demethylases is dependent on the methylation status of the specific K residue, with some enzymes removing mono- or dimethyl groups but not trimethylated groups.

Recently the first histone demethylase mutated or deleted in MM, UTX, was identified [104]. UTX is responsible for demethylating K27 residue on histone H3 [105] and its overexpression decreases endogenous H3K27 methylation. It should therefore promote gene expression through eliminating a repressor mark. Very recently it has been shown to regulate the expression of several RB-binding proteins thus inducing cell-cycle arrest [106]. The frequency of inactivation of this gene due to truncating mutations in MM was close to 10% [104]. Others mechanisms such as homozygous deletions or aberrant methylation of the promoter further increases to up to 30% the inactivation of this gene in MM, suggesting a strong pathogenetic role (Frenquelli M. and Tonon G., unpublished data).

Very few data are available on histone demethylases and histone demethylase inhibitors. Treatment of MM cell lines with the natural compound Triptolide decreases methylation levels of H3K9 and H3K27 residues and induces cell cycle arrest and caspase-dependent apoptosis [107].

The most studied histone modification is the acetylation of specific lysine residues on histone tails, regulated by the opposing effects of histone acetylases (HATs) and histone deacetylases (HDACs). Old studied associated increased histone acetylation with transcriptionally active chromatin [108] while the action of HDACs is responsible for gene silencing [109]. Human cancers are frequently showing high levels of histone acetylation [110], resulting from deregulated activity of HDACs. Numerous examples attest the involvment of different HDACs in several types of solid tumors, and HDAC inhibitors are effective in the treatment of both solid and haematological tumors and several clinical trials are ongoing to test the efficacy of new inhibitory molecules [111].

So far there are not experimental data showing abnormal expression of HDAC in myeloma, but there are several reports supporting the role of HDAC inhibitors as anti-proliferative agents both *in vitro* and *in vivo*. This effects on cell growth are not fully elucidated, and seems to depend on both cell cycle arrest, caused by upregulation of p21 and p53, and on induction of apoptosis. Heller *et al.* reported that treatment with the HDAC inhibitors Trichostatin A (TSA) alone or in combination with the DNA demethylating agent 5-Aza induce down-regulation of several MM proliferation-associated genes, like MAF, CCND1/2, FGFR3 and MMSET [112]. HDAC inhibitors exhert their action not only on myeloma cells directly, but also modifying the bone marrow microenvironment. Treatment with HDAC inhibitors in fact lowers the levels of IL-6 and VEGF, both representing survival/proliferation factors for myeloma cells and are produced by both malignant cells and bone marrow stromal cells [135-139].

Beside being of crucial importance in the regulation of histone modifications, HDAC have also several non-histone targets. The HDAC member with the more pronounced non-histone activity is HDAC6. Its activity is principally related to mechanism involved in cellular stress from misfolded proteins, a process of well-known importance for myeloma cells. Misfolded proteins are degraded by the proteasome, but have also the tendency to accumulate in insoluble aggregates that would be toxic if not degraded by fusion with lysosomes and HDAC6 is involved in this alternative mechanism of misfolded protein clearence. HDAC6 has also been shown to regulate the activity of the chaperone molecule HSP90, acetylating and thus activating it. These additional activities od HDAC6 make its inhibition an attractive means to interfere with myeloma cells survival and proliferation. The connection with misfolded protein response provided the rationale for combining HDAC inhibitors with proteasomal inhibitors [113, 114] or HSP90 inhibitors[141-143] that resulted to significantly increase the efficacy.

2.3. microRNAs

microRNAs (miRNAs) are endogenous 19-23 nt RNAs that play important roles in plant and animal development acting at post-transcriptional level by either targeting mRNA for degradation or controlling translation. They are one of the most abundant classes of regulatory molecules and control every biological mechanism (development, differentiation, cell growth and apoptosis). Taking part in almost all biological processes, it is not surprising their documented role in the development of most, if not all, type of cancers. Increasing evidences support the role of miRNAs in cancer, as a general deregulation of miRNA profile is found in cancer in respect to normal tissue, and often the miRNA profile reflect the developmental origin of tissue (epithelial vs non-epithelial tumors) [35, 41, 45, 54, 64-66, 113, 115, 116], leading to the definition of a specific miRNA signature. Mapping miRNA genes in the whole genome revealed that they are not randomly distributed: they are often found in cluster and in some cases share the same regulatory region, and most importantly they are frequently located in genomic region involved in cancer: fragile sites, loss of heterozygosity regions, minimal regions of amplification or common chromosal breakpoints, generally referred to as CAGRs [117].

Deregulated miRNAs expression can occur because of changes in the gene copy number, mutations, transcriptional activation, epigenetic silencing and altered processing. In this context miRNA may represent a level of regulation in between genetic and epigenetic.

Despite the great number of publication regarding miRNA and cancer, there are few published data concerning miRNAs'involvement in myeloma.

In a pioneristic study Loffler *et al.* have shown that IL-6 regulates *miR-21* transcription in IL-6-dependent MM cell lines [118]. This regulation goes through a STAT-3-related mechanism, and ectopic *miR-21* expression can sustain the growth of IL-6-dependent cells in the absence of IL-6 [118]. Oncogenic role for miR-21 in MM has been confirmed in a subsequent work by Pichiorri, *et al.*, in which they have also reported a set of miRNAs that are differentially expressed in MGUS and MM when compared to normal plasma cells and that can be associated with neoplastic transformation and progression in MM [119]. A role for oncogenic miR-21, miR-106b-25 and miR-181a and b was suggested in inducing a pre-malignant state (being overexpressed already in MGUS) and expression of miR-19, miR-17-92 cluster, miR-32 as clear markers of MM. The proposed oncogenic mechanism is mediated by regulation of p300-CBP-Associated Factor (PCAF) by miR-181 and mir-106 in initial stages. miR-19a and b are involved in the regulation of SOCS-1, important in the negative regulation of STAT-3 with consequent up-regulation of IL-6 transcription. The other miRNAs studied in this work, that is the miR-17-92 cluster, have a well established oncogenic role (reviewed in [120]). In the context of MM it could exert pro-survival activity by regulating the expression of the pro-apoptotic gene BIM. More recently, Roccaro *et al.* reported the downregulation of *miR-15a* and *miR-16* in a small cohort of relapsed-refractory MM patients, showing that they may regulate the proliferation and growth of MM cells *in vitro* and *in vivo* [121]. A recent extensive analysis on miRNA expression in both MM cell lines and primary tumors have identified a set of deregulated miRNAs that correlate with copy number (CN) alterations or gene expression patterns [122, 123] but a clear biological role for these miRNAs has not been established yet. This group also analyzed the global miRNA expression profile and through unsupervised analysis found specific pattern of expression in different groups of patients classified according to the TC classification [124], identifying 26 miRNAs capable of discriminating patients belonging to different TC groups. It has also been proposed an association between miRNA expression and the occurrence of recurrent chromosomal abnormalities. For example miR-99b and miR-125a-5p are highly expressed in patients with t(4;14) compared to the ones without this specific translocation, miR-133b expression is upregulated in patients carrying t(14;16)/t(14;20) and miR-582-5p is associated with the presence of t(11;14) [124].

3. SUMMARY

- Multiple myeloma (MM) is a malignant disorder due to clonal proliferation of plasma cells in the bone marrow in association with elevated serum or urine monoclonal paraprotein levels.

MM is associated, particularly in the most advanced stages of the disease, with severe complication, like lytic bone lesion, anemia, immunodeficiency and renal failure.

- MM development is a multistep process characterized by the presence of a series of chromosomal abnormalities and complex translocation. Genomic aberrations are present with increasing frequency as disease progress.

- MM patients can be subdivided in different groups according to genetic criteria. Approximately 55–60% of patients have a hyperdiploid karyotype, which confers a better prognosis than those with non-hyperdiploid disease. Most non-hyperdiploid tumours have IgH translocations (primary translocations) that involve several recurrent chromosomal loci, including 11q13 (cyclin D1), 6p21 (cyclin D3), 4p16 (*FGFR3* and *MMSET*), 16q23 (*MAF*) and 20q11 (*MAFB*).

- Primary translocations are early and initiating events in the pathogenesis of MM, whereas secondary translocations contribute to progression by dysregulating other oncogenes, for example c-*MYC*. Moreover because of the presence of activating mutations of *NRAS* or *KRAS2*, and also a higher incidence of monosomy 13, myeloma demonstrates higher proliferation at a late stage of progression.

- In addition to genetic events, epigenetic mechanisms have an increasingly significant role in the pathogenesis and progression of MM. DNA methylation of CpG islands in the promoter of important genes like VHL, CDKN2A-p16, CDKN2B, TP53, IRF8 and DAPK has been reported.

- Histone modification is involved in myeloma pathogenesis as well. Histone methyltransferase (MMSET) and demethylases (UTX) are dysregulated in myeloma patients. *In vitro* and *in vivo* studies demonstrated that HAT and HDAC inhibitors have anti-proliferative capacity and represent a new potential avenues in the treatment of myeloma patients.

- miRNAs represent another important oncogenic mechanism, as miRNA signatures characterize MGUS and MM patients and miRNA expression profiles are able to distinguish between subgroups of patients. Clear biological targets of dysregulated miRNAs have not been identified as yet, but some deregulated miRNAs seem to be involved in IL-6 signaling, a key survival factor for myeloma cells.

REFERENCES

[1] Tonon G. Molecular pathogenesis of multiple myeloma. Hematol Oncol Clin North Am 2007; 21(6): 985-1006, vii.

[2] Hideshima T, Bergsagel PL, Kuehl WM, Anderson KC. Advances in biology of multiple myeloma: clinical applications. Blood 2004; 104(3): 607-18.

[3] Chng WJ, Glebov O, Bergsagel PL, Kuehl WM. Genetic events in the pathogenesis of multiple myeloma. Best Pract Res Clin Haematol 2007; 20(4): 571-96.

[4] Lai JL, Zandecki M, Mary JY, *et al.* Improved cytogenetics in multiple myeloma: a study of 151 patients including 117 patients at diagnosis. Blood 1995; 85(9): 2490-7.

[5] Sawyer JR, Waldron JA, Jagannath S, Barlogie B. Cytogenetic findings in 200 patients with multiple myeloma. Cancer Genet Cytogenet 1995; 82(1): 41-9.

[6] Smadja NV, Fruchart C, Isnard F, *et al.* Chromosomal analysis in multiple myeloma: cytogenetic evidence of two different diseases. Leukemia 1998; 12(6): 960-9.

[7] Fonseca R, Debes-Marun CS, Picken EB, *et al.* The recurrent IgH translocations are highly associated with nonhyperdiploid variant multiple myeloma. Blood 2003; 102(7): 2562-7.

[8] Smadja NV, Bastard C, Brigaudeau C, Leroux D, Fruchart C. Hypodiploidy is a major prognostic factor in multiple myeloma. Blood 2001; 98(7): 2229-38.

[9] Bergsagel PL, Kuehl WM, Zhan F, *et al.* Cyclin D dysregulation: an early and unifying pathogenic event in multiple myeloma. Blood 2005; 106(1): 296-303.

[10] Chng WJ, Kumar S, Vanwier S, *et al.* Molecular dissection of hyperdiploid multiple myeloma by gene expression profiling. Cancer Res 2007; 67(7): 2982-9.

[11] Agnelli L, Fabris S, Bicciato S, *et al.* Upregulation of translational machinery and distinct genetic subgroups characterise hyperdiploidy in multiple myeloma. Br J Haematol. 2007; 136(4): 565-73.

[12] Calasanz MJ, Cigudosa JC, Odero MD, *et al.* Hypodiploidy and 22q11 rearrangements at diagnosis are associated with poor prognosis in patients with multiple myeloma. Br J Haematol 1997; 98(2): 418-25.

[13] Fassas AB, Spencer T, Sawyer J, *et al.* Both hypodiploidy and deletion of chromosome 13 independently confer poor prognosis in multiple myeloma. Br J Haematol 2002; 118(4): 1041-7.

[14] Chng WJ, Santana-Davila R, Van Wier SA, *et al.* Prognostic factors for hyperdiploid-myeloma: effects of chromosome 13 deletions and IgH translocations. Leukemia 2006; 20(5): 807-13.

[15] Carrasco DR, Tonon G, Huang Y, *et al.* High-resolution genomic profiles define distinct clinico-pathogenetic subgroups of multiple myeloma patients. Cancer Cell. 2006; 9(4): 313-25.

[16] Zhan F, Huang Y, Colla S, *et al.* The molecular classification of multiple myeloma. Blood 2006; 108(6): 2020-8.

[17] Chng WJ, Ketterling RP, Fonseca R. Analysis of genetic abnormalities provides insights into genetic evolution of hyperdiploid myeloma. Genes Chromosomes Cancer 2006; 45(12): 1111-20.

[18] Potter M, Wiener F. Plasmacytomagenesis in mice: model of neoplastic development dependent upon chromosomal translocations. Carcinogenesis 1992; 13(10): 1681-97.

[19] Bergsagel PL, Chesi M, Nardini E, *et al.* Promiscuous translocations into immunoglobulin heavy chain switch regions in multiple myeloma. Proc Natl Acad Sci U S A 1996; 93(24): 13931-6.

[20] Bergsagel PL, Kuehl WM. Chromosome translocations in multiple myeloma. Oncogene 2001; 20(40): 5611-22.

[21] Kuehl WM, Bergsagel PL. Multiple myeloma: evolving genetic events and host interactions. Nat Rev Cancer 2002; 2(3): 175-87.

[22] Kobayashi H, Saito H, Kitano K, *et al.* Overexpression of the PRAD1 oncogene in a patient with multiple myeloma and t(11;14)(q13;q32). Acta Haematol 1995; 94(4): 199-203.

[23] Akiyama N, Tsuruta H, Sasaki H, *et al.* Messenger RNA levels of five genes located at chromosome 11q13 in B-cell tumors with chromosome translocation t(11;14)(q13;q32). Cancer Res 1994; 54(2): 377-9.

[24] Chesi M, Bergsagel PL, Brents LA, *et al.* Dysregulation of cyclin D1 by translocation into an IgH gamma switch region in two multiple myeloma cell lines. Blood 1996 Jul 15; 88(2): 674-81.

[25] Seto M, Yamamoto K, Iida S, *et al.* Gene rearrangement and overexpression of PRAD1 in lymphoid malignancy with t(11;14)(q13;q32) translocation. Oncogene 1992; 7(7): 1401-6.

[26] Avet-Loiseau H, Facon T, Daviet A, *et al.* 14q32 translocations and monosomy 13 observed in monoclonal gammopathy of undetermined significance delineate a multistep process for the oncogenesis of multiple myeloma. Intergroupe Francophone du Myelome. Cancer Res 1999; 59(18): 4546-50.

[27] Fonseca R, Bailey RJ, Ahmann GJ, *et al.* Genomic abnormalities in monoclonal gammopathy of undetermined significance. Blood 2002; 100(4): 1417-24.

[28] Fonseca R, Blood EA, Oken MM, *et al.* Myeloma and the t(11; 14)(q13; q32); evidence for a biologically defined unique subset of patients. Blood 2002; 99(10): 3735-41.

[29] Avet-Loiseau H, Facon T, Grosbois B, *et al.* Oncogenesis of multiple myeloma: 14q32 and 13q chromosomal abnormalities are not randomly distributed, but correlate with natural history, immunological features, and clinical presentation. Blood 2002; 99(6): 2185-91.

[30] Shaughnessy J, Jr., Gabrea A, Qi Y, *et al.* Cyclin D3 at 6p21 is dysregulated by recurrent chromosomal translocations to immunoglobulin loci in multiple myeloma. Blood 2001; 98(1): 217-23.

[31] Keats JJ, Reiman T, Maxwell CA, *et al.* In multiple myeloma, t(4;14)(p16;q32) is an adverse prognostic factor irrespective of FGFR3 expression. Blood 2003; 101(4): 1520-9.

[32] Avet-Loiseau H, Li JY, Facon T, *et al.* High incidence of translocations t(11;14)(q13;q32) and t(4;14)(p16;q32) in patients with plasma cell malignancies. Cancer Res 1998; 58(24): 5640-5.

[33] Chesi M, Brents LA, Ely SA, *et al.* Activated fibroblast growth factor receptor 3 is an oncogene that contributes to tumor progression in multiple myeloma. Blood 2001; 97(3): 729-36.

[34] Intini D, Baldini L, Fabris S, *et al.* Analysis of FGFR3 gene mutations in multiple myeloma patients with t(4;14). Br J Haematol 2001; 114(2): 362-4.

[35] Keats JJ, Maxwell CA, Taylor BJ, *et al.* Overexpression of transcripts originating from the MMSET locus characterizes all t(4;14)(p16;q32)-positive multiple myeloma patients. Blood 2005; 105(10): 4060-9.

[36] Stewart JP, Thompson A, Santra M, *et al.* Correlation of TACC3, FGFR3, MMSET and p21 expression with the t(4;14)(p16.3;q32) in multiple myeloma. Br J Haematol 2004; 126(1): 72-6.

[37] Santra M, Zhan F, Tian E, Barlogie B, Shaughnessy J, Jr. A subset of multiple myeloma harboring the t(4;14)(p16;q32) translocation lacks FGFR3 expression but maintains an IGH/MMSET fusion transcript. Blood 2003; 101(6): 2374-6.

[38] Plowright EE, Li Z, Bergsagel PL, *et al.* Ectopic expression of fibroblast growth factor receptor 3 promotes myeloma cell proliferation and prevents apoptosis. Blood 2000; 95(3): 992-8.

[39] Ronchetti D, Greco A, Compasso S, *et al.* Deregulated FGFR3 mutants in multiple myeloma cell lines with t(4;14): comparative analysis of Y373C, K650E and the novel G384D mutations. Oncogene 2001; 20(27): 3553-62.

[40] Li Z, Zhu YX, Plowright EE, *et al.* The myeloma-associated oncogene fibroblast growth factor receptor 3 is transforming in hematopoietic cells. Blood 2001; 97(8): 2413-9.

[41] Hudlebusch HR, Theilgaard-Monch K, Lodahl M, Johnsen HE, Rasmussen T. Identification of ID-1 as a potential target gene of MMSET in multiple myeloma. Br J Haematol 2005; 130(5): 700-8.

[42] Todoerti K, Ronchetti D, Agnelli L, *et al.* Transcription repression activity is associated with the type I isoform of the MMSET gene involved in t(4;14) in multiple myeloma. Br J Haematol 2005; 131(2): 214-8.

[43] Rosati R, La Starza R, Veronese A, *et al.* NUP98 is fused to the NSD3 gene in acute myeloid leukemia associated with t(8;11)(p11.2;p15). Blood 2002; 99(10): 3857-60.

[44] Angrand PO, Apiou F, Stewart AF, *et al.* NSD3, a new SET domain-containing gene, maps to 8p12 and is amplified in human breast cancer cell lines. Genomics 2001; 74(1): 79-88.

[45] Tonon G, Wong KK, Maulik G, *et al.* High-resolution genomic profiles of human lung cancer. Proc Natl Acad Sci U S A 2005; 102(27): 9625-30.

[46] Jaju RJ, Fidler C, Haas OA, *et al.* A novel gene, NSD1, is fused to NUP98 in the t(5;11)(q35;p15.5) in de novo childhood acute myeloid leukemia. Blood 2001; 98(4): 1264-7.

[47] Marango J, Shimoyama M, Nishio H, *et al.* The MMSET protein is a histone methyltransferase with characteristics of a transcriptional corepressor. Blood 2008; 111(6): 3145-54.

[48] Lauring J, Abukhdeir AM, Konishi H, *et al.* The multiple myeloma associated MMSET gene contributes to cellular adhesion, clonogenic growth, and tumorigenicity. Blood 2008; 111(2): 856-64.

[49] Fonseca R, Blood E, Rue M, *et al.* Clinical and biologic implications of recurrent genomic aberrations in myeloma. Blood 2003; 101(11): 4569-75.

[50] Rasmussen T, Knudsen LM, Dahl IM, Johnsen HE. C-MAF oncogene dysregulation in multiple myeloma: frequency and biological relevance. Leuk Lymphoma 2003; 44(10): 1761-6.

[51] Chesi M, Nardini E, Lim RS, *et al.* The t(4;14) translocation in myeloma dysregulates both FGFR3 and a novel gene, MMSET, resulting in IgH/MMSET hybrid transcripts. Blood 1998; 92(9): 3025-34.

[52] Hanamura I, Iida S, Akano Y, *et al.* Ectopic expression of MAFB gene in human myeloma cells carrying (14;20)(q32;q11) chromosomal translocations. Jpn J Cancer Res 2001; 92(6): 638-44.

[53] Hurt EM, Wiestner A, Rosenwald A, *et al.* Overexpression of c-maf is a frequent oncogenic event in multiple myeloma that promotes proliferation and pathological interactions with bone marrow stroma. Cancer Cell 2004; 5(2): 191-9.

[54] Suzuki A, Iida S, Kato-Uranishi M, *et al.* ARK5 is transcriptionally regulated by the Large-MAF family and mediates IGF-1-induced cell invasion in multiple myeloma: ARK5 as a new molecular determinant of malignant multiple myeloma. Oncogene 2005; 24(46): 6936-44.

[55] Tian E, Zhan F, Walker R, *et al.* The role of the Wnt-signaling antagonist DKK1 in the development of osteolytic lesions in multiple myeloma. N Engl J Med 2003; 349(26): 2483-94.

[56] Robbiani DF, Colon K, Ely S, *et al.* Osteopontin dysregulation and lytic bone lesions in multiple myeloma. Hematol Oncol 2007; 25(1): 16-20.

[57] Wullich B, Riedinger S, Brinck U, *et al.* Evidence for gains at 15q and 20q in brain metastases of prostate cancer. Cancer Genet Cytogenet 2004; 154(2): 119-23.

[58] Fujita Y, Sakakura C, Shimomura K, *et al.* Chromosome arm 20q gains and other genomic alterations in esophageal squamous cell carcinoma, as analyzed by comparative genomic hybridization and fluorescence in situ hybridization. Hepatogastroenterology 2003; 50(54): 1857-63.

[59] Corradini P, Inghirami G, Astolfi M, *et al.* Inactivation of tumor suppressor genes, p53 and Rb1, in plasma cell dyscrasias. Leukemia 1994; 8(5): 758-67.
[60] Mazars GR, Portier M, Zhang XG, *et al.* Mutations of the p53 gene in human myeloma cell lines. Oncogene 1992; 7(5): 1015-8.
[61] Chng WJ, Price-Troska T, Gonzalez-Paz N, *et al.* Clinical significance of TP53 mutation in myeloma. Leukemia 2007; 21(3): 582-4.
[62] Avet-Loiseau H, Attal M, Moreau P, *et al.* Genetic abnormalities and survival in multiple myeloma: the experience of the Intergroupe Francophone du Myelome. Blood 2007; 109(8): 3489-95.
[63] Avet-Loiseau H, Li JY, Godon C, *et al.* P53 deletion is not a frequent event in multiple myeloma. Br J Haematol 1999; 106(3): 717-9.
[64] Chang H, Qi C, Yi QL, Reece D, Stewart AK. p53 gene deletion detected by fluorescence in situ hybridization is an adverse prognostic factor for patients with multiple myeloma following autologous stem cell transplantation. Blood 2005; 105(1): 358-60.
[65] Gertz MA, Lacy MQ, Dispenzieri A, *et al.* Clinical implications of t(11;14)(q13;q32), t(4;14)(p16.3;q32), and -17p13 in myeloma patients treated with high-dose therapy. Blood 2005;106(8): 2837-40.
[66] Rasmussen T, Kuehl M, Lodahl M, Johnsen HE, Dahl IM. Possible roles for activating RAS mutations in the MGUS to MM transition and in the intramedullary to extramedullary transition in some plasma cell tumors. Blood 2005; 105(1): 317-23.
[67] Skopelitou A, Hadjiyannakis M, Tsenga A, *et al.* Expression of C-myc p62 oncoprotein in multiple myeloma: an immunohistochemical study of 180 cases. Anticancer Res 1993; 13(4): 1091-5.
[68] Palumbo AP, Pileri A, Dianzani U, *et al.* Altered expression of growth-regulated protooncogenes in human malignant plasma cells. Cancer Res 1989; 49(17): 4701-4.
[69] Selvanayagam P, Blick M, Narni F, *et al.* Alteration and abnormal expression of the c-myc oncogene in human multiple myeloma. Blood 1988; 71(1): 30-5.
[70] Pope B, Brown R, Luo XF, Gibson J, Joshua D. Disease progression in patients with multiple myeloma is associated with a concurrent alteration in the expression of both oncogenes and tumour suppressor genes and can be monitored by the oncoprotein phenotype. Leuk Lymphoma 1997; 25(5-6): 545-54.
[71] Avet-Loiseau H, Gerson F, Magrangeas F, *et al.* Rearrangements of the c-myc oncogene are present in 15% of primary human multiple myeloma tumors. Blood 2001; 98(10): 3082-6.
[72] Shou Y, Martelli ML, Gabrea A, *et al.* Diverse karyotypic abnormalities of the c-myc locus associated with c-myc dysregulation and tumor progression in multiple myeloma. Proc Natl Acad Sci U S A 2000; 97(1): 228-33.
[73] Hollis GF, Gazdar AF, Bertness V, Kirsch IR. Complex translocation disrupts c-myc regulation in a human plasma cell myeloma. Mol Cell Biol 1988; 8(1): 124-9.
[74] Fabris S, Storlazzi CT, Baldini L, *et al.* Heterogeneous pattern of chromosomal breakpoints involving the MYC locus in multiple myeloma. Genes Chromosomes Cancer 2003; 37(3): 261-9.
[75] Annunziata CM, Davis RE, Demchenko Y, *et al.* Frequent engagement of the classical and alternative NF-kappaB pathways by diverse genetic abnormalities in multiple myeloma. Cancer Cell 2007; 12(2): 115-30.
[76] Keats JJ, Fonseca R, Chesi M, *et al.* Promiscuous mutations activate the noncanonical NF-kappaB pathway in multiple myeloma. Cancer Cell 2007; 12(2): 131-44.
[77] Demchenko YN, Glebov OK, Zingone A, *et al.* Classical and/or alternative NF{kappa}B pathway activation in multiple myeloma. Blood 2010; 113(17); 3541-52.
[78] Iida S, Rao PH, Butler M, *et al.* Deregulation of MUM1/IRF4 by chromosomal translocation in multiple myeloma. Nat Genet 1997; 17(2): 226-30.
[79] Heintel D, Zojer N, Schreder M, *et al.* Expression of MUM1/IRF4 mRNA as a prognostic marker in patients with multiple myeloma. Leukemia 2008; 22(2): 441-5.
[80] Shaffer AL, Emre NC, Lamy L, *et al.* IRF4 addiction in multiple myeloma. Nature 2008; 454(7201): 226-31.
[81] Shaffer AL, Emre NC, Romesser PB, Staudt LM. IRF4: Immunity. Malignancy! Therapy? Clin Cancer Res 2009; 15(9): 2954-61.
[82] Feinberg AP, Ohlsson R, Henikoff S. The epigenetic progenitor origin of human cancer. Nat Rev Genet 2006; 7(1): 21-33.
[83] Moving AHEAD with an international human epigenome project. Nature 2008; 454(7205): 711-5.
[84] Feinberg AP, Vogelstein B. Hypomethylation distinguishes genes of some human cancers from their normal counterparts. Nature 1983; 301(5895): 89-92.

[85] Baylin SB, Herman JG. DNA hypermethylation in tumorigenesis: epigenetics joins genetics. Trends Genet 2000; 16(4): 168-74.
[86] Costello JF, Fruhwald MC, Smiraglia DJ, *et al.* Aberrant CpG-island methylation has non-random and tumour-type-specific patterns. Nat Genet 2000; 24(2): 132-8.
[87] Hatzimichael E, Dranitsaris G, Dasoula A, *et al.* Von Hippel-Lindau methylation status in patients with multiple myeloma: a potential predictive factor for the development of bone disease. Clin Lymphoma Myeloma 2009; 9(3):239-42.
[88] de Carvalho F, Colleoni GW, Almeida MS, Carvalho AL, Vettore AL. TGFbetaR2 aberrant methylation is a potential prognostic marker and therapeutic target in multiple myeloma. Int J Cancer 2009; 125(8): 1985-91.
[89] Hodge DR, Peng B, Cherry JC, *et al.* Interleukin 6 supports the maintenance of p53 tumor suppressor gene promoter methylation. Cancer Res 2005; 65(11): 4673-82.
[90] Chen G, Wang Y, Huang H, *et al.* Combination of DNA methylation inhibitor 5-azacytidine and arsenic trioxide has synergistic activity in myeloma. Eur J Haematol 2009; 82(3): 176-83.
[91] Tshuikina M, Jernberg-Wiklund H, Nilsson K, Oberg F. Epigenetic silencing of the interferon regulatory factor ICSBP/IRF8 in human multiple myeloma. Exp Hematol 2008; 36(12): 1673-81.
[92] Ng MH, To KW, Lo KW, *et al.* Frequent death-associated protein kinase promoter hypermethylation in multiple myeloma. Clin Cancer Res 2001; 7(6): 1724-9.
[93] Jost E, Gezer D, Wilop S, *et al.* Epigenetic dysregulation of secreted Frizzled-related proteins in multiple myeloma. Cancer Lett 2009; 281(1): 24-31.
[94] Cheng SH, Ng MH, Lau KM, *et al.* 4q loss is potentially an important genetic event in MM tumorigenesis: identification of a tumor suppressor gene regulated by promoter methylation at 4q13.3, platelet factor 4. Blood 2007; 109(5): 2089-99.
[95] Peng B, Hurt EM, Hodge DR, Thomas SB, Farrar WL. DNA hypermethylation and partial gene silencing of human thymine- DNA glycosylase in multiple myeloma cell lines. Epigenetics 2006; 1(3): 138-45.
[96] Chim CS, Kwong YL, Fung TK, Liang R. Methylation profiling in multiple myeloma. Leuk Res 2004; 28(4): 379-85.
[97] Yuregir OO, Yurtcu E, Kizilkilic E, *et al.* Detecting methylation patterns of p16, MGMT, DAPK and E-cadherin genes in multiple myeloma patients. Int J Lab Hematol 2010; 32(2): 142-9.
[98] Ullmannova-Benson V, Guan M, Zhou X, *et al.* DLC1 tumor suppressor gene inhibits migration and invasion of multiple myeloma cells through RhoA GTPase pathway. Leukemia 2009; 23(2): 383-90.
[99] Kiziltepe T, Hideshima T, Catley L, *et al.* 5-Azacytidine, a DNA methyltransferase inhibitor, induces ATR-mediated DNA double-strand break responses, apoptosis, and synergistic cytotoxicity with doxorubicin and bortezomib against multiple myeloma cells. Mol Cancer Ther 2007; 6(6): 1718-27.
[100] Khong T, Sharkey J, Spencer A. The effect of azacitidine on interleukin-6 signaling and nuclear factor-kappaB activation and its *in vitro* and *in vivo* activity against multiple myeloma. Haematologica 2008; 93(6): 860-9.
[101] Zhu WG, Hileman T, Ke Y, *et al.* 5-aza-2'-deoxycytidine activates the p53/p21Waf1/Cip1 pathway to inhibit cell proliferation. J Biol Chem 2004; 279(15): 15161-6.
[102] Chesi M, Nardini E, Brents LA, *et al.* Frequent translocation t(4;14)(p16.3;q32.3) in multiple myeloma is associated with increased expression and activating mutations of fibroblast growth factor receptor 3. Nat Genet 1997; 16(3): 260-4.
[103] Kim JY, Kee HJ, Choe NW, *et al.* Multiple-myeloma-related WHSC1/MMSET isoform RE-IIBP is a histone methyltransferase with transcriptional repression activity. Mol Cell Biol 2008; 28(6): 2023-34.
[104] van Haaften G, Dalgliesh GL, Davies H, *et al.* Somatic mutations of the histone H3K27 demethylase gene UTX in human cancer. Nat Genet 2009; 41(5): 521-3.
[105] Hong S, Cho YW, Yu LR, *et al.* Identification of JmjC domain-containing UTX and JMJD3 as histone H3 lysine 27 demethylases. Proc Natl Acad Sci U S A 2007; 104(47): 18439-44.
[106] Wang JK, Tsai MC, Poulin G, *et al.* The histone demethylase UTX enables RB-dependent cell fate control. Genes Dev 2010; 24(4): 327-32.
[107] Zhao F, Chen Y, Li R, *et al.* Triptolide alters histone H3K9 and H3K27 methylation state and induces G0/G1 arrest and caspase-dependent apoptosis in multiple myeloma *in vitro*. Toxicology 12; 267(1-3): 70-9.
[108] Adler AJ, Fasman GD, Wangh LJ, Allfrey VG. Altered conformational effects of naturally acetylated histone f2al (IV) in f2al-deoxyribonucleic acid complexes. Circular dichroism studies. J Biol Chem 1974; 10; 249(9): 2911-4.

[109] Hassig CA, Tong JK, Fleischer TC, *et al.* A role for histone deacetylase activity in HDAC1-mediated transcriptional repression. Proc Natl Acad Sci U S A 1998 31; 95(7): 3519-24.

[110] Fraga MF, Ballestar E, Villar-Garea A, *et al.* Loss of acetylation at Lys16 and trimethylation at Lys20 of histone H4 is a common hallmark of human cancer. Nat Genet 2005; 37(4): 391-400.

[111] Lane AA, Chabner BA. Histone deacetylase inhibitors in cancer therapy. J Clin Oncol 2009; 27(32): 5459-68.

[112] Heller G, Schmidt WM, Ziegler B, *et al.* Genome-wide transcriptional response to 5-aza-2'-deoxycytidine and trichostatin a in multiple myeloma cells. Cancer Res 2008; 68(1): 44-54.

[113] Hideshima T, Bradner JE, Wong J, *et al.* Small-molecule inhibition of proteasome and aggresome function induces synergistic antitumor activity in multiple myeloma. Proc Natl Acad Sci U S A 2005 14; 102(24): 8567-72.

[114] Catley L, Weisberg E, Kiziltepe T, *et al.* Aggresome induction by proteasome inhibitor bortezomib and alpha-tubulin hyperacetylation by tubulin deacetylase (TDAC) inhibitor LBH589 are synergistic in myeloma cells. Blood 2006; 108(10): 3441-9.

[115] Rahmani M, Reese E, Dai Y, *et al.* Cotreatment with suberanoylanilide hydroxamic acid and 17-allylamino 17-demethoxygeldanamycin synergistically induces apoptosis in Bcr-Abl+ Cells sensitive and resistant to STI571 (imatinib mesylate) in association with down-regulation of Bcr-Abl, abrogation of signal transducer and activator of transcription 5 activity, and Bax conformational change. Mol Pharmacol 2005; 67(4): 1166-76.

[116] Trudel S, Li ZH, Wei E, *et al.* CHIR-258, a novel, multitargeted tyrosine kinase inhibitor for the potential treatment of t(4;14) multiple myeloma. Blood 2005; 105(7): 2941-8.

[117] Calin GA, Sevignani C, Dumitru CD, *et al.* Human microRNA genes are frequently located at fragile sites and genomic regions involved in cancers. Proc Natl Acad Sci U S A 2004; 101(9): 2999-3004.

[118] Loffler D, Brocke-Heidrich K, Pfeifer G, *et al.* Interleukin-6 dependent survival of multiple myeloma cells involves the Stat3-mediated induction of microRNA-21 through a highly conserved enhancer. Blood 2007; 110(4): 1330-3.

[119] Pichiorri F, Suh SS, Ladetto M, *et al.* MicroRNAs regulate critical genes associated with multiple myeloma pathogenesis. Proc Natl Acad Sci U S A 2008; 105(35): 12885-90.

[120] van Haaften G, Agami R. Tumorigenicity of the miR-17-92 cluster distilled. Genes Dev 2010; 24(1): 1-4.

[121] Roccaro AM, Sacco A, Thompson B, *et al.* MicroRNAs 15a and 16 regulate tumor proliferation in multiple myeloma. Blood 2009; 113(26): 6669-80.

[122] Ronchetti D, Lionetti M, Mosca L, *et al.* An integrative genomic approach reveals coordinated expression of intronic miR-335, miR-342, and miR-561 with deregulated host genes in multiple myeloma. BMC Med Genomics 2008; 1: 37.

[123] Lionetti M, Agnelli L, Mosca L, *et al.* Integrative high-resolution microarray analysis of human myeloma cell lines reveals deregulated miRNA expression associated with allelic imbalances and gene expression profiles. Genes Chromosomes Cancer 2009; 48(6): 521-31.

[124] Lionetti M, Biasiolo M, Agnelli L, *et al.* Identification of microRNA expression patterns and definition of a microRNA/mRNA regulatory network in distinct molecular groups of multiple myeloma. Blood 2009; 114(25): e20-6.

CHAPTER 4

Guideline to Multiple Myeloma Treatment Strategies

Klaus Podar[1,2,*], Jonathan L. Kaufmann[3], Jacob P. Laubach[1], Sagar Lonial[3], Paul G. Richardson[2] and Kenneth C. Anderson[2]

[1]Department of Medical Oncology, Dana-Farber Cancer Institute, Harvard Medical School, Boston, MA, USA; [2]National Center for Tumor Diseases (NCT)/ University of Heidelberg, Heidelberg, Germany and [3]Winship Cancer Institute, Emory University, Atlanta, GA, USA

Abstract: Multiple Myeloma (MM) is a clonal plasma cell malignancy with a highly heterogeneous genetic background, characterized by bone marrow (BM) plasmacytosis, production of monoclonal proteins, osteolytic bone lesions, renal disease, anemia, hypercalcemia, and immunodeficiency. The inclusion of thalidomide, bortezomib, and lenalidomide into conventional cytotoxic and transplantation regimens, first in relapsed and refractory and now also in newly diagnosed MM, has fundamentally changed treatment in MM during the last decade and steadily improved MM patient outcome.

Keywords: Clinical features, monoclonal gammopathy of unknown significance (MGUS), smoldering multiple myeloma (SMM), CRAB, staging (Durie-Salmon, International Staging System), upfront therapy, autologous stem cell transplantation (ASCT), maintenance therapy, salvage therapy, bone disease.

1. INTRODUCTION

Initially described in the mid 1850s, successful treatment for multiple myeloma (MM) using Melphalan and prednisone was not begun until the late 1960s and achieved a median overall survival of 3-4 years. The introduction of both combination chemotherapy and high-dose therapy (HDT) with autologous stem cell transplantation (ASCT) in the 1980s improved overall survival to 3-5 years. During the last decade, exciting advances in understanding MM pathogenesis within the bone marrow (BM) microenvironment have led to the identification of multiple novel therapeutic targets and derived targeted agents (see Chapter 14). Indeed, thalidomide (Thal), immunomodulatory drugs (IMiDs), as well as the first-in-class proteasome inhibitor bortezomib (Bort), have rapidly translated from the bench to the bedside and derived clinical trials. First approved for treatment in the relapsed/ refractory setting these agents have now also fundamentally changed treatment in newly diagnosed MM. Improved survival triggered by the introduction of novel agents, with extension of the median survival of MM patients from three to seven years especially in patients less than age 50 years, has been recently reported [1]. Remarkably, some of the novel agents are also active in high- risk MM patients. Despite these dramatic therapeutic advances, disease relapse is inevitable and MM remains incurable. Besides the continued search for new targeted therapies, ongoing clinical studies aim: to further optimize treatment regimens by determining patient- specific sequence and combination regimens; and to further reduce dose- limiting adverse side effects. Here we give a brief overview of current treatment strategies in the upfront setting (see also Chapter 6 for more detail) as well as in the relapsed/ refractory setting.

2. CLINICAL FEATURES

At first diagnosis the majority of MM patients presents with symptoms secondary to: (1) myelosuppression with anemia (*e.g.* pallor, dyspnoea, weakness, fatigue); thrombocytopenia (increased bruising, and bleeding); and immunodeficiency (recurrent infections); (2) bone lesions (*e.g.* tenderness, pain, loss of height, kyphosis due to vertebral compression fractures); (3) hypercalcemia (weakness, fatigue, confusion, altered menatal status, polyuria, polydipsia, constipation); (4) hyperviscosity (visual symptoms, headaches); (5) renal failure; (6) neural lesions due to vertebral collapse and cord compression (paraplegic or quadriplegic symptoms and peripheral neuropathy) as well as polyneuropathy. Alternatively MM patients may present without symptoms following the incidental discovery of an M protein in serum or urine.

***Address correspondence to Klaus Podar:** National Center for Tumor Diseases, Im Neuenheimer Feld #410; Tel: ++49 06221 (0) 56-38689; Fax: ++49 06221 (0) 56-8815; E-mail: klaus.podar@med.uni-heidelberg.de or klaus_podar@dfci.harvard.edu

3. DIAGNOSIS

Initial diagnostic workup of patients with suspected MM includes: CBC, differential and platelets; BUN/ creatinine, electrolytes; LDH; calcium/ albumin; β2-M; serum free light chain assay; serum quantitative immunoglobulins, serum/24h urine protein electrophoresis (SEP/UPEP), serum/urine immunofixation electrophoresis (SIFE/ UIFE); skeletal survey (whole body CT in low-dose technique or whole body MRT); bone marrow aspirate and biopsy, including bone marrow immunohistocehmistry and/ or bone marrow flow cytometry; cytogenetics; FISH[del13, del17,t(4;14),t(11;14),t(14;16),1q21 amplification].

Active MM is distinguished from monoclonal gammopathy of undetermined significance (MGUS), and smoldering MM (SMM)/ indolent/ asymptomatic MM based on (1) serum M protein levels, (2) extent of bone marrow plasmacytosis and (3) related organ or tissue impairment (ROTI), also referred to as increases in calcium levels, renal insufficiency, anemia, and bone lesions (CRAB). **MGUS is defined as** <30g/L paraprotein, BM clonal plasma cells <10%, and no evidence of MM, other B-cell disorders, or light-chain (AL) amyloidosis). **SMM** is characterized by paraprotein ≥ 30g/L and/or clonal BM plasma cells ≥ 10% without ROTI and does not require treatment; observation at 3 to 6 months intervals is recommended. A subgroup of patients with SMM with small lytic lesions and a slow clinical course is referred to as **indolent myeloma**, also does not require treatment. Finally, a small group (2%) of **non- secretory MM** patients displays BM plasmacytosis and ROTI with no serum or urine M- protein (**non-secretory MM**). The transition rate of **MGUS** to MM approximates 1%, with a maximum risk in patients with a non-IgG M protein of ≥1.5g/dL, an abnormal free light chain ratio, the presence of urinary M protein, and circulating plasma cells. The transition rate of **SMM** to active MM approximates 5 to 10% each year for 5 years, with a decreasing risk in subsequent years; and increased risk in SMM patients with an abnormal serum free light chain ratio [2-4].

4. STAGING

The clinical **Durie- Salmon** staging system, which is based on indirect tumor estimation (hemoglobin, serum calcium, M-protein levels as well as bone lesions), has now been largely replaced by the simplified but powerful **International Staging System (ISS),** which is based on serum β2-M and serum albumin levels [6,7]. In addition to disease stage, also **genetic abnormalities** and the **plasma labeling index** (PLI) represent prognostic factors which influence the determination of further treatment regimens. Specifically, high-risk MM to conventional low and high dose therapy is defined by non-hyperdiploidy and IgH translocations t(4;14), t(11;14), t(14;16), progression- associated deletions of chromosome 13 and 17, and abnormalities of chromosome 1 (1p deletion, 1q amplification); as well as a PLI of ≥ 3% [1,8,9]. In these patients median overall survival (OS), even with tandem autologous stem cell transplantation (ASCT) is only 2-3 years vs. more than 5 years for patients with standard-risk disease. In contrast, more indolent forms of MM are associated with hyperdiploidy and trisomies. Importantly, novel therapies such as bortezomib can, at least in part, overcome these abnormalities.

5. TREATMENT REGIMENS

5.1. Treatment of Newly Diagnosed MM- Upfront Therapy

Once the decision of treatment initiation has been made, the initial choice of current treatment options depends on whether the patient is eligible for stem cell transplantation (SCT) or not. The decision to undergo ASCT should be based on the patient's physiologic age and preference. In young patients, high dose therapy (HDT)/ ASCT is still considered the standard therapy.

5.1.1. Treatment of Transplant- Eligible Patients: Induction Therapy, Conditioning Therapy, ASCT, Tandem ASCT, and Allo- SCT

In potential candidates for ASCT, **induction therapy** regimens aim to maximize tumor control, minimize drug toxicity, facilitate collection of peripheral blood stem cells (PBSCs), and increase the quality of life (QOL). Regimens last 4 to 6 months and are followed by **peripheral blood stem cell collection** and **conditioning** HDT.

Induction Therapy

Until the introduction of novel agents Thal, Len, and Bort, *single-agent dexamethasone* or a combination of vincristine, doxorubicin, and dexamethasone (*VAD*) have been the initial MM therapies most commonly used since the 1990s [10]. The addition of novel agents before and/ or after HDT/ ASCT has recently dramatically changed upfront treatment regimens by improving both CR/ VGPR rates and duration of response.

To date most MM centers predominantly have used one of three **combination regimens** dependent on patient- specific pre-morbidities: (1) thalidomide *plus* dexamethasone [11,12]; (2) bortezomib *plus* dexamethasone; and most recently (3) lenalidomide *plus* low-dose dexamethasone [13,14]. Efforts to improve two- drug combinations by inclusion of a third agent (*e.g.* thalidomide plus doxorubicine plus dexamethasone, TAD; bortezomib *plus* doxorubicin *plus* dexamethasone, PAD [15,16]; bortezomib *plus* cyclophosphamide *plus* dexamethasone; Len *plus* cyclophosphamide *plus* Dex, RCd [17]. VCD [18]; most popular bortezomib *plus* thalidomide *plus* dexamethasone, VTD; lenalidomide *plus* bortezomib *plus* dexamethasone, RVD) [19] and most recently low-dose Bort *plus* low-dose Thal *plus* dexamethasone (Decadron) (vTD) [20] indicate the superiority of **triple combinations** in achieving high rates of overall complete response (CR) and very good partial responses (VGPR). Importantly, benefits of Bort- and Len-based regimens were also observed in MM patients with adverse cytogenetic abnormalities including t(4;14) and del(13), whereas del(17) remains an adverse feature. Based on these data three combination induction regimens are currently changing upfront treatment strategies once again. In addition, preliminary results of **quadruple combinations** including Len *plus* Bort *plus* cyclophosphamid *plus* Dex (RVCD, EVOLUTION- trial; [21]); and Len *plus* Bort *plus* peg liposomal doxorubicin (peg Dox) *plus* Dex [22] are providing support for their continued evaluation. The combination of Thal with Dex, cisplatin, Dox, cyclophosphamide, and etoposide (DTPACE) has been incorporated into induction therapy, especially for patients with high- risk features [23].

Stem Cell Collection and Consolidation Therapy

Stem cells (adequate for 2 transplants) are collected generally after 4 cycles of induction therapy using granulocyte stimulating factors (G-CSF or GM-CSF) alone or following initial priming with cyclophosphamide and collection during recovery. Based on results of the IFM95-02 trial, Melphalan 200mg/m^2 is the most widely used conditioning regimen; dose reduction to 140mg/m^2 or 100mg/m^2 may be considered, dependent on age and comorbidities [24,25,26,27]. Efforts to improve Melphalan ablative conditioning have included: increasing the Melphalan dose alone or in combination with cytoprotectants such as amifostine as well as novel agents Samarium, Holmium, Bort, and Len [14,28,29-34].

Initial Thal and Bort therapy do not negatively influence stem cell yield [35-37]. To overcome Len-induced decreases of CD34+ SC, collection and harvesting early after Len induction therapy using cyclophosphamide and G-CSF mobilization is recommended [38,39].

Double ASCT

The NCCN Guidelines recommend a second ASCT within 6 months of the initial ASCT for those MM patients without at least VGPR after the first ASCT [3]. The use of novel therapies during the first transplant is increasing the ≥ VGPR rate, thereby decreasing the patient population eligible for second transplant.

Allogenic Stem Cell Transplantation

Although allogeneic stem cell transplantation (allo- SCT) following preparative myeloablative regimens can induce molecular remissions, toxicity and transplant- related mortality is excessively high and has been limited to MM patients with high- risk features or to those patients who relapse within 12 months of ASCT who are less than 55 years of age [40-45]. Attempts to improve the efficacy of allografting (*e.g.* by exploiting alloimmune graft-*versus*-MM effects) and minimize high transplant- related mortality (*e.g.* graft-*versus*-host disease) include: T cell depletion from allografts [46,47] and reduced- intensity conditioning (RIC; mini- allogeneic, non- myeloablative) SCT [48,49]. Indeed, ASCT followed by allo- RIC achieved dramatic reduction of transplant- related mortality with potent anti- tumor activity [50,51]. However, in contrast to the French IFM99-04 trial and a prospective PETHMA trial which reported inferiority of tandem ASCT *plus* allo- RIC vs. tandem ASCT [52,53]. Only the study by Bruno *et al.* strongly indicated survival benefits of tandem- ASCT – allo- RIC vs. tandem ASCT [54]. Differences in these studies include conditioning and patient selection. Finally, non- myeloablative allografting following ASCT as consolidation immunotherapy significantly reduces the incidence of disease progression compared to tandem ASCT [55]. In summary, RIC- regimens represent the most promising clinical research area for allo- SCT. However they should be done primarily in the context of a clinical trial.

5.1.2. Maintenance Therapy

Maintenance therapy after single or tandem ASCT in MM patients with VGPR or CR has been evaluated in order to prolong remission and to reduce the risk of relapse [56]. Three agents, interferon- α, glucocorticoids, and thalidomide have been studied in greater detail. If at all, only marginal benefit has been reported with interferon- α after either standard therapy or ASCT; it therefore has been abandoned as a maintenance therapy option for MM [5]. In contrast to interferon- α, steroids prolonged OS and PFS significantly both after standard therapy and ASCT[57-59]. However further studies are needed to support these data obtained in small patient groups.

Three clinical trials have used maintenance with either thalidomide alone (category 1) or thalidomide in combination with prednisone (category 2A)[60-62]. Importantly, results indicate an additional antitumor effect post- ASCT. The optimal duration of maintenance therapy remains to be determined.

More clinical trials are ongoing to evaluate the potential role of Bort and Len in maintenance therapy both in the transplantation setting as well as non- transplantation setting. Both the French and CALGB studies support the use of maintenance Len to prolong PFS post-ASCT [60,63]. Palumbo *et al.* have shown prolonged PFS in non- ASCT candidates treated with Melphalan plus prednisone plus Len followed by Len maintenance [64].

5.2. Treatment of Transplant- Ineligible Patients

It is emphasized that age (> 65 years) alone is no longer a determinant for transplant eligibility. Rather, performance status and comorbidities represent determinants of ASCT eligibility. Specifically, patients with Eastern Cooperative Oncology Group (ECOG) performance status > 3, and New York Heart Association (NYHA) class > 3 have higher morbidity and mortality if offered HDT-ASCT [65]. Moreover, patients in renal failure with serum creatinine > 2.5 mg/dl have increased transplant-related mortality, but are still transplant eligible as long as other criteria for HDT are met [66].

Nevertheless, because nearly two-thirds of MM patients are older than 65 years at diagnosis, the management of elderly patients in general warrants particular attention This is underscored by the fact that while overall clinical outcomes in MM have improved substantially in the past decade, outcomes for the elderly have not [1]. Various factors may contribute to this discrepancy in outcomes between older and younger patients, including the higher incidence of significant co-morbid conditions among the elderly, an increase in therapy-related toxicities, and treatment patterns that favour less intensive, and perhaps less effective, therapeutic regimens. Indeed whether there are distinct differences in the tumor biology of elderly vs. younger MM patients is unknown. In some instances, intensive therapy aimed at maximum reduction of tumor burden may be appropriate, whereas in others less intensive therapy aimed disease control is preferred.

When should therapy be initiated? As is true for all patients with MM, treatment should be initiated when symptoms develop and/ or there is evidence of disease-related organ impairment (ROTI). Consideration should be given to the use of intravenous bisphosphonate therapy even in the absence of symptoms or organ impairment if bone imaging suggests decreased bone density. Patients with SMM or early stage disease should be monitored closely so that in the event of progression, treatment can be initiated before disease related complications develop.

As for the initial treatment of transplant eligible MM patients, the development of Thal, Len, and Bort has also dramatically altered the management of transplant- ineligible MM patients. Doublet and triplet combinations of these agents and conventional therapies have already largely replaced previous standards such as Melphalan *plus* prednisone (MP) in the treatment of transplant- ineligible MM patients. Ongoing clinical trials aim to further improve patient outcome utilizing quadruplet regimens.

Doublet treatment regimens include TD and Rd. (1) MP vs. TD. With median PFS of 14.5 months vs. 6.5 months, median TTP of 22.6 months vs. 6.5 months, and ORR of 63% vs. 46% (CR 7.7% vs. 2.6%), TD was superior to dexamethasone alone [67]. TD has been compared with MP in elderly patients [68]: no survival benefit was seen (41.5 months vs. 49.4 months), though the TD group showed a significantly higher rate of CR and VGPR. Median OS in patients > age 75 was 41.3 months in MP arm vs. 19.8 months in TD arm (HR 1.85; P = 0.71) due to the poor tolerability of TD with higher numbers of toxicity-related deaths. (2) RD vs. Rd. An ECOG trial randomized 445 patients to receive Rd or RD [69]. The PFS and TTP rates were similar between the two arms, possibly due to better tolerability of low-dose and higher efficacy of high-dose dexamethasone. Importantly, the OS was significantly longer for the low-dose dexamethasone arm; 2-year OS was 75% for high-dose dexamethasone arm and 87% in the low-dose dexamethasone arm (P = 0.0002). Len *plus* low-dose dexamethasone achieves higher overall and extent of response, better tolerability, and prolonged OS.

Triplet treatment regimens include MPT, VMP, VTP, MPR/m.

(1) MPT* vs. *MP. In 2006 the oral regimen of MP- Thal replaced the standard combination of Melphalan and prednisone for the treatment of newly diagnosed patients older than 65 years or transplant- ineligible patients younger than 65 years [74]. Specifically, as suggested by the preclinical trials advocating synergy between thalidomide/ IMiDs and Melphalan [75], a meta-analysis of five clinical phase 3 trials demonstrated improved response rates with addition of thalidomide to MP (MPT) vs. MP. However, differences in OS were demonstrated only in some studies. Two studies from IFM offered both improvement in PFS as well as OS in the MPT arm [71,76]. In contrast, the "Stichting Hemato-Oncologie voor Volwassenen Nederland" (HOVON) study [77] and the "Gruppo Italiano Malattie Ematologiche dell'Adulto" (GIMEMA) study [78] showed improved PFS, but not OS, in the MPT arm. In both the GIMEMA and HOVON studies, Thal was given as maintenance until further evidence of progression of the disease. In the trial by GIMEMA, 331 patients were randomly assigned to receive oral MPT or MP. The overall response rates were 68.9% vs. 47.6% (CR rates of 15.6% vs. 3.7%) in favour of MPT. After a median follow-up of 38.1 months, the median PFS was 21.8 months for MPT vs. 14.5 months for MP (P = 0.004); however, the median OS was 45 months for MPT and 47.6 months for MP (P = 0.79). An increased incidence of drug- resistant relapse with Thal maintenance or more effective salvage regimen in the control group may be the reason for lack of overall survival advantage. Moreover, grade 3 or 4 adverse events were more common with MPT (55%) than MP (22%). Similar results were shown with the HOVON study: the overall response rates for MPT vs. MP were 66% vs. 47% (CR rates of 2% vs. 2%).

Table 1. Response rates with IMiD containing regimens in transplant-ineligible patients

Study Year	Regimen	N	Median age (yr)	Median follow up (m)	RR			Survival		Comments
					CR %	≥VGPR %	≥PR%	Median EFS	Median OS	
Ludwig H[68] (2009)	MP→IFNm/Tm TD→IFNm/Tm	141 142	72	28.1	2 2	26 13	68 50	20.7 m 16.7 m HR 1.30, *P* = *0.1*	49.4 m 41.5 m HR 1.55, *P* = *0.024*	Post- maintenance, median OS for TD 41.1 months; MP 53.1 months; *P* = *0.41*)
Facon[72] (2006)	MP Dex M-Dex Dex-IFN	122 118 127 121	70	82.8	1 3 1 1		41 70 40 42	21.1 m 22.9 m 12.2 m 15.2 m	34 m 39.6 m 33.4 m 32 m	No difference in OS was observed between the 4 treatment groups
Palumbo[78] GIMEMA (2008)	MPT→ Tm MP	159 160	72	38.1	15.6 3.7	29.3 11	68.9 47.6	21.8 m 14.5 m HR 0.63, *P* = *0.0004*	45.0 m 47.6 m HR 1.04, *P* = *0.79*	

Table 1. cont....

Facon[71] IFM 99-06 (2007)	MPT (No Tm) MP MEL100	125 196 126	<70	51.5	13 2 18	47 7 43	76 35 65	27.5 m 17.8 m 19.4 m HR* 0.51, *P* = *0*.0001	51.6 m 33.2 m 38.3 m HR* 0.59, *P* = *0*.006	*MPT vs. MP MPT vs. MEL100 - HR OS 0.69, *P* = *0*.027; HR PFS 0.59, *P* = *0*.002. MP vs. MEL100 NS
Hulin[76] IFM 01-01 (2009)	MPT (No Tm) MP	107 112	78.5	NRe	7 1	21 7	62 31	24.1m 18.5 m HR 0.62, *P* = *0*.001	44.0 m 29.1 m HR 0.68, *P* = *0*.028	
Wijermans[77] HOVON 49 (ASCO 2010)	MPT→Tm MP	165 168	NRe	NRe	2 2	30 10	66 47	13 m 10 m *P* < 0.02	37 m 30 m *P* = *0*.16	
Waage[70] NORDIC	MPT→Tm MP	182 181	75	36	6 3	15 6	42 28	16 m 14 m *P* = NS	29 m 32 m *P* = NS	
Palumbo[83] (2007)	MPR	54	71		23.8	47.6	81			
Palumbo[64] (ASH 2009)	MPR→Rm MPR MP	152 153 154	71	9.4	18 13 5	32 33 11	77 67 49	NR 13.2 13	92%	HR PFS 0.499 MPR+Rm vs. MP *P* = *0*.001; HR PFS 0.530 MPR+Rm vs. MPR; *P* = *0*.002 *1 yr OS MPR+Rm vs. MP NS
Rajkumar[69] EA403 (2009)	RD Rd	223 222	65	35.8	5 4	71 26	81 70	63% 65%	75% ± 87%	2 yr PFS ±2 yr OS

Tm – Thalidomide maintenance; Rm – Revlimid maintenance; VPm – Maintenance with Bortezomib and Prednisone; VTm – Maintenance with Bortezomib and Thalidomide.

The median PFS was 13 months for MPT and 10 months for MP (P<0.02) with median OS of 37 months for MPT and 30 months for MP (P =0.16). In the NORDIC study, the overall response rates were 42% vs. 28% (CR rates of 6 vs. 3%). After a median follow-up of 36 months, the median PFS was 16 months for MPT vs. 14 months for MP (P=NS), with the median OS was 29 months for MPT and 32 months for MP (P=NS).

Table 2. Response rates with bortezomib containing regimens in transplant-ineligible patients

Study Year	Regimen	N	Median age (yr)	Median follow up (m)	RR			Survival		Comments
					CR %	≥VGPR %	≥PR%	Median EFS	Median OS	
San Miguel[82] VISTA	VMP MP	344 338	71	36.7	33 4			17.6 m 8.4 m HR 0.543, *P* < 0.0001	NR 43.1 m HR 0.653, *P* = *0*.0008	TFS (Treatment Free Survival)
Palumbo[80] (ASCO 2010)	VMPT →VTm MPV	254 257	71	21.6	38 24	59 50	89 81	60% 42% *P* = *0*.007	89.2%± 88.8% *P* = NS	3 yr PFS ±3 yr OS
Mateos[81] PETHEMA	VMP →VTm/VPm VTP →VTm/VPm	130 130	73	24	20 27	32 37	80 83	34 m 23 m HR 1.3 *P* = *0*.1	80% 64% HR 1.4 *P* = *0*.1	3 yr OS; CR increased from 27%→44% in VMP+VTm. VTP+VPm vs. VMP+VTm HR PFS 1.6; *P* = *0*.008

In the IFM 99-06 [71], 447 patients were randomized to MPT vs. MP vs. reduced intensity ASCT using Melphalan 100 mg/m2 (MEL 100). MPT arm prolonged survival advantage compared to MP (MPT vs. MP - hazards ratio[HR] for PFS 0.51, P = 0.0001; HR OS 0.59, P = 0.006) and MEL 100 arm (MPT vs. MEL100 - HR PFS 0.59, P = 0.002; HR OS 0.69, P = 0.027). In the IFM study 01/01 [76], 219 patients were randomized to MPT vs. MP. The overall response rates were 62% vs. 31% (CR rates of 7% vs. 1%) with median PFS of

24.1 months for MPT and 18.5 months for MP (P = 0.001). However, the median OS was 44 months for MPT and 29.1 months for MP (P = 0.79). A meta-analysis of these randomized control trials comparing MPT vs. MP as initial therapy for transplant-ineligible patients demonstrated that MPT has superior RR, superior PFS and marginally improved OS, with minimal additional toxicity, compared with MP alone [79].

(2) VMP* vs. *MP. In the phase 3 VISTA trial comparing VMP (bortezomib, Melphalan and prednisone) vs. MP, VMP was superior in ORR, PFS, and OS [82]. Among 337 patients randomized to VMP vs. 331 patients to MP arms, IFx-neg CR rate was 33% vs. 4% (P<0.001), respectively. At a median follow up of 36.7 months, median OS was not estimable vs. 43.1 months, and 3-year OS rates were 68.5% vs. 54.0% with VMP vs. MP, respectively. Median treatment- free survival was 17.6 vs. 8.4 months in the (HR, 0.543; P<0.0001), and median time to next therapy (TTNT) was 28.1 vs. 19.2 months (HR 0.527: p<0.0001). Median survival from start of subsequent therapy following VMP and MP was 30.2 vs. 21.9 months (HR 0.815, P = 0.21), despite crossover and 50% MP patients being rescued with bortezomib-based therapy at relapse.

(3) VMP* vs. *VTP. The Spanish Myeloma Group also evaluated the combination of VMP vs. VTP (bortezomib, thalidomide and prednisone) [81]. In the 1st randomization, 260 patients were randomized to VMP vs. VTP to evaluate whether an alkylating agent or an IMiD is the best combination with bortezomib during induction. Post- induction, RR was 80% vs. 83% for VMP vs. VTP arms. Overall IFx-neg CR rate was 23% (20% vs. 27% for VMP vs. VTP). VMP was associated with more hematological toxicities, whereas VTP had more cardiac toxicities. In the 2nd randomization, 178 patients were randomized to receive VTm (bortezomib administered at 1.3 mg/m^2 on days 1, 4,8,11 every 90 days and thalidomide 50 mg orally daily up to 3 years) or VPm (bortezomib administered at 1.3 mg/m^2 on days 1, 4,8,11 every 90 days and prednisone 50 mg orally every 48 hours up to 3 years) as maintenance therapy. Overall IFx-neg CR rate increased from 23% to 42% suggesting that maintenance therapy improves the depth of responses, but there was no statistically significant difference between the two maintenance groups.

(4) MPRm* vs. *MPR* vs. *MP. Data from a clinical phase 1/2 study by GIMEMA suggests that lenalidomide in combination with MP (MPR) [83] may be a promising upfront treatment in transplant ineligible patients. Of the 54 patients that were enrolled, ORR was achieved by 81%, VGPR by 47.6% and IFx-neg CR by 23.8% of the patients. Palumbo and colleagues evaluated the efficacy and safety of lenalidomide in combination with Melphalan and prednisone (MPR) followed by lenalidomide maintenance (MPRm) in elderly patients in a phase III trial [64]. 459 patients were randomized to MP and MPR and MPRm for 9 cycles during the double-blind treatment phase. From cycle 10 onwards MPRm arm received lenalidomide maintenance at a dose of 10 mg/day on days 1-21 of 28 day cycle until disease progression. The other two arms received placebo during the maintenance phase. The RR for MPRm vs. MPR vs. MP were 77% vs. 67% vs. 49% (CR rate of 18% vs. 13% vs. 5%). At a median follow up of 9.4 months, median PFS for MPRm was not reached, for MP was 13 months (HR 0.499; P<0.001), and for MPR was 13.2 months (HR PFS MPRm vs. MPR 0.530; P = 0.002). Longer follow up is needed to draw adequate conclusions on overall survival, as the follow up is quite short.

Finally, the **quadruple treatment** regimen VMPT is under evaluation. ***VMPT* vs. *VMP*.** VMP along with thalidomide (VMPT) followed by maintenance with VT resulted in RR of 89% (CR rate of 38%) compared to VMP with RR 81% (CR rate of 24%). At a median follow up of 21.6 months, VMPT had superior TTNT (75% vs. 60% at 3 yrs, P = 0.0029) and superior PFS (60% vs. 42% at 3 yrs, P = 0.007); OS at 3 yrs was 89.2% vs. 88.8% (p=NS). This study suggested superior results with VTm maintenance regimen, as was demonstrated by the Spanish Myeloma Group study. Importantly, this trial also reported that Bort can be safely administered as weekly infusion without losing efficacy, but minimizing peripheral neuropathy.

5.3. Salvage Therapy

Salvage therapy is considered for: (1) MM patients with relapsed disease (defined as 25% increase from the lowest response value of serum or urine M- protein, BM plasma cell percentage, or kappa and lambda FLC; new bone or soft lesions; serum calcium > 11.5mg/dl) after initial ASCT or allo- SCT; (2) MM patients with relapsed-and-refractory or primary refractory disease; or (3) MM patients with progressive disease (*e.g.* following initial ASCT or allo- SCT); and (4) MM patients ineligible for SCT with progressive or relapsing disease after initial induction therapy [3]. Patients with relapsed/ refractory MM, if possible, should be enrolled into a clinical trial. Outside a clinical trial the choice of therapy depends on previous therapies, duration of response to previous therapies, presence of high-risk cytogenetic features, and previous toxicities. Treatment options include HD- therapy with ASCT [84,85,86] and allo- SCT [87], rechallenge with the initial treatment regimen, or the switch to a new regimen. Most importantly, salvage therapy has been significantly changed by the introduction of Thal, Len, and Bort. Regimens containing novel therapies have now replaced standard therapy regimens established in the late 1960s to 1980s; *e.g.* high- dose Dex as well as combinations of various chemotherapeutic agents (*e.g.* VAD) with or without ASCT or allo- SCT [88,89].

If relapse occurs after 6 months of initial induction therapy, patients may be retreated with the same induction regimen, if relapse occurs on or within 6 months of discontinuing therapy novel therapies should be initiated. In MM patients with cytogenetic adverse features Bort- or Len- based regimens should be used due to the ability of these agents to, at least in part, overcome their negative effects.

Ongoing studies are evaluating: efficacy of single, doublet, and triplet combination regimens; how prior therapies including SCT may influence their efficacy; and whether novel therapies overcome negative prognostic risk.

Specifically, based on promising preclinical studies [90], and from two multicenter clinical phase II trials (SUMMIT and the CREST trial) [91,92] Bort was approved by the FDA and EMEA for the treatment of relapsed refractory MM in 2003. Subsequently, the international, randomized clinical phase III APEX trial revealed superior response rate and prolonged median PFS and OS after Bort vs. high dose Dex therapy in relapsed MM patients [93,94]. Indeed, Bortezomib achieved survival benefit and high overall response rate of 43% (PR+CR) in the setting of relapsed MM, leading to the FDA approval of Bort in 2005 for treatment of MM in patients with at least one prior therapy in 2005. Importantly, also patients with poor prognostic factors (*e.g.* del 13) may also benefit from Bort [92].

Subsequently, the combination of Bort with pegylated liposomal doxorubicin (PLD) has been FDA approved in 2007 for the treatment of MM patients who have not previously received Bort and have had at least one prior line of anti- MM therapy [95]. Additional clinical trials evaluate the efficacy of bortezomib with cyclophosphamide and steroids [96,97,98]. Common Bort- associated dose- limiting adverse side effects include peripheral neuropathy, gastrointestinal toxicity, and thrombocytopenia.

Based on promising single agent activity in MM refractory to Thal [99], two clinical phase II trials, and two large, randomized, multicenter, double- blind, placebo- controlled clinical phase III trials, Len in combination with high- dose Dex was FDA- approved (2006) as therapy for relapsed and refractory MM in patients with at least one prior therapy. The NCCN panel considers this regimen as a category 1 recommendation. Adverse side effects in MM patients receiving Len/ Dex include neutropenia and thromboembolic events (DVT and pulmonary emboli) [11,100]; therefore, the use of antithrombotic prophylaxis is recommended. Other regimens that combine Len with other agents include: Len with DVd; Len plus adriamycin and Dex; and Len plus Dex and cyclophosphamide [101,102]; as well as Len *plus* Bort and Dex in relapsed and/ or refractory MM.

Empirically tested as a single agent in relapsed/ refractory MM patients, Thal achieved responses in approximately one- third of patients as monotherapy[103-105]. To enhance efficacy and reduce toxicity Thal has been combined with a variety of agents including Dex, cisplatin, cyclophosphamide, etoposide (DT- PACE) and PLD[23,106-110]. Despite high response rates, responses are transient and associated with significant toxicity (constipation, weakness, fatigue, dose- dependent neuropathy, thrombosis, grad 1 and 2 leukopenia, unexplained hyperkalemia, dermatologic side effects).

In addition to Bort, Len, and Thal, a retrospective analysis suggested that bendamustin is effective and tolerable in patients with advanced progressive myeloma [111].

5.4. Choice of Treatment

The presence of comorbidities and toxicities of previous treatment regimens influences the choice of treatment of relapsed or relapsed/ refractory disease.

Renal impairment. Elimination of Bort is independent of renal clearance and Bort may even help to normalize MM- associated renal dysfunction in selected patients. Therefore, Bort- containing regimens are recommended in MM patients with renal disease. In contrast to Bort, Len is primarily excreted by the kidneys; therefore careful monitoring and dose adaptation to creatinine clearance is indicated.

Thromboembolic events. Thal and Len increase risk of DVT, especially with high-dose Dex can trigger DVT [112,113]. To overcome this risk prophylaxis with aspirin is recommended in patients with one additional risk factor (age, central catheter, diabetes, cardiac disease, immobilization, hyperviscosity), with full dose warfarin or LMWH recommended in patients with more than one additional risk factor [114].

Aggressive relapse and cytogenetic abnormalities. Subanalysis data from several clinical trials both in the upfront as well as in the relapsed/ refractory setting indicate efficacy of bortezomib[82,92,115] and lenalidomide [79,116] in MM patients carrying an adverse cytogenetic feature.

Polyneuropathy. Due to bortezomib- and thalidomide- induced neuropathies dose reduction or discontinuation of treatment may be necessary [117]. Lenalidomide- containing treatment regimens are recommended in MM patients with pre-existing disease- or treatment- associated neuropathy.

Reactivation of Herpes zoster. Treatemnt with bortezomib is associated with reactivation of herpes zoster [82,118]. Antiviral prophylaxis is successfully preventing this adverse side effect [118].

6. TREATMENT FOR MM- INDUCED BONE DISEASE

Common approaches to treat MM bone disease include radiotherapy, surgery and medical management. Radiotherapy is mainly used to control bone fracture- related pain. Surgery, vertebroplasty and kyphoplasty in particular, aim to restore vertebral integrity and height as well as offer pain relief. The medical management of MM bone disease is based on the clinical use of amino-bisphosphonates (BP), including zoledronic acid and pamidronate. Based on the significant reduction in the incidence of skeletal related events (hypercalcemia, compression fractures, pain and the necessity of radiotherapy/ surgical intervention), pamidronate and zoledronate received FDA approval for the treatment of MM- associated osteolytic lesions in 1996 and 2002, respectively [119,120]. Importantly, recent data also indicate that zolendronic acid improves MM patient survival when compared to clodronate [121]. However, patients on bisphosphonates must be monitored for both renal toxicity as well as osteonecrosis of the jaw (ONJ) [122]. New guidelines to avoid ONJ include maintenance of optimal dental health and recommendations on duration of BP treatment [123]. Novel agents, *i.e.* demosumab are under evaluation to similarly decrease related complications.

REFERENCES

[1] Kumar SK, Rajkumar SV, Dispenzieri A, *et al.* Improved survival in multiple myeloma and the impact of novel therapies. Blood 2008; 111: 2516-2520.

[2] Kyle RA, Rajkumar SV. Criteria for diagnosis, staging, risk stratification and response assessment of multiple myeloma. Leukemia 2009; 23: 3-9.

[3] Network NCC. NCCN Clinical Practice Guidelines in Oncology: Multiple Myeloma. www.nccn.org/professionals/physicians_gls/PDF/myeloma.pdf 2010; Version 1.2011:

[4] Kyle RA, Rajkumar SV. Multiple myeloma. N Engl J Med 2004; 351: 1860-1873.

[5] Kyle RA, Rajkumar SV. Multiple myeloma. Blood 2008; 111: 2962-2972.

[6] Greipp PR, San Miguel J, Durie BG, *et al.* International staging system for multiple myeloma. J Clin Oncol 2005; 23: 3412-3420.

[7] Palumbo A, Gay F, Falco P, *et al.* Bortezomib as induction before autologous transplantation, followed by lenalidomide as consolidation-maintenance in untreated multiple myeloma patients. J Clin Oncol 2010; 28: 800-807.

[8] Stewart AK, Bergsagel PL, Greipp PR, *et al.* A practical guide to defining high-risk myeloma for clinical trials, patient counseling and choice of therapy. Leukemia 2007; 21: 529-534.

[9] Qazilbash MH, Saliba RM, Ahmed B, *et al.* Deletion of the short arm of chromosome 1 (del 1p) is a strong predictor of poor outcome in myeloma patients undergoing an autotransplant. Biol Blood Marrow Transplant 2007; 13: 1066-1072.

[10] Alexanian R, Barlogie B. New treatment strategies for multiple myeloma. Am J Hematol 1990; 35: 194-198.

[11] Weber D, Rankin K, Gavino M, Delasalle K, Alexanian R. Thalidomide alone or with dexamethasone for previously untreated multiple myeloma. J Clin Oncol 2003; 21: 16-19.

[12] Rajkumar SV, Blood E, Vesole D, Fonseca R, Greipp PR. Phase III clinical trial of thalidomide plus dexamethasone compared with dexamethasone alone in newly diagnosed multiple myeloma: a clinical trial coordinated by the Eastern Cooperative Oncology Group. J Clin Oncol 2006; 24: 431-436.

[13] Rajkumar SV, Jacobus S, Callander NS, *et al.* Lenalidomide plus high-dose dexamethasone vs. lenalidomide plus low-dose dexamethasone as initial therapy for newly diagnosed multiple myeloma: an open-label randomised controlled trial. Lancet Oncol 2010; 11: 29-37.

[14] Lacy MQ, Gertz MA, Dispenzieri A, *et al.* Long-term results of response to therapy, time to progression, and survival with lenalidomide plus dexamethasone in newly diagnosed myeloma. Mayo Clin Proc 2007; 82: 1179-1184.

[15] Harousseau JL, Attal M, Leleu X, *et al.* Bortezomib plus dexamethasone as induction treatment prior to autologous stem cell transplantation in patients with newly diagnosed multiple myeloma: results of an IFM phase II study. Haematologica 2006; 91: 1498-1505.

[16] Oakervee HE, Popat R, Curry N, *et al.* PAD combination therapy (PS-341/bortezomib, doxorubicin and dexamethasone) for previously untreated patients with multiple myeloma. Br J Haematol 2005; 129: 755-762.

[17] Kumar S, Hayman S, Buadi F, *et al.* Phase II trial of lenalidomide (RevlimidTM) with cyclophosphamide and dexamethasone (RCd) for newly diagnosed myeloma. Blood 2009; 112: Abstract 91

[18] Reeder CB, Reece DE, Kukreti V, *et al.* Cyclophosphamide, bortezomib and dexamethasone induction for newly diagnosed multiple myeloma: high response rates in a phase II clinical trial. Leukemia 2009; 23: 1337-1341.

[19] Richardson PG, Weller E, Lonial S, *et al.* Lenalidomide, bortezomib, and dexamethasone combination therapy in patients with newly diagnosed multiple myeloma. Blood 2010; 116: 679-686.

[20] Moreau P, Facon T, Attal M, *et al.* Comparison of reduced-dose bortezomib plus thalidomide plus dexamethasone (vTD) to bortezomib plus dexamethasone (VD) as induction treatment prior to ASCT in de novo multiple myeloma (MM): Results of IFM2007-02 study. J Clin Oncol 2010; 28:15s, 2010 (suppl; abstr 8014)

[21] Kumar S, Flinn I, Hari P, *et al.* Novel three– and four–drug combinations of bortezomib, dexamethasone, cyclophosphamide, and lenalidomide, for newly diagnosed multiple myeloma: encouraging results from the multi-center, randomized, phase 2 EVOLUTION study. Blood 2009; 114: Abstract 127:

[22] Jakubowiak A, Reece D, Hofmeister C, *et al.* Lenalidomide, bortezomib, pegylated liposomal doxorubicin, and dexamethasone in newly diagnosed multiple myeloma: updated results of phase I/II MMRC trial. Blood 2009; 114: Abstract 132

[23] Lee CK, Barlogie B, Munshi N, *et al.* DTPACE: an effective, novel combination chemotherapy with thalidomide for previously treated patients with myeloma. J Clin Oncol 2003; 21: 2732-2739.

[24] Moreau P, Facon T, Attal M, *et al.* Comparison of 200 mg/m(2) Melphalan and 8 Gy total body irradiation plus 140 mg/m(2) Melphalan as conditioning regimens for peripheral blood stem cell transplantation in patients with newly diagnosed multiple myeloma: final analysis of the Intergroupe Francophone du Myelome 9502 randomized trial. Blood 2002; 99: 731-735.

[25] Palumbo A, Triolo S, Argentino C, *et al.* Dose-intensive Melphalan with stem cell support (MEL100) is superior to standard treatment in elderly myeloma patients. Blood 1999; 94: 1248-1253.

[26] Palumbo A, Bringhen S, Bertola A, *et al.* Multiple myeloma: comparison of two dose-intensive Melphalan regimens (100 vs 200 mg/m(2)). Leukemia 2004; 18: 133-138.

[27] Palumbo A, Bringhen S, Petrucci MT, *et al.* Intermediate-dose Melphalan improves survival of myeloma patients aged 50 to 70: results of a randomized controlled trial. Blood 2004; 104: 3052-3057.

[28] Spencer A, Horvath N, Gibson J, *et al.* Prospective randomised trial of amifostine cytoprotection in myeloma patients undergoing high-dose Melphalan conditioned autologous stem cell transplantation. Bone Marrow Transplant 2005; 35: 971-977.

[29] Thieblemont C, Dumontet C, Saad H, *et al.* Amifostine reduces mucosal damage after high-dose Melphalan conditioning and autologous peripheral blood progenitor cell transplantation for patients with multiple myeloma. Bone Marrow Transplant 2002; 30: 769-775.

[30] Dispenzieri A, Wiseman GA, Lacy MQ, *et al.* A Phase II study of (153)Sm-EDTMP and high-dose Melphalan as a peripheral blood stem cell conditioning regimen in patients with multiple myeloma. Am J Hematol 2010; 85: 409-413.

[31] Christoforidou AV, Saliba RM, Williams P, *et al.* Results of a retrospective single institution analysis of targeted skeletal radiotherapy with (166)Holmium-DOTMP as conditioning regimen for autologous stem cell transplant for patients with multiple myeloma. Impact on transplant outcomes. Biol Blood Marrow Transplant 2007; 13: 543-549.

[32] Desikan KR, Tricot G, Dhodapkar M, *et al.* Melphalan plus total body irradiation (MEL-TBI) or cyclophosphamide (MEL-CY) as a conditioning regimen with second autotransplant in responding patients with myeloma is inferior compared to historical controls receiving tandem transplants with Melphalan alone. Bone Marrow Transplant 2000; 25: 483-487.

[33] Roussel M, Moreau P, Huynh A, *et al.* Bortezomib and high-dose Melphalan as conditioning regimen before autologous stem cell transplantation in patients with de novo multiple myeloma: a phase 2 study of the Intergroupe Francophone du Myelome (IFM). Blood 2010; 115: 32-37.

[34] Lonial S, Kaufman J, Tighiouart M, *et al.* A Phase I/II Trial Combining High Dose Melphalan and Autologous Transplant with Bortezomib for Multiple Myeloma: A Dose and Schedule Finding Study. Clin Cancer Res 2010:

[35] Breitkreutz I, Lokhorst HM, Raab MS, *et al.* Thalidomide in newly diagnosed multiple myeloma: influence of thalidomide treatment on peripheral blood stem cell collection yield. Leukemia 2007; 21: 1294-1299.

[36] Oakervee H, Popat R, Cavenagh JD. Use of bortezomib as induction therapy prior to stem cell transplantation in frontline treatment of multiple myeloma: impact on stem cell harvesting and engraftment. Leuk Lymphoma 2007; 48: 1910-1921.

[37] Kumar S, Giralt S, Stadtmauer EA, *et al.* Mobilization in myeloma revisited: IMWG consensus perspectives on stem cell collection following initial therapy with thalidomide-, lenalidomide-, or bortezomib-containing regimens. Blood 2009; 114: 1729-1735.

[38] Kumar S, Dispenzieri A, Lacy MQ, *et al.* Impact of lenalidomide therapy on stem cell mobilization and engraftment post-peripheral blood stem cell transplantation in patients with newly diagnosed myeloma. Leukemia 2007; 21: 2035-2042.

[39] Paripati H, Stewart AK, Cabou S, *et al.* Compromised stem cell mobilization following induction therapy with lenalidomide in myeloma. Leukemia 2008; 22: 1282-1284.

[40] Osserman EF, DiRe LB, DiRe J, *et al.* Identical twin marrow transplantation in multiple myeloma. Acta Haematol 1982; 68: 215-223.

[41] Fefer A. Current status of syngeneic marrow transplantation and its relevance to autografting. Clin Haematol 1986; 15: 49-65.

[42] Thomas ED. Landmarks in the development of hematopoietic cell transplantation. World J Surg 2000; 24: 815-818.

[43] Groth CG, Brent LB, Calne RY, *et al.* Historic landmarks in clinical transplantation: conclusions from the consensus conference at the University of California, Los Angeles. World J Surg 2000; 24: 834-843.

[44] Gahrton G. Autologous stem-cell transplantation in multiple myeloma. Wien Med Wochenschr 1995; 145: 52-54.

[45] Bensinger WI, Appelbaum FA, Demirer T, *et al.* Transplantation of allogeneic peripheral blood stem cells. Stem Cells 1995; 13 Suppl 3: 63-70.

[46] Alyea E, Weller E, Schlossman R, *et al.* T-cell--depleted allogeneic bone marrow transplantation followed by donor lymphocyte infusion in patients with multiple myeloma: induction of graft-versus-myeloma effect. Blood 2001; 98: 934-939.

[47] Lokhorst HM, Segeren CM, Verdonck LF, *et al.* Partially T-cell-depleted allogeneic stem-cell transplantation for first-line treatment of multiple myeloma: a prospective evaluation of patients treated in the phase III study HOVON 24 MM. J Clin Oncol 2003; 21: 1728-1733.

[48] Maloney DG, Sandmaier BM, Mackinnon S, Shizuru JA. Non-myeloablative transplantation. Hematology Am Soc Hematol Educ Prog 2002: 392-421.

[49] Badros A, Barlogie B, Siegel E, *et al.* Improved outcome of allogeneic transplantation in high-risk multiple myeloma patients after nonmyeloablative conditioning. J Clin Oncol 2002; 20: 1295-1303.

[50] Kroger N, Sayer HG, Schwerdtfeger R, *et al.* Unrelated stem cell transplantation in multiple myeloma after a reduced-intensity conditioning with pretransplantation antithymocyte globulin is highly effective with low transplantation-related mortality. Blood 2002; 100: 3919-3924.

[51] Maloney DG, Molina AJ, Sahebi F, *et al.* Allografting with nonmyeloablative conditioning following cytoreductive autografts for the treatment of patients with multiple myeloma. Blood 2003; 102: 3447-3454.

[52] Moreau P, Garban F, Attal M, *et al.* Long-term follow-up results of IFM99-03 and IFM99-04 trials comparing nonmyeloablative allotransplantation with autologous transplantation in high-risk de novo multiple myeloma. Blood 2008; 112: 3914-3915.

[53] Rosinol L, Perez-Simon JA, Sureda A, *et al.* A prospective PETHEMA study of tandem autologous transplantation vs. autograft followed by reduced-intensity conditioning allogeneic transplantation in newly diagnosed multiple myeloma. Blood 2008; 112: 3591-3593.

[54] Bruno B, Rotta M, Patriarca F, *et al.* A comparison of allografting with autografting for newly diagnosed myeloma. N Engl J Med 2007; 356: 1110-1120.

[55] Carella AM, Beltrami G, Corsetti MT, *et al.* Reduced intensity conditioning for allograft after cytoreductive autograft in metastatic breast cancer. Lancet 2005; 366: 318-320.

[56] Badros AZ. The role of maintenance therapy in the treatment of multiple myeloma. J Natl Compr Canc Netw 2010; 8 Suppl 1: S21-27.

[57] Berenson JR, Crowley JJ, Grogan TM, *et al.* Maintenance therapy with alternate-day prednisone improves survival in multiple myeloma patients. Blood 2002; 99: 3163-3168.

[58] Salmon SE, Crowley JJ, Balcerzak SP, *et al.* Interferon vs. interferon plus prednisone remission maintenance therapy for multiple myeloma: a Southwest Oncology Group Study. J Clin Oncol 1998; 16: 890-896.

[59] Palumbo A, Giaccone L, Bertola A, *et al.* Low-dose thalidomide plus dexamethasone is an effective salvage therapy for advanced myeloma. Haematologica 2001; 86: 399-403.

[60] Attal M, Cristini C, Marit G, *et al.* Lenalidomide maintenance after transplantation for myeloma. J Clin Oncol 2010; 28: 15s

[61] Barlogie B, Tricot G, Anaissie E, *et al.* Thalidomide and hematopoietic-cell transplantation for multiple myeloma. N Engl J Med 2006; 354: 1021-1030.

[62] Spencer A, Prince HM, Roberts AW, *et al.* Consolidation therapy with low-dose thalidomide and prednisolone prolongs the survival of multiple myeloma patients undergoing a single autologous stem-cell transplantation procedure. J Clin Oncol 2009; 27: 1788-1793.

[63] McCarthy P, Owzar K, Anderson K, *et al.* Phase III intergroup study of lenalidomide vs. placebo maintenance therapy following single autologous stem cell transplant (ASCT) for multiple myeloma (MM): CALGB 100104. J Clin Oncol 2010; 28:15s

[64] Palumbo A, Dimopoulos M, Delforge M, *et al.* A phase III study to determine the efficacy and safety of lenalidomide in combination with Melphalan and prednisone (MPR) in elderly patients with newly diagnosed multiple myeloma. Blood 2009; 114: Abstract 613

[65] Kristinsson SY, Bjorkholm M, Andersson TM, *et al.* Patterns of survival and causes of death following a diagnosis of monoclonal gammopathy of undetermined significance: a population-based study. Haematologica 2009; 94: 1714-1720.

[66] Badros A, Barlogie B, Siegel E, *et al.* Results of autologous stem cell transplant in multiple myeloma patients with renal failure. Br J Haematol 2001; 114: 822-829.

[67] Rajkumar SV, Rosinol L, Hussein M, *et al.* Multicenter, randomized, double-blind, placebo-controlled study of thalidomide plus dexamethasone compared with dexamethasone as initial therapy for newly diagnosed multiple myeloma. J Clin Oncol 2008; 26: 2171-2177.

[68] Ludwig H, Hajek R, Tothova E, *et al.* Thalidomide-dexamethasone compared with Melphalan-prednisolone in elderly patients with multiple myeloma. Blood 2009; 113: 3435-3442.

[69] Rajkumar S, Jacobus S, Callander N, *et al.* A randomized trial of lenalidomide plus high-dose dexamethasone (RD) vs. lenalidomide plus low-dose dexamethasone (Rd) in newly diagnosed multiple myeloma (E4A03): a trial coordinated by the eastern cooperative oncology group. Blood 2007; 110: Abstract 74:

[70] Waage A, Gimsing P, Fayers P, *et al.* Melphalan and prednisone plus thalidomide or placebo in elderly patients with multiple myeloma. Blood 2010; 116: 1405-1412.

[71] Facon T, Mary JY, Hulin C, *et al.* Melphalan and prednisone plus thalidomide vs. Melphalan and prednisone alone or reduced-intensity autologous stem cell transplantation in elderly patients with multiple myeloma (IFM 99-06): a randomised trial. Lancet 2007; 370: 1209-1218.

[72] Facon T, Mary JY, Pegourie B, *et al.* Dexamethasone-based regimens vs. Melphalan-prednisone for elderly multiple myeloma patients ineligible for high-dose therapy. Blood 2006; 107: 1292-1298.

[73] Facon T, San Miguel J, Mateos MV, Hulin C. Frontline treatment in elderly patients with multiple myeloma. Semin Hematol 2009; 46: 133-142.

[74] Palumbo A, Bringhen S, Caravita T, *et al.* Oral Melphalan and prednisone chemotherapy plus thalidomide compared with Melphalan and prednisone alone in elderly patients with multiple myeloma: randomised controlled trial. Lancet 2006; 367: 825-831.

[75] Mitsiades N, Mitsiades CS, Richardson PG, *et al.* The proteasome inhibitor PS-341 potentiates sensitivity of multiple myeloma cells to conventional chemotherapeutic agents: therapeutic applications. Blood 2003; 101: 2377-2380.

[76] Wij C, Facon T, Rodon P, *et al.* Efficacy of Melphalan and prednisone plus thalidomide in patients older than 75 years with newly diagnosed multiple myeloma: IFM 01/01 trial. J Clin Oncol 2009; 27: 3664-3670.

[77] Wijermans P, Schaafsma M, Termorshuizen F, *et al.* Phase III study of the value of thalidomide added to Melphalan plus prednisone in elderly patients with newly diagnosed multiple myeloma: the HOVON 49 study. J Clin Oncol 2010; 28 3160-3166.

[78] Palumbo A, Bringhen S, Liberati AM, *et al.* Oral Melphalan, prednisone, and thalidomide in elderly patients with multiple myeloma: updated results of a randomized controlled trial. Blood 2008; 112: 3107-3114.

[79] Kapoor P, Kumar S, Fonseca R, *et al.* Impact of risk stratification on outcome among patients with multiple myeloma receiving initial therapy with lenalidomide and dexamethasone. Blood 2009; 114: 518-521.

[80] Palumbo AP, Bringhen S, Rossi D, *et al.* A phase III study of VMPT vs. VMP in newly diagnosed elderly myeloma patients. J Clin Oncol 2010; 27: 15s:

[81] Mateos M, Oriol A, Martínez-López J, *et al.* Bortezomib, Melphalan, and prednisone vs. bortezomib, thalidomide, and prednisone as induction therapy followed by maintenance treatment with bortezomib and thalidomide vs. bortezomib and prednisone in elderly patients with untreated multiple myeloma: a randomised trial. Lancet Oncol, 2010 Oct; 11(10): 934-41.

[82] San Miguel JF, Schlag R, Khuageva NK, *et al.* Bortezomib plus Melphalan and prednisone for initial treatment of multiple myeloma. N Engl J Med 2008; 359: 906-917.

[83] Palumbo A, Falco P, Corradini P, *et al.* Melphalan, prednisone, and lenalidomide treatment for newly diagnosed myeloma: a report from the GIMEMA--Italian Multiple Myeloma Network. J Clin Oncol 2007; 25: 4459-4465.

[84] Mehta J, Tricot G, Jagannath S, *et al.* Salvage autologous or allogeneic transplantation for multiple myeloma refractory to or relapsing after a first-line autograft? Bone Marrow Transplant 1998; 21: 887-892.

[85] Elice F, Raimondi R, Tosetto A, *et al.* Prolonged overall survival with second on-demand autologous transplant in multiple myeloma. Am J Hematol 2006; 81: 426-431.

[86] Olin RL, Vogl DT, Porter DL, *et al.* Second auto-SCT is safe and effective salvage therapy for relapsed multiple myeloma. Bone Marrow Transplant 2009; 43: 417-422.

[87] de Lavallade H, El-Cheikh J, Faucher C, *et al.* Reduced-intensity conditioning allogeneic SCT as salvage treatment for relapsed multiple myeloma. Bone Marrow Transplant 2008; 41: 953-960.

[88] Alexanian R, Barlogie B, Dixon D. High-dose glucocorticoid treatment of resistant myeloma. Ann Intern Med 1986; 105: 8-11.

[89] Barlogie B, Hall R, Zander A, Dicke K, Alexanian R. High-dose Melphalan with autologous bone marrow transplantation for multiple myeloma. Blood 1986; 67: 1298-1301.

[90] Hideshima T, Richardson P, Chauhan D, *et al.* The proteasome inhibitor PS-341 inhibits growth, induces apoptosis, and overcomes drug resistance in human multiple myeloma cells. Cancer Res 2001; 61: 3071-3076.

[91] Richardson PG, Barlogie B, Berenson J, *et al.* A phase 2 study of bortezomib in relapsed, refractory myeloma. N Engl J Med 2003; 348: 2609-2617.

[92] Jagannath S, Richardson PG, Sonneveld P, *et al.* Bortezomib appears to overcome the poor prognosis conferred by chromosome 13 deletion in phase 2 and 3 trials. Leukemia 2007; 21: 151-157.

[93] Richardson PG, Sonneveld P, Schuster MW, *et al.* Bortezomib or high-dose dexamethasone for relapsed multiple myeloma. N Engl J Med 2005; 352: 2487-2498.

[94] Richardson PG, Sonneveld P, Schuster M, *et al.* Extended follow-up of a phase 3 trial in relapsed multiple myeloma: final time-to-event results of the APEX trial. Blood 2007; 110: 3557-3560.

[95] Orlowski RZ, Nagler A, Sonneveld P, *et al.* Randomized phase III study of pegylated liposomal doxorubicin plus bortezomib compared with bortezomib alone in relapsed or refractory multiple myeloma: combination therapy improves time to progression. J Clin Oncol 2007; 25: 3892-3901.

[96] Kropff M, Bisping G, Schuck E, *et al.* Bortezomib in combination with intermediate-dose dexamethasone and continuous low-dose oral cyclophosphamide for relapsed multiple myeloma. Br J Haematol 2007; 138: 330-337.

[97] Davies FE, Wu P, Jenner M, *et al.* The combination of cyclophosphamide, velcade and dexamethasone induces high response rates with comparable toxicity to velcade alone and velcade plus dexamethasone. Haematologica 2007; 92: 1149-1150.

[98] Reece DE, Rodriguez GP, Chen C, *et al.* Phase I-II trial of bortezomib plus oral cyclophosphamide and prednisone in relapsed and refractory multiple myeloma. J Clin Oncol 2008; 26: 4777-4783.

[99] Richardson PG, Schlossman RL, Weller E, *et al.* Immunomodulatory drug CC-5013 overcomes drug resistance and is well tolerated in patients with relapsed multiple myeloma. Blood 2002; 100: 3063-3067.

[100] Dimopoulos M, Spencer A, Attal M, *et al.* Lenalidomide plus dexamethasone for relapsed or refractory multiple myeloma. N Engl J Med 2007; 357: 2123-2132.

[101] Baz R, Walker E, Karam MA, *et al.* Lenalidomide and pegylated liposomal doxorubicin-based chemotherapy for relapsed or refractory multiple myeloma: safety and efficacy. Ann Oncol 2006; 17: 1766-1771.

[102] Morgan GJ, Schey SA, Wu P, *et al.* Lenalidomide (Revlimid), in combination with cyclophosphamide and dexamethasone (RCD), is an effective and tolerated regimen for myeloma patients. Br J Haematol 2007; 137: 268-269.

[103] Singhal S, Mehta J, Desikan R, *et al.* Antitumor activity of thalidomide in refractory multiple myeloma. N Engl J Med 1999; 341: 1565-1571.

[104] Barlogie B, Desikan R, Eddlemon P, *et al.* Extended survival in advanced and refractory multiple myeloma after single-agent thalidomide: identification of prognostic factors in a phase 2 study of 169 patients. Blood 2001; 98: 492-494.

[105] Rajkumar SV, Fonseca R, Dispenzieri A, *et al.* Thalidomide in the treatment of relapsed multiple myeloma. Mayo Clin Proc 2000; 75: 897-901.

[106] Alexanian R, Weber D, Anagnostopoulos A, *et al.* Thalidomide with or without dexamethasone for refractory or relapsing multiple myeloma. Semin Hematol 2003; 40: 3-7.

[107] Dimopoulos MA, Zervas K, Kouvatseas G, *et al.* Thalidomide and dexamethasone combination for refractory multiple myeloma. Ann Oncol 2001; 12: 991-995.

[108] Dimopoulos MA, Hamilos G, Zomas A, *et al.* Pulsed cyclophosphamide, thalidomide and dexamethasone: an oral regimen for previously treated patients with multiple myeloma. Hematol J 2004; 5: 112-117.

[109] Moehler TM, Neben K, Benner A, *et al.* Salvage therapy for multiple myeloma with thalidomide and CED chemotherapy. Blood 2001; 98: 3846-3848.

[110] Offidani M, Corvatta L, Piersantelli MN, *et al.* Thalidomide, dexamethasone, and pegylated liposomal doxorubicin (ThaDD) for patients older than 65 years with newly diagnosed multiple myeloma. Blood 2006; 108: 2159-2164.

[111] Knop S, Straka C, Haen M, *et al.* The efficacy and toxicity of bendamustine in recurrent multiple myeloma after high-dose chemotherapy. Haematologica 2005; 90: 1287-1288.

[112] Harousseau JL. Thalidomide in multiple myeloma: past, present and future. Future Oncol 2006; 2: 577-589.

[113] Menon SP, Rajkumar SV, Lacy M, Falco P, Palumbo A. Thromboembolic events with lenalidomide-based therapy for multiple myeloma. Cancer 2008; 112: 1522-1528.

[114] Palumbo A, Rajkumar SV, Dimopoulos MA, *et al.* Prevention of thalidomide- and lenalidomide-associated thrombosis in myeloma. Leukemia 2008; 22: 414-423.

[115] Sagaster V, Ludwig H, Kaufmann H, *et al.* Bortezomib in relapsed multiple myeloma: response rates and duration of response are independent of a chromosome 13q-deletion. Leukemia 2007; 21: 164-168.

[116] Avet-Loiseau H, Soulier J, Fermand JP, *et al.* Impact of high-risk cytogenetics and prior therapy on outcomes in patients with advanced relapsed or refractory multiple myeloma treated with lenalidomide plus dexamethasone. Leukemia 2010; 24: 623-628.

[117] Palumbo A, Sezer O, Kyle R, *et al.* International Myeloma Working Group guidelines for the management of multiple myeloma patients ineligible for standard high-dose chemotherapy with autologous stem cell transplantation. Leukemia 2009; 23: 1716-1730.

[118] Chanan-Khan A, Sonneveld P, Schuster MW, *et al.* Analysis of herpes zoster events among bortezomib-treated patients in the phase III APEX study. J Clin Oncol 2008; 26: 4784-4790.

[119] Berenson JR, Lichtenstein A, Porter L, *et al.* Efficacy of pamidronate in reducing skeletal events in patients with advanced multiple myeloma. Myeloma Aredia Study Group. N Engl J Med 1996; 334: 488-493.

[120] Berenson JR. Recommendations for zoledronic acid treatment of patients with bone metastases. Oncologist 2005; 10: 52-62.

[121] Morgan G, Davies F, Gregory W, *et al.* Evaluating the effects of zoledronic acid (ZOL) on overall survival (OS) in patients (Pts) with multiple myeloma (MM): Results of the Medical Research Council (MRC) Myeloma IX study. J Clin Oncol 2010; 28:15s.

[122] Ruggiero SL, Woo SB. Biophosphonate-related osteonecrosis of the jaws. Dent Clin North Am 2008; 52: 111-128, ix.

[123] Kyle RA, Yee GC, Somerfield MR, *et al.* American Society of Clinical Oncology 2007 clinical practice guideline update on the role of bisphosphonates in multiple myeloma. J Clin Oncol 2007; 25: 2464-2472.

CHAPTER 5

The Role of Stem Cell Transplantation in Multiple Myeloma

Jean-Luc Harousseau*

René Gaudicheau Cancer Center, Nantes /St Herblain, France

Abstract: High-dose therapy plus autologous stem-cell transplantation (ASCT) is currently the standard of care for patients with multiple myeloma up to the age of 65 without severe comorbidities. The introduction of novel agents (thalidomide, bortezomib, lenalidomide) has already dramatically improved the ASCT results. Two or three-drug bortezomib-based induction treatments are superior to the classical VAD. Post-ASCT treatment with thalidomide and probably in the near future with lenalidomide further improves the response rate and the progression-free survival. The use of novel agents both before and after ASCT yields unprecedented complete plus very good partial response rates and progression-free survival. These new strategies partially overcome poor prognosis related to t(4;14) and/or del(17p).

At the same time, novel agents without ASCT have also improved the outcome in patients who are not candidates for ASCT and yield complete plus very partial response rates that are comparable to those achieved with high-dose therapy. Therefore the place of ASCT in the treatment of MM (upfront or after progression) should be addressed in future randomized trials

In this context, the role of allogeneic stem-cell transplantation remains limited since it still induces a high incidence of treatment-related morbidity and mortality despite the use of reduced conditioning regimens.

Keywords: Autologous stem cell transplantation (ASCT), allogeneic stem cell transplantation

1. AUTOLOGOUS STEM CELL TRANSPLANTATION

1.1 Before the Era of Novel therapies

Until now, High-dose therapy (HDT) supported by Autologous Stem-Cell Transplantation (ASCT) has been the standard frontline therapy for patients with newly diagnosed multiple myeloma (MM) up to the age of 65 and without severe comorbidities [1]. This strategy has been based on a number of randomized trials, showing a benefit compared to conventional chemotherapy, at least in terms of response rate and progression-free survival (PFS) [2], and in some trials in terms of overall survival (OS) as well [3,4]

The superiority of HDT/ASCT compared to conventional chemotherapy was mostly due to a better quality of response, with more complete responses (CR) or very good partial responses (VGPR). It has been clearly shown that, in the field of HDT, CR or at least VGPR achievement is significantly associated with a better outcome [5,6]. Overall, with HDT/ASCT the CR plus VGPR rates is 40-50%, the median PFS is 24-36 months and the median OS is 5-6 years [1]. In randomized trials, more intensive treatment with double ASCT improves the PFS compared to single ASCT but OS benefit is controversial [7-9]. Moreover, only patients who are not at least in VGPR after one ASCT appear to benefit from the second [7,6]. Finally, patients with poor-risk cytogenetic abnormalities still do poorly even with double HDT/ASCT [10,11].

1.2 Integrating Novel Agents in the ASCT Paradigm

The introduction of novel agents (thalidomide, bortezomib and more recently lenalidomide) in the frontline therapy of MM patients is changing the scenario. The addition of novel agents before and/or after

***Address coreespondence to Jean-Luc Harousseau:** René Gaudicheau Cancer Center, Bd J Monod, 44805 Nantes /St Herblain, France; Tel: 33 (0) 240 679 987; E-mail: jl-harousseau@nantes.fnclcc.fr

Klaus Podar and Kenneth C. Anderson (Eds)

HDT/ASCT is improving dramatically the CR/VGPR rates and consequently the duration of response and might overcome the negative impact of some poor-prognostic factors. Moreover prolonged treatment with novel agents without HDT/ASCT might yield response rates that are comparable to those achieved with HDT/ASCT and that might translate into prolonged PFS as well

Induction therapy prior to HDT/ASCT

The objectives of induction therapy prior to HDT/ASCT are

- To reduce tumour burden and to increase the post ASCT CR/VGPR rate
- To decrease the plasma cell bone marrow infiltration (*in vivo* purging)

Before the era of novel therapies, the standard induction was dexamethasone-based, either dexamethasone alone or mostly vincristine-adriamycin-dexamethasone (VAD). Although high-dose dexamethasone induced adverse events including infections, these regimens were preferred to Melphalan-prednisone based regimens due to a better quality of stem-cell collection. However, the CR/VGPR rate after 3-4 cycles remained low (<10%CR and <20% CR plus VGPR)

All randomized studies comparing dexamethasone or VAD to induction treatment with thalidomide or bortezomib have shown a superiority of the recent combinations [12-18] and VAD should no longer be considered the standard induction treatment prior to HDT/ASCT.

Double Combinations

All three novel agents have been tested in combination with dexamethasone. Results are shown in Table **1**.

Table 1. Induction therapy with novel agents prior to ASCT. Two-drug combinations (comparative studies). CR: complete remission

	VAD (13-18)	TD (12-13, 20, 21)	VD (15)	RD (19)	Rd (19)
Post-Induction (%)					
CR	2-9	7-14	6	42	24
≥ VGPR	15-17	26-35	39	79	68
≥ PR	54-65	62-76	82		
Post –ASCT (%)					
CR	9-14	33-37	16	NA	NA
≥ VGPR	32-44	44-64	54	NA	NA

VGPR: very good partial remission, PR: partial remission, V: Vincristin, T: Thalidomide, d: low-dose dexamethasone, A: Adriamycin, B: Bortezomib, ASCT: autologous stem cell transplantation, D: Dexamethasone, L : Lenalidomide

With thalidomide-dexamethasone (TD), although the post-induction response rate is superior to dexamethasone alone or to VAD, there is no significant benefit in terms of post induction CR or of post-HDT/ASCT CR plus VGPR rate [12-14]

With bortezomib-dexamethasone (VD), the CR plus VGPR rate is significantly increased compared to VAD, both before and after HDT/ASCT [15].

With lenalidomide-dexamethasone, in only one study the response rate after 4 cycles of induction therapy is available [19] In this study, CR plus VGPR rate is superior with lenalidomide plus high-dose dexamethasone compared to low-dose dexamethasone. Lenalidomide-dexamethasone has not yet been compared to other induction regimens.

Triple Combinations

Thalidomide and bortezomib have been combined with dexamethasone and a third drug:cyclophosphamide [17,20],anthracycline [16,18] or together (VTD) [21-23]. Results achieved with these combinations are in

Table 2. Three-drug combinations appear to be superior to two-drug combinations and yield CR plus VGPR rates of 32-62 % prior to HDT/ASCT and up to 49-76 % after HDT/ASCT. In three randomized studies, the three-drug combination of bortezomib-thalidomide-dexamethasone (VTD) is significantly superior to TD [21,22] and VD [23].

Table 2. Induction Therapy with novel therapies prior to ASCT. Three-drug combinations.

	Thalidomide-Based		**Bortezomib-Based**		**VTD**		
	TAD vs VAD	**TCD vs c-VAD**	**BCD**	**PAD vs VAD**	**VTD vs TD**	**VTD vs TD**	**VTD vs VD**
Author Nb of patients	Lokhorst (16) 402	Morgan (17) 251	Einsele (20) 300	Sonneveld (18) 300	Cavo (21) 460	Rosinol (22) 299	Harousseau (23)
Post-Induction CR or CR/nCR ≥ VGPR ≥ PR	- 32% vs 15% 72% vs 54%	19% vs 9% 29% vs 27% -	10% 84%	- 42% vs 15% 83% vs 59%	- 62% vs 29% 94% vs 79%	- 29% vs 25% 82% vs 75%	14%vs 12% 50%vs 36% 90%vs 81%
Post-ASCT CR ≥ VGPR	16% vs 11% 49% vs 32%	51% vs 40% 67% vs 43%	- -	23% vs 9% 55% vs 50%	43% vs 23% 76% vs 58%	59% vs 48% -	20%vs26% 66%vs 54%

Although no randomized study has compared three-drug combinations, the most effective appears to be the combination containing 2 novel agents (VTD). The addition of a fourth agent does not apparently increase further the efficacy and may increase toxicity [24,25].

Questions Regarding Induction Therapy

Safety of Induction Therapy

The first issue is feasibility of stem-cell collection. In randomized trials comparing TD or VD and VAD, the number of CD34+ cells was superior in the VAD groups, but without significant clinical consequence (proportion of collection failures or time to post-ASCT hematopoietic recovery) [15,26]. With lenalidomide dexamethasone, stem-cell collection is less easy, due to the myelosuppressive effect of lenalidomide [27,28] and should be performed after cyclophosphamide priming [29,30].

Thalidomide and lenalidomide may increase the risk of deep-vein thrombosis when they are used in combination with dexamethasone, and especially for induction treatment since the tumor burden is higher. Therefore some form of prophylaxis is justified, at least aspirin or low-molecular weight heparin in patients at higher-risk.

Thalidomide and bortezomib are associated with peripheral neuropathy. However, with thalidomide, the risk is related to cumulative dose and with short treatment (3-4 months), is limited. With bortezomib, peripheral neuropathy may occur rapidly and in studies on bortezomib-containing induction treatments, the incidence of Grade >1 and Grade >2 peripheral neuropathy was respectively 25-30% and 7-9% [15,18,21]. Reduced doses of bortezomib ($1mg/m^2$ instead of $1.3mg/m^2$) in combination with thalidomide and dexamethasone (vTD) were more active and less neurotoxic than conventional doses of bortezomib plus dexamethasone [23].

Will the better CR rate achieved with novel induction regimens translate into longer PFS?

Since there is a statistical correlation with CR or CR plus VGPR achievement and PFS, one can hope that the better post HDT/ASCT CR/VGPR achieved with novel agents will translate into longer PFS. However, in most randomized trials addressing the question of induction therapy, it will be difficult to answer this question since post HDT/ASCT treatment was not the same in the two induction groups. In the IFM 2005-01, post HDT/ASCT maintenance was comparable in the VAD and VD arms. Median PFS was 36 months in the VD arm versus 30 months in the VAD arm (p=0.057) [31].

An indirect way to address this question is to look at the prognostic impact of achieving CR /VGPR after induction treatment. In the past, it has been very difficult to show that it was better to achieve CR prior to HDT/ASCT than after, mostly because CR was a are event [6] While the IFM failed to show a benefit of achieving CR after VAD induction therapy [5], the Spanish group showed a trend in favour of a better outcome inpatients achieving CR prior to HDT/ASCT [32].

In the IFM 2005-01, patients achieving at least VGPR after induction therapy had a significantly longer PFS than patients having less than VGPR or even than patients achieving PR [31].

Which patients benefit more from induction treatment with novel agents?

In the IFM 2005-01 trial, VD was equally effective and significantly superior to VAD across all prognostic subgroups [15]. Patients with t(4;14) and/or del(17p) had the same response rate than patients without these abnormalities, which is found as well in other studies evaluating induction treatment with bortezomib [20-22].

1.3 High-Dose Therapy Regimen

Until now the standard high-dose therapy regimen is Melphalan IV 200 mg/m^2 which is superior to Melphalan 140mg/m^2 plus total body irradiation [33] and to Melphalan 100mg/m^2 [34]. Attempts to improve results by adding another cytotoxic agent have not been convincing, due to higher toxicity.

Recently the addition of bortezomib to high-dose Melphalan yielded promising results. In a Phase II study from the IFM group, 70% of patients achieved at least VGPR after ASCT and a matched-controlled analysis suggested that this combination was superior to Melphalan 200mg/m^2 [35].

1.4 Post-ASCT Therapy

Maintenance with Thalidomide

Thalidomide has been tested in this setting by several groups. Five randomised studies have been completed and are summarized in Table **3**. [36-40]. Although the study design and the dose and duration of thalidomide treatment were variable, all studies showed a significant benefit in terms of CR (or CR+VGPR) rate and PFS. However, OS was significantly prolonged in only 2/5 studies, due to a shorter OS after relapse in the thalidomide groups. It should be noted that since salvage therapies at relapse are becoming more effective, differences in OS may appear late [41].

Table 3. Maintenance Therapy after ASCT. Randomized studies.

Author	*Attal (36)*	*Barlogie (37)*	*Spencer (38)*	*Lokhorst (39)*	*Morgan (40)*
Nb of patients	597	668	269	556	NA
Induction	No Thal	Thal 50%	No Thal	50% Thal	50% Thal
ASCT	Double	Double	Single	Double	Single
Thal administration	Starting dose 400mg/D until relapse	Starting dose 400mg/D until relapse	200mg/D 1 year	200mg/D until relapse	100mg/D until relapse
Date of randomisation	After ASCT (if no progression)	Initial	After ASCT (if no progression)	Initial	After ASCT
Randomisation	No treatment vs Pamidronate vs Thal + Pamidronate	Thal vs no Thal	Thal-Pred vs Pred	TAD → Thal VAD → IFN	Thal vs no Thal
Median follow-up	40 m	42m	33m	52m	32m

Table 3. cont....

Complete response rate	67% vs 57% or 55%* p=0.03	62% vs 43% p< 0.001	65% vs 44%* p<0.001	66% vs 54% * p=0.005	NA
PFS of EFS	3-yr 52% vs 37% p=0.002	5-yr 56% vs 44% p=0.01	3-yr 42% vs 23% p<0.001	median 3m vs 22m p< 0.001	Better in patients with < VGPR p<0.007
OS	4-yr 87% vs 75% p=0.04	5-yr 65% vs 65% NS	3-yr 26% vs 75% p=0.004	73m vs 60m p=0.77	NS
		updated analysis 8-yr 57% vs 44% p=0.09** (41)			

* CR + VGPR

** Significant in patients with cytogenetic abnormalities

Therefore post-ASCT treatment with thalidomide appears to improve the outcome

However a number of questions still persist

- What is the optimal duration of treatment? Prolonged treatment with thalidomide increases the risk of severe peripheral neuropathy and might select resistant clones and reduce the efficacy of salvage treatment at relapse.
- Does maintenance therapy benefit to all patients and especially to patients with poor-risk cytogenetics? In the Arkansas group study, with long-term follow-up, it appeared that patients with translocations by conventional cytogenetics had a better OS in the thalidomide group [41]. On the other hand, the British group suggest that OS might be shorter in the thalidomide group for patients with del (17p) [42].

Maintenance with other Novel Agents

Lenalidomide appears to be an better drug than thalidomide for long-term maintenance treatment since it is much better tolerated and, particularly, induces very rarely peripheral neuropathy very rarely. Two randomized studies (from the CALGB and from the IFM) have compared lenalidomide to placebo as post HDT/ASCT maintenance therapy. Results are pending.

Bortezomib every 2 weeks has also been evaluated as maintenance after HDT/ASCT and preliminary results show an increase in the CR plus VGPR rate [18].

Consolidation

In two of these studies the better outcome was observed only in patients achieving <VGPR after ASCT [36,40]. This might mean that post-ASCT thalidomide acts more by increasing the depth of response and by increasing the CR/VGPR rate (consolidation effect) than by a long-term control of the malignant clone (maintenance effect).

Recent studies have shown that consolidation with lenalidomide or bortezomib increase the CR or CR plus VGPR rates [43,44]. If consolidation is needed, a combination might be more active than thalidomide alone. The Italian group has shown that post-ASCT consolidation with a combination of bortezomib, thalidomide and dexamethasone (VTD) may upgrade the level of remission and yield molecular remissions [45].

The respective role of consolidation and maintenance in PFS is unknown

1.5 The Role of HDT/ASCT in the Era of Novel Therapies

A number of groups are currently evaluating novel therapies both before and after HDT/ASCT but the only mature results come from the Arkansas group investigators. They have integrated novel agents in their complex approach including tandem ASCT called total therapy programs. In the total therapy 2 program, patients were randomly assigned to receive thalidomide throughout their treatment. Thalidomide appeared to increase the response rate, the PFS and the long-term OS [37,41]. More recently in the total therapy 3 program, the same group has added bortezomib to induction and consolidation. Current results show impressive CR rate of more than 90% and 5-year PFS and OS rates of 71% and 78 % [46,47]. The addition of bortezomib appears to partially overcome the poor prognosis related to t(4;14) and del(17p) [47,48]. These results appear to be the best ever achieved in MM. Whether such a complex and potentially toxic strategy is needed in all patients will be clarified by the recently completed trials

But at the same time, frontline therapy with novel agents is markedly improving the outcome in patients who are not candidates for HDT/ASCT, especially older patients. Several European groups have evaluated the combination of Melphalan-prednisone (MP) with thalidomide, bortezomib or lenalidomide in elderly patients [49-52]. Combinations with lenalidomide plus dexamethasone have been evaluated by US investigators both in young patients who did not wish to undergo HDT/ASCT and in older patients [53,54]. These studies show CR plus VGPR rates (up to 45 % with MP-based regimens, up to 70% with prolonged lenalidomide-dexamethasone) and median PFS (20-28 months) that are quite comparable to those achieved with HDT/ASCT. It is not easy to compare these results with those currently achieved with HDT/ASCT since the populations of patients are not comparable and since in the US studies younger and older patients were mixed.

Moreover, in some studies with novel agents without HDT/ASCT, the median follow-up is still short. Although PFS obtained with HDT/ASCT plus novel agents appear to be longer, randomized studies comparing novel agents plus upfront HDT/ASCT with novel agents plus HDT/ASCT at progression/relapse are mandatory [55]. One important question to be addressed by these ongoing or planned studies will be to determine in which subgroups of patients upfront HDT/ASCT is necessary.

2. ALLOGENEIC STEM-CELL TRANSPLANTATION

Allogeneic stem cell transplantation (SCT) following myeloablative conditioning regimen can induce molecular remissions and before the era of novel therapies was the only therapy with a potential for cure or long-term disease control in at least some patients [56]. However toxicity is excessively high with transplant-related mortality of up to 50% in some studies. Therefore, myeloablative conditioning is abandoned by a large majority of investigators.

Much of the clinical impact of allogeneic SCT has been attributed to the immunologic effect of donor lymphoid cells, the so called graft-versus-myeloma effect (GVM). This antitumor effect of donor cells, which is unfortunately linked to graft-versus-host-disease (GVHD) is the basis of reduced intensity conditioning (RIC) allogeneic SCT. The principle of RIC allogeneic SCT is to reduce transplant-related toxicity while harnessing GVM effect. Preliminary experience showed that RIC allogeneic SCT is feasible in MM even in older patients, older than 60 years of age and with matched-unrelated donors [57]. However, in patients with a high tumor burden, the allogeneic GVM is not sufficient and relapses are more frequent than with standard myeloablative regimens [58]. Therefore currently RIC allogeneic SCT is mostly performed after HDT/ASCT. The Seattle group recently updated their results with this approach [59] and reported 5-year PFS and OS of respectively 36% and 64%. However toxicity remained high with 11% transplant-related mortality, 42% grades 2-4 acute GVHD and 72% chronic GVHD. Three studies have prospectively compared tandem ASCT-RIC allotransplantation with double ASCT. [60-62]. The Italian is the only one to show a significant benefit in favour of RIC allogeneic SCT. Even in this study, the PFS is only x % at years, due to both toxic deaths and relapses [63]. Considering the results currently achieved novel agents with or without ASCT, this strategy should not be proposed in the upfront setting out of a clinical trial in selected patients with poor-risk features. The most attractive clinical research area is the evaluation of novel agents after RIC allogeneic SCT with the objective of upgrading the level of remission [64].

REFERENCES

[1] Harousseau J-L, Moreau P Autologous stem-cell transplantation in multiple myeloma. N Engl J Med 2009; 360: 2645-2654.

[2] Koreth J, Cutler CS, Djulbegovic B, *et al.* High-dose therapy with single autologous transplantation versus chemotherapy for newly diagnosed multiple myeloma. A systematic review and meta-analysis of randomized controlled trials. Biol Blood Marrow Transplant 2007; 13: 183-196.
[3] Attal M, Harousseau JL, Stoppa AM, *et al.* A prospective randomized trial of autologous bone marrow transplantation and chemotherapy in multiple myeloma. N Engl J Med 1996; 335: 91-97.
[4] Child JA, Morgan GJ, Davies FE, *et al.* High-dose chemotherapy with hematopoietic stem-cell rescue for multiple myeloma. N Engl J Med 2003; 348: 1875-1883.
[5] Harousseau JL, Avet-Loiseau, Attal M, *et al.* Achieving at least very good partial remission is a simple and robust prognostic factor in patients with multiple myeloma treated with high-dose therapy. Long-term results of the IFM 99-02 and 99-94 trials J Clin Oncol 2009; 27: 5720-5726.
[6] Harousseau J-L, Attal M, Avet-Loiseau H The role of complete remission in multiple myeloma. Blood 2009; 114: 3139-3146.
[7] Attal M, Harousseau J-L, Facon T, *et al.* Single versus double autologous stem cell transplantation for multiple myeloma. N Engl J Med 2003; 349: 2495-2.
[8] Cavo M, Tosi P, Zamagni E, *et al.* Prospective randomized study of single compared with double autologous stem cell transplantation for multiple myeloma: Bologna 96 clinical study. J Clin Oncol 2007; 25: 2434-2441.
[9] Sonneveld P, van der Holt B, Segeren CM, *et al.* Intermediate-dose Melphalan compared with myeloablative treatment in multiple: long-term results of the Dutch Cooperative Group Hovon 24 trial. Haematologica 2007; 92: 298-935.
[10] Avet-Loiseau H, Attal M, Moreau P, *et al.* Genetic abnormalities and survival in multiple myeloma: the experience of the Intergroupe Francophone du Myélome. Blood 2007; 109: 3489-3495.
[11] Barlogie B, Shaughnessy J, Tricot G, *et al.* Treatment of multiple myeloma Blood 2004; 103: 20-32.
[12] Rajkumar SV, Blood E, Vesole D, *et al.* Phase III clinical trial of Thalidomide plus Dexamethasone compared with Dexamethasone alone in newly diagnosed multiple myeloma: a clinical trial coordinated by the Eastern Cooperative Oncology Group. J Clin Oncol 2006; 24: 431-436.
[13] Cavo M, Zamagni E, Tosi P, *et al.* Superiority of Thalidomide and Dexamethsone over Vincristine-Doxorubicine-Dexamethasone (VAD) as primary therapy in preparation for autologous transplantation for multiple myeloma. Blood 2005; 106: 35-39.
[14] Macro M, Divine M, Uzunban Y, *et al.* Dexamethasone plus thalidomide compared to VAD as pre-transplant treatment in newly diagnosed multiple myeloma: a randomized trial. Blood 2006; 108: 22a (abstract).
[15] Harousseau J-L, Mathiot C, Attal M, *et al.* Bortezomib/Dexamethasone versus VAD as induction prior to autologous stem-cell transplantation in previously untreated multiple myeloma. Updated results from IFM 2005/01 trial. J Clin Oncol 2008; 26: 455s (abstract).
[16] Lokhorst HM, Schmidt- Wolf I, Sonneveld P, *et al.* Thalidomide in induction treatment increases the very good partial remission rate before and after high-dose therapy in previously untreated multiple myeloma. Haematologica 2008; 93: 124-127
[17] Morgan GJ, Davies FE, Owen RG, *et al.* Thalidomide combinations improve response rates: results from the MRC IX study. Blood 2007; 110: 1051a (abstract).
[18] Sonneveld P, van der Holt B, Schmidt-Wolf I, *et al.* First analysis of Hovon 65/GMMG-HD4 randomized Phase III trial comparing bortezomib, adriamycine, dexamethasone (PAD) vs VAD as induction prior to high dose Melphalan in patients with newly diagnosed multiple myeloma. Blood 2008; 112: 243-244 (abstract).
[19] Rajkumar SV, Jacobus S, Callander NS, *et al.* Lenalidomide plus high-dose dexamethasone versus lenalidomide plus low-dose dexamethasone as initial therapy for newly diagnosed multiple myeloma:an open-label randomized controlled trial. Lancet Oncol 2010 Jan 11(1): 29-37.
[20] Einsele H, Liebisch P, Langer C, *et al.* Velcade, intravenous cyclophosphamide and dexamethasone induction for przviously untreated multiple myeloma (German DSMM Xia trial) Blood 2009; 114: 59-60 Abstract.
[21] Cavo M, Tacchetti P, Patriarca F, *et al.* Superior complete response rate and progression-free survival after autologous transplantation with upfront Velcade-Thalidomide- Dexamethasone compared with Thalidomide-Dexamethasone in newly diagnosed multiple myeloma. Blood 2008; 112: 65 Abstract.
[22] Rosinol L, Cibeira T, Martinez J, *et al.* Thalidomide/Dexamethasone (TD) versus Bortezomib (Velcade)/ Thalidomide/ Dexamethasone (VTD) versus VBMCP/VBAD Velcade as induction regimen prior to autologous stem-cell transplantation in multiple myeloma. Results of a Phase III Pethema/ Gemm trial. Blood 2009; 114: 58-59, Abstract 129.

[23] Harousseau J-L, Avet-Loiseau H, Facon T, *et al.* Bortezomib plus dexamethasone versus reduced-dose of bortezomib plus thalidomide plus dexamethasone as induction treatment prior to autologous stem-cell transplantation in newly diagnosed patients with multiple myeloma Blood 2009; 114: 150 Abstract 354.

[24] Ludwig H, Viterbo L, Greil R, *et al.* Bortezomib, thalidomide and dexamethasone (VTD) versus VTD plus cyclophosphamide as induction therapy in previously untreated multiple myeloma patients eligible for HDY-ASCT: a randomized Phase 2 trial. Blood 2009; 114 Abstract 2312.

[25] Kumar S, Fin IW, Hari PN, *et al.* Novel three and four combinations of bortezomib, dexamethasone, cyclophosphamide and lenalidomide for newly diagnosed multiple myeloma: encouraging results from multicenter, randomized, Phase 2 Evolution trial. Blood 2009; 114: Abs 127.

[26] Breitkreutz I, Lokhorst HW, Raab MS, *et al.* Thalidomide in newly diagnosed multiple myeloma: influence of thalidomide treatment on peripheral blood stem cell collection yield. Leukemia 2007; 21: 1294-1299.

[27] Mazumder A, Kaufman J, Niesvizky R, Lonial S, Vesole D, Jagannath S. Effect of lenalidomide therapy on mobilization of peripheral blood stem cells in previously untreated multiple myeloma patients. Leukemia 2008; 22(6): 1280-1.

[28] Paripati H, Stewart AK, Cabou S, *et al.* Compromised stem cell mobilization following induction therapy with lenalidomide in myeloma. Leukemia 2008; 22(6): 1282-4

[29] Mark T, Stern J, Furst JR, *et al.* Stem cell mobilization with cyclophosphamide overcomes the suppressive effect of lenalidomide therapy on stem cell collection in multiple myeloma. Biol Blood Marrow Transplant 2008; 14: 795-798.

[30] Giralt S, Stadtmauer EA, Harousseau J-L, *et al.* International Working group –IMWG) consensus statement and guidelines regarding the current status of stem cell collection and high-dose therapy in multiple myeloma and the role of plerixafor. Leukemia 2009; 23: 1904-1912.

[31] Harousseau J-L, Avet-Loiseau H, Attal M, *et al.* High complete and very good partial remission response rates with bortezomib- dexamethasone as induction prior to ASCT in newly diagnosed patients with high-risk myeloma: results of the IFM 2005-01 Phase 3 trial. Blood 2009; 114; 149-150 Abstract 353.

[32] Lahuerta JJ, Mateos MV, Rosinol L, *et al.* Influence of pre- and post-transplantation outcomes of patients with multiple myeloma: sequential improvement of response and achievement of complete response are associated with longer survival. J Clin Oncol 2008; 26: 5775-5782.

[33] Moreau P, Facon T, Attal M, *et al.* Comparison of 200mg/m2 Melphalan and 8 Gy total body irradiation plus 140mg/m2 Melphalan as conditioning regimen for perripheral blood stem cell transplantation in patients with newly diagnosed multiple myeloma; final analysis of the Intergroupe Francophone du Myelome 95002 randomized trial. Blood 2002; 99:73-735

[34] Palumbo A, Brighen S, Bruno B, *et al.* Melphalan 200mg/m2 versus Melphalan 100mg/m2 in newly diagnosed myeloma patients: a prospective, multicenter phase II study. Blood 2010; 115(10): 1873-9

[35] Roussel M, Moreau P, Huinh A, *et al.* Bortezomib and high-dose Melphalan as conditioning regimen before autologous stem-cell transplantation in patients with de novo multiple myeloma: a phase 2 study of the Intergroupe Francophone du Myelome (IFM) Blood 2010; 115: 32-37

[36] Attal M, Harousseau JL, Leyvraz S, *et al.* Maintenance therapy with thalidomide improves survival in multiple myeloma patients. Blood 2006; 15: 3289-3294

[37] Barlogie B,Tricot G, Anaissie E, *et al.* Thalidomide and hematopoietic stem cell transplantation for multiple myeloma.N Engl J Med 2006; 354 :1021-1030

[38] Spencer A, Prince HM, Roberts A, *et al.* Consolidation therapy with thalidomide and prednisolone prolongs the survival of multiple myeloma patients undergoing a single ASCT procedure. J Clin Oncol 2009; 27: 1788-1793.

[39] Lokhorst H, van der Holt B, Zweegman S, *et al.* A randomized phase III study on the effect of thalidomide combined with adriamycin, dexamethasone (TAD) and high-dose Melphalan followed by thalidomide maintenance in patients with multiple myeloma. Blood 2010; 115(6): 1113-20

[40] Morgan GJ, Jackson GH, Davies FE, *et al.* Maintenance thalidomide may improve progression free but not overall survival: results from the Myeloma IX maintenance randomization [abstract]. Blood 2008; 112: Abstract 656.

[41] Barlogie B, Pineda-Roman M, van Rhee F, *et al.* Thalidomide arm of Total Therapy 2 improves complete remission duration and survival in myeloma patients with interphase cytogenetic abnormalities. Blood 2008; 112: 2999-3000.

[42] Morgan GJ, Davies FR, Gregory WM, *et al.* The addition of thalidomide to the induction treatment of newly presenting myeloma patients increases the CR rate which is likely to translate into improved PFS and OS. Blood 2009; 114: Abs 352.

[43] Mellqvist UH, Westin J, Gimsing P, *et al.* Improved response rate with consolidation after high-dose Melphalan: first results of a Nordic Myeloma Study Group randomized Phase III TRIAL 536 Blood 2009; 114: Abstract.

[44] Attal M, Harousseau J-L Marit G, *et al.* Lenalidomide after autologous transplantation for myeloma. First analysis of a prospective randomized study of the Intergroupe Francophone du Myelome (IFM 2005602) Blood 2009,114: Abstract 529.

[45] Ladetto M, Pagliano G, Ferrero, *et al.* Major shrinking of residual tumor cell burden and achievement of molecular remissions in myeloma patients undergoing post-transplant consolidation with bortezomib, thalidomide and dexamethasone: a qualitative and quantitative PCR study. Blood 2008; 112: Abstract 3683.

[46] Barlogie B, Attal M, Crowley J, *et al.* Long- term follow-up of autologous transplantation trials for multiple myeloma: update of protocols conducted by the Intergroupe Francophone du Myelome, Southwest Oncology Group and University of Arkansas Medical Sciences. J Clin Oncol 2010; 28(7): 1209-14

[47] Pineda Roman M, Zangari M, Haessler J, *et al.* Sustained complete remissions in multiple myeloma linked to bortezomib in total therapy 3:comparison with total therapy 2 Br J Haematol 2008; 140: 625-634

[48] Shaughnessy JD, Zhou Y, Haessler J, *et al.* TP53 deletion is not an adverse feature in multiple myeloma treated with total therapy 3. Br J Haematol 2009; 147: 347-351

[49] Facon T, Mary JY, Hulin C, *et al.* Intergroupe Francophone du Myélome. Melphalan and prednisone plus thalidomide versus Melphalan and prednisone alone or reduced-intensity autologous stem cell transplantation in elderly patients with multiple myeloma (IFM 99-06): a randomised trial. Lancet. 2007; 307: 1209-121837

[50] Palumbo A, Bringhen S, Liberati A, *et al.* Oral Melphalan, prednisone, and thalidomide in elderly patients with multiple myeloma:updated results of a randomized, controlled trial Blood 2008; 112: 3107-3114

[51] San Miguel JF, Schlag R, Khuageva NK, *et al.* Bortezomib plus Melphalan and prednisone for initial treatment of multiple myeloma. N Engl J Med 2008; 35: 906-17.

[52] Palumbo A, Falco P, Corradini P, *et al.* Melphalan, Prednisone, Lenalidomide treatment for newly diagnosed myeloma:a report from the GIMEMA-Italian Multiple Myeloma Network. J Clin Oncol 2007; 25:4459-4465

[53] Niesvizky R, Jayabalan DS, Christos PJ, *et al.* BiRD (Biaxin/ Revlimid/ Dexamethasone) combination therapy results in high complete and overall response rates in treatment-naïve symptomatic multiple myeloma. Blood 2008; 111: 1101-1109.

[54] Richardson PG, Lonial S, Jakubowiak AT, *et al.* High response rate and encouraging time to event data with lenalidomide, bortezomib and dexamethasone in newly diagnosed multiple myeloma. Final results of a phase 1/2 study. Blood 2009: 114: 501-502, Abstract 1218.

[55] San Miguel J, Harousseau J-L, Joshua D, Anderson KC Individualizing treatment of patients with myeloma in the era of novel therapies J Clin Oncol 2008; 26: 2761-2766.

[56] Harousseau J-L. The allogeneic dilemma. Bone Marrow Transplant 2007; 40: 1123-1128

[57] Crawley C, Lalancette M, Szydlo R, *et al.* Outcomes of reduced-intensity allogeneic transplantation for multiple myeloma: an analysis of prognostic factors from the Chronic Leukemia Working Party of the EBMT. Blood 2005; 105: 4532-4539.

[58] Crawley C, Iacobelli S, Björkstrand B, *et al.* Reduced-intensity conditioning for myeloma: lower nonrelapse mortality but higher relapse rates compared with myeloablative conditioning. Blood 2007; 109: 3588-3594

[59] Rotta M, Storer BE, Sahebi F, *et al.* Long-term outcome of patients with multiple myeloma after autologous hematopietic cell transplantation and nonmyeloablative allografting. Blood 2009; 113: 3383-3391.

[60] Bruno B, Rotta M, Patriarca F, *et al.* A comparison of allografting with autografting for newly diagnosed myeloma. N Engl J Med 2007; 356: 1110-1120.

[61] Moreau P, Garban F, Attal M, *et al.* Long-term follow-up results of IFM 99-03 and IFM 99-04 trials comparing nonmyeloablative allotransplantation with autologous transplantation in high-risk de novo multiple myeloma. Blood 2008; 112: 3914-3915.

[62] Rosinol L, Perez-Simon JA, Sureda A, *et al.* A prospective Pethema study of tandem autologous transplantation versus autograft followed by reduced-intensity conditioning allogeneic transplantation in multiple myeloma. Blood 2008; 112: 3591-3592.

[63] Bruno B, Rotta M, Patriarca F, *et al.* Nonmyeloablative allografting for newly diagnosed multiple myeloma: the experience of the Gruppo Italiano Trapianti di Midolla. Blood 2009; 113: 3375-3382.

[64] Kroger N, Zabelina T, Ayuk T, *et al.* Bortezomib after dose-reduced allogeneic stem cell transplantation for multipe myeloma to enhance or maintain remission status; Exp Hematol 2006; 34: 770-775.

CHAPTER 6

Pathogenesis and Treatment of Bone Disease in Multiple Myeloma

Sonia Vallet and Noopur Raje*

Division of Hematology-Oncology, Massachusetts General Hospital Cancer Center, Harvard Medical School, Massachusetts General Hospital, Boston, MA

Abstract: More than 80% of multiple myeloma (MM) patients present with bone involvement frequently develop serious complications that negatively affect both quality of life and overall survival. Bone disease in MM is a consequence of unbalanced remodeling resulting in the development of osteolytic lesions. Generalized osteoclast (OC) activation is the underlying mechanism coupled with osteoblast (OB) inhibition. The molecular events leading to this imbalance of the OC/OB axis is a result of the interaction of MM cells with bone cells within the bone marrow milieu and consequent cytokine deregulation. Here we will discuss the pathogenesis, clinical sequelae and therapeutic strategies for the treatment of MM bone disease. We will focus on novel therapeutic strategies under investigation to restore bone homeostasis. Such approaches are being studied not only with the goal of alleviating morbidity from bone disease but also for their resultant anti-MM activity.

Keywords: Osteoclasts (OCs), osteoblasts (OBs), receptor activator of NF-κB ligand (RANKL), osteoprotegerin (OPG), OC activating factors (OAFs), dickkopf (DKK) 1, bisphosphonates, denosumab, osteonecrosis of the jaw (ONJ), activin A, B-cell activating factor (BAFF)

1. INTRODUCTION

Multiple myeloma (MM) is a hematological malignancy of clonogenic plasma cells proliferating in the bone marrow (BM) milieu, where they interfere with the delicate balance of bone homeostasis. The resulting excessive bone resorption not balanced by new bone formation translates clinically in the development of osteolytic lesions.

Bone disease develops in more than 80% of MM patients and is complicated by severe pain in 75%, vertebral body compression fractures in 54% and pathologic fractures in 40-50% of MM patients. This impacts patients'quality of life and also affects overall survival. Pathologic fractures due to bone disease increase the risk of death by more than 20% compared to patients without fractures [1,2].

Common treatment strategies to overcome bone pain and neurological sequelae by vertebral compression include local radiation, surgical fixation and medical treatment including treatment of the underlying disease and bisphosphonates use. Ongoing studies are aimed at unraveling the pathogenesis of bone lesions in MM with the goal of developing treatment strategies that reverse the osteolytic process and restore physiologic bone remodeling. Based on recent findings on tumor and bone cell interactions, novel targeted therapies are currently under clinical investigation.

2. PATHOGENESIS OF MYELOMA BONE DISEASE

The BM niche is a highly regulated environment, consisting of a network of bone, immune, endothelial and hematopoietic cells, modulated by cytokines and extracellular matrix. MM cells home to the BM and disrupt this balance to create a permissive environment for their proliferation and survival. As a result, extensive bone damage occurs resulting in the classical osteolytic lesions. Insight into the signaling pathways involved in tumor-bone interactions is critical to the identification of novel therapeutically relevant targets and the development of effective treatment strategies.

***Address correspondence to Noopur Raje:** POB 216, MGH Cancer Center, Massachusetts General Hospital, 55 Fruit Street, Boston, MA 02114; Tel: 617 726 0711 ; Fax: 617 724 6801; E-mail: nraje@partners.org,

Klaus Podar and Kenneth C. Anderson (Eds)

Bone Homeostasis

Bone is an extremely active organ undergoing extensive remodeling, that relies on balanced activity of bone-resorption by osteoclasts (OCs) and bone-formation by osteoblasts (OBs) [3].

OCs are terminally-differentiated cells of the monocytic-macrophagic lineage, that resorb bone and regulate OB number. They differentiate *via* three main steps: 1) proliferation of progenitor cells, 2) formation of multinucleated precursors and 3) functional activation of mature cells. This process is regulated by cytokines, such as monocyte-colony stimulating factor (M-CSF), receptor activator of NF-κB ligand (RANKL) and chemokines, as well as interactions with OBs and T lymphocytes.

OBs differentiate from mesenchymal cells, into active bone-forming cells, quiescent bone-lining cells and bone-embedded osteocytes. They regulate bone formation *via* matrix deposition and mineralization. They also regulate bone homeostasis by modulating OC function. OB differentiation and function is under the influence of systemic and local regulation. Parathyroid hormone (PTH) stimulates OB differentiation and inhibits apoptosis, whereas locally secreted inhibitory factors, such as osteocyte-derived sclerostin and dickkopf (DKK)1 regulate OB activity by interfering with Wnt and (bone morphogenetic proteins) BMP signaling pathways [4].

In the bone remodeling process, OC and OB activities are coupled *via* secreted cytokines, mainly RANKL and osteoprotegerin (OPG), and cell-to-cell signaling, depending on bidirectional Ephrin/Eph signaling. OCs express the membrane-bound ligand ephrinB2 that activates its receptor EphB4 on OBs surface to promote osteoblastogenesis. In turn, the reverse signaling *via* ephrinB2 inhibits OC differentiation [5], thus regulating bone remodeling.

Molecular Basis of MM Bone Disease

Homing and migration of MM cells to the BM is mediated by several signals, including chemokine (C-C motif) ligand (CCL)12/ stromal-derived factor 1 (SDF1) and CXCR4, CCL3 and CCR1, vascular endothelial growth factor (VEGF) and its receptors[6-8]. In the bone milieu, tumor cells modify cell composition and function to create a cancer niche permissive to their propagation (Fig. **1**). MM cells stimulate osteoclastogenesis directly and indirectly *via* BM stromal cell (BMSC)-mediated release of OC activating factors (OAFs). BMSC and OCs in turn support tumor proliferation and mediate chemoresistance [9]. Conversely, OBs have an overall inhibitory effect on the proliferation of MM cells [10], that in turn inhibit their differentiation [11]. Indeed, BM biopsies from MM patients show a correlation among tumor burden, OC number and resorption surface [12,13] implying a generalized OC activation. In addition, decrease in trabecular thickness and low calcification rates suggest that OBs activity is also impaired [14]. Therefore, the pathogenesis of bone disease in MM relies on a deregulated OC/OB axis.

OC-MM interactions. Several OAFs are secreted in the MM niche, by tumor cells and BMSC (Fig. **1**). In particular, the RANKL/OPG balance regulating OC differentiation is disrupted in MM. The BM levels of RANKL are notably increased in MM patients, in comparison to normal control and monoclonal gammopathy of undetermined significance (MGUS) [15]. Moreover, the expression of its inhibitor, the soluble decoy receptor OPG, is downregulated and low serum levels of OPG correlated with advanced osteolytic bone disease in MM [16]. Malignant plasma cells up-regulate RANKL expression and strongly down-regulate OPG production in OB, BMSCs and T lymphocytes [17-19]. In particular, the signaling pathways activated by MM to BMSC interactions include p38 and nuclear factor-kappa B (NF-κB), both regulated by the sequestrosome p62. p62 represents a novel promising target in MM-bone disease, since its inhibition in BMSC represses OC differentiation and MM cell proliferation [20]. Moreover, OPG is degraded by MM cells *via* CD138 contributing to a further decrease in its serum levels [21]. Studies in *in-vivo* models of MM bone disease demonstrated that OPG and OPG-like molecules prevent bone destruction and tumor growth [15,22]. In patients, anti-MM strategies such as thalidomide and autologous bone marrow transplantation normalize the RANKL/OPG ratio and inhibit bone resorption [23,24]. Targeted therapies against the RANKL/OPG axis are currently under clinical investigation.

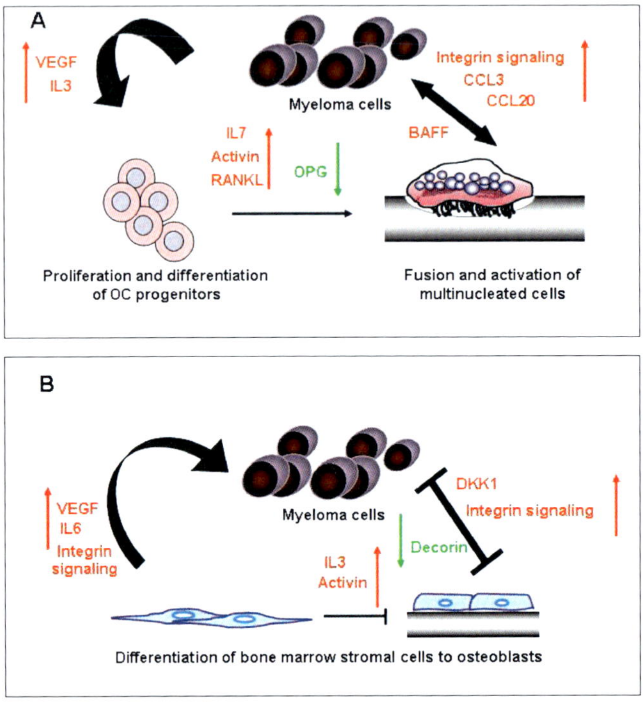

Fig. (1). Pathogenesis of bone disease. The interactions of multiple myeloma (MM) cells with bone cells within the bone marrow microenvironment lead to unbalance of the osteoclast (OC)/osteoblast (OB) axis and alter the bone remodeling process. (A) OC differentiation and function is enhanced in the MM niche due to a deregulated cytokine network, mainly RANKL/OPG unbalance and chemokines upregulation. In turn, OC stimulate tumor cell proliferation and confer resistance to chemotherapies. (B) MM cells impair OB differentiation by cell-to-cell contact and release of cytokines, in particular DKK1 and activin. As a result the inhibitory signal of OB on MM cell proliferation is removed.

MM cells are also a source for CCL3, a chemokine important to OC differentiation, mediating precursor cell migration and fusion [25]. CCL3 levels correlate with osteolytic burden and MM patients'survival [26]. *In vitro* studies demonstrate that blocking CCL3 activity impairs osteoclastogenesis and OC-induced MM cell proliferation. *In-vivo*, CCL3 inhibition prevents bone damage and delays tumor growth [27,28], therefore the CCL3 pathway represents a promising target in MM bone disease [29].

Other than RANKL and CCL3, several cytokines are upregulated in BM serum of MM patients and promote OC activation either directly or indirectly *via* RANKL expression, including interleukin (IL)-1,-6,-3,-7, CCL20 and activin. Tumor cells and T-lymphocyte-derived IL-3 synergizes with RANKL to induce OC differentiation [30,31]. MM-derived IL-7 promotes OC differentiation by inducing RANKL secretion from T lymphocytes [17]. MM cells also stimulate OBs and BMSCs to release CCL20, that directly promotes osteoclastogenesis [32], and activin, a transforming growth factor (TGF)β family member that activates OCs while inhibiting OB differentiation [33]. Importantly, impaired OB differentiation removes an inhibitory stimulus to OC, further promoting their function.

A consequence of OC up-regulation other than increased bone resorption is enhanced MM cell growth. Both OC and BMSC promote tumor cell survival and proliferation *via* direct contact and cytokine secretion. Cell adhesion mediated by integrin signaling, such as very late antigen (VLA)-4/ vascular cell adhesion molecule (VCAM)-1 and lymphocyte function-associated antigen (LFA)-1/ intercellular adhesion molecule (ICAM)-1, activates drug resistance mechanisms (CAM-DR) [34]. Important pro-survival cytokines include IL-6, B-cell activating factor (BAFF), CCL3 and VEGF [6,7,35,36].

OB-MM interactions. The molecular mechanism responsible for OB impairment in MM has been recently investigated and two relevant OB inhibitors identified, DKK1 and activin. (Fig. **1**). DKK1 is a MM-derived Wnt signaling antagonist, upregulated in BM plasma of MM patients with osteolytic lesions [37]. The signaling pathway activated by DKK1 in MM has yet to be clarified. Although DKK1 downregulates RUNX2 activity, a direct effect on β-catenin has always been elusive and β-catenin expression in BM biopsies of MM patients did not correlate with osteolytic lesions and DKK1 levels [38]. Studies relating DKK1 to the non-canonical Wnt signaling pathway are ongoing.

Activin A is upregulated in MM patients with high osteolytic burden and its main sources have been identified in BMSC and OCs. MM cells do not produce activin but up-regulate its secretion by BMSC. Activin-mediated OB inhibition depends on SMAD2 upregulation and subsequent DLX5 inhibition, a critical OB transcription factor. The *in-vivo* relevance of this pathway is demonstrated by the correlation between DLX5 downregulation in BM biopsies of MM patients with bone disease and high BM plasma activin A levels [33]. Other OB inhibitors are soluble frizzle-related protein (sFRP) 2, sFRP3, IL3 and IL7, but their role has yet to be fully clarified.

In addition to secreted factors, MM cells'inhibitory effects on osteogenesis are mediated by VLA4/VCAM-1 interactions, leading to downregulation of RUNX2 activity in OBs progenitor cells [39].

In contrast to OCs and BMSC, OBs negatively affect MM cell survival, as shown *in-vivo* by tumor growth inhibition resulting from up-regulation of the β-catenin signaling pathway [40]. Although the mechanism of MM inhibition has still to be clarified, small leucine-rich proteoglycans are probably involved. Decorin, in particular, is an OB-derived extracellular matrix component that induces MM cell apoptosis *via* p21 activation and inhibits angiogenesis and osteoclastogenesis [41].

In summary, MM cells interfere with different steps of both osteoclastogenesis and OB differentiation disrupting the physiologic balance of OC and OB activity. This results in not only the development of bone disease, but also promotes MM cell growth.

3. TREATMENT OF MULTIPLE MYELOMA BONE DISEASE

Recent advances in MM treatment have resulted in improved patient overall survival, and targeting bone disease has taken on a new relevance as the focus is now largely on quality of life. Indeed, current therapies, including medical treatment, mainly bisphosphonates (BPs), radiotherapy and surgery, aim at preventing skeletal complications as well as the development of new bone lesions. Although these strategies effectively inhibit bone resorption and decrease the incidence of morbidity from skeletal disease, none of them restore normal bone architecture. With our improved understanding of the BM niche and the identification of novel targets, several studies suggest that manipulating this BM niche may result in balanced bone homeostasis and consequent tumor growth inhibition (Fig. **2**). Therefore the identification of novel agents to overcome bone disease and, eventually, treat MM is an important clinical challenge.

Bisphosphonates. BPs are the standard of care in the treatment of cancer-related bone disease. They exert an anti-catabolic effect by interfering with the OC-bone interface, and forcing OCs to a pre-apoptotic, non-functional state [42]. Nitrogen-containing BPs, such as pamidronate and zoledronic acid have been widely used in the clinical setting for their greater anti-resorbtive activity. Compared to placebo, BP treatment significantly decreases skeletal-related events (SREs), namely fracture, radiation to bone, surgery to bone, or spinal cord compression [43]. When pamidronate was compared directly to zoledronic acid, they were noted to be equally efficacious forming the basis for guidelines proposed by the American Society of Clinical Oncolgy (ASCO) for the use of either agent for the treatment of MM related bone disaeese. Despite *in vitro* data suggesting anti-tumor effects by BPs [44]; no clinical trial to date has demonstrated a survival benefit in the MM setting [45]. Serious adverse events associated with BPs include renal impairment and osteonecrosis of the jaw (ONJ) [46]. ONJ is defined as an area of exposed bone in the maxillofacial region that did not heal within 8 weeks after its diagnosis [47]. The identification of ONJ has led to revised ASCO guidelines suggesting reassessing the value of continued BP use beyond 2 years in MM. The profound effects of long-term BPs exposure on bone remodeling, that is a long-lasting inhibition of bone resorption associated with a reversible decrease in bone formation [42,48], may in part contribute to ONJ development by changing the mechanical properties of bone [49,50]. Based on these data several clinical trials have been designed to optimize BPs administration using bone marker-directed (like urine N-telopeptide of type 1 collagen, NTX) schedules. In addition, up to 20 to 30% of patients do not respond to BPs, underscoring the need for novel alternative treatment approaches [51].

Denosumab. The RANKL/OPG axis regulates OC differentiation and function and plays a key role in the pathogenesis of MM-bone disease. Several studies show that OPG-like molecules and neutralizing antibodies against RANKL are effective inhibitors of osteolysis in murine models of MM-bone disease [52]. In clinical trials, subcutaneous administrations of RANKL neutralizing antibody, Denosumab (AMG165, Amgen Pharmaceutical), induces a sustained long-lasting inhibition of bone resorption markers with minimal toxicity, mainly asthenia and peripheral edema [53]. In a large phase III study involving MM patients, denosumab demonstrated non-inferiority to ZA in delaying time to first SRE (Amgen, Thousand Oaks, CA), and the side effect profile was comparable. Importantly, no difference in ONJ incidence was noted lending credence to the theory that this is indeed a consequence of altered bone remodeling as a result of anti-resorptive strategies. Importantly, denosumab prevents SREs even in BPs-refractory patients [54], indicating that RANKL inhibition may be a valid alternative to BPs. With respect to effects on tumor burden, a recent study reported that single agent denosumab did not induce any complete or partial responses, but 20% of relapsed patients and 46% of plateau-phase patients maintained stable disease status. These results set the stage for future combination strategies with anti-MM therapies [55].

DKK1 antagonists. DKK1, a negative regulator of OB differentiation is overexpressed in MM patients [37] and strategies to block DKK1 activity have been investigated. Neutralizing antibodies against DKK1 promote OB differentiation *in vitro* and reverse the negative effect of MM cells on OB formation [56]. *In-vivo* studies using both murine and humanized models of MM-bone disease demonstrated bone-anabolic properties of DKK1 inhibition, with increased bone formation, increased OB number and improvement of osteolytic lesions [57,58]. Importantly, blocking DKK1 resulted in reduced tumor growth, mainly as an indirect effect *via* modification of the tumor microenvironment [56]. Clinical trials combining DKK1 neutralizing antibody and BPs are ongoing to confirm these promising preclinical data.

ACE-011. Activin A is a bone-targeting cytokine with dual activity; stimulation of OC differentiation and inhibition of OB formation. MM patients with advanced bone disease have high levels of activin A suggesting it may play a pathogenetic role in MM-bone disease. Inhibition of activin A with a chimeric antibody, RAP-011 (Acceleron Pharma, Cambridge, MA) stimulated OB differentiation and inhibited OC development *in vitro* [59]. In animal models of osteoporosis and MM-bone disease, RAP-011 treatment improved bone density, prevented osteolytic bone disease and reduced tumor growth [33]. ACE-011, its clinical grade counterpart, downregulated bone resorption and upregulated bone formation markers in post-menopausal women. Ongoing clinical trials are evaluating its role in the MM setting.

BAFF inhibition. OC-MM interactions are characterized by bi-directional signaling that enhances each others'growth and survival. An important mediator of this interplay is the tumor necrosis factor (TNF) family member, B-cell activating factor (BAFF). BAFF is an OC and BMSC derived MM growth factor that stimulates MM cell survival and MM-BMSC adhesion [35,60]. *In-vivo* studies using a neutralizing antibody against BAFF (Ely Lilly, Indianapolis) significantly reduced tumor burden and inhibited OC differentiation as well as development of lytic lesions [36]. Based on these promising results, a clinical trial combining BAFF neutralizing antibody with bortezomib is currently ongoing.

Chemokine inhibition. CCL3 mediates mononuclear cell fusion *via* activation of the AKT and mitogen-activated protein kinase (MAPK) signaling pathways after binding to G-protein coupled receptors, CCR1 and CCR5. CCL3 is also involved in MM cell survival and migration, and its inhibition using antisense strategies prevents the development of osteolytic lesions and inhibits tumor growth *in-vivo* [27]. Blocking its receptor CCR1 impairs osteoclastogenesis and overcomes the proliferative advantage conferred by OC to MM cells [29]. These preclinical studies set the stage for future clinical trials using CCR1 inhibition strategies in patients with MM-bone disease. Similarly, targeting the CXCR4/CXCL12 pathway may block OC recruitment and inhibit osteolysis as shown in murine model of MM [61].

Anti-MM therapies with bone effects. Several novel anti-MM agents have demonstrated anti-catabolic or anabolic effects, specifically the thalidomide analogues, lenalidomide and pomalidomide, and the proteasome inhibitor bortezomib.

Immunomodulatory derivatives of thalidomide (IMiDs) have a broad range of activities affecting tumor growth directly and indirectly by alteration of the tumor microenvironment. Lenalidomide and pomalidomide regulate immune response, inhibit angiogenesis and, recent studies suggest their ability to impair OC development[62-65]. In particular, they downregulate PU.1 an early transcription factor involved in monocytic cell commitment to OC differentiation. In addition, lenalidomide inhibits RANKL secretion by BMSCs. Indeed, lenalidomide-treated patients show a restored RANKL/OPG balance.

Bortezomib has a direct cytotoxic effect on MM cells *via* proteasome and NF-κB signaling pathway inhibition and also indirectly by inhibition of MM-BMSC interactions. Several studies have identified bone effects resulting from OC inhibition and enhancement of OB differentiation. The suggested mechanism for the anti-OC effects of bortezomib consists of early p38 inhibition followed by a late impairment of NF-κB signaling and AP1 [66]. In contrast, the anabolic properties rely on the inhibition of proteasome activity and resultant RUNX2 upregulation, an early transcription factor modulating the expression of OB-specific genes, like osterix [67,68]. In MM patients, bortezomib treatment with or without dexamethasone induces upregulation of OB activation markers and downregulation of bone-resorption markers [69,70]. Notably, combination with alkylating agents and thalidomide (VMTD) diminishes benefits of bortezomib on OB differentiation [71]. Therefore, continued assessment of the effects of anti-MM strategies on bone remodeling are needed and may help identify optimal combination strategies.

Several signaling pathways involved in MM cell growth also modulate OC differentiation and their specific inhibitors demonstrate anti-catabolic effects. Extracellular signal-regulated kinases (ERK) and p38 inhibitors block early OC differentiation and control tumor growth as well as reduce OCs number in *in-vivo* models of MM [72,73]. Heat shock protein (HSP)90 inhibitors have a broad range of effects on the MM microenvironment [74] and inhibit OC *via* ERK and PU.1 down-regulation. Similarly, HDAC inhibitors prevent bone disease *in-vivo* when used alone or in combination with bortezomib [75,76].

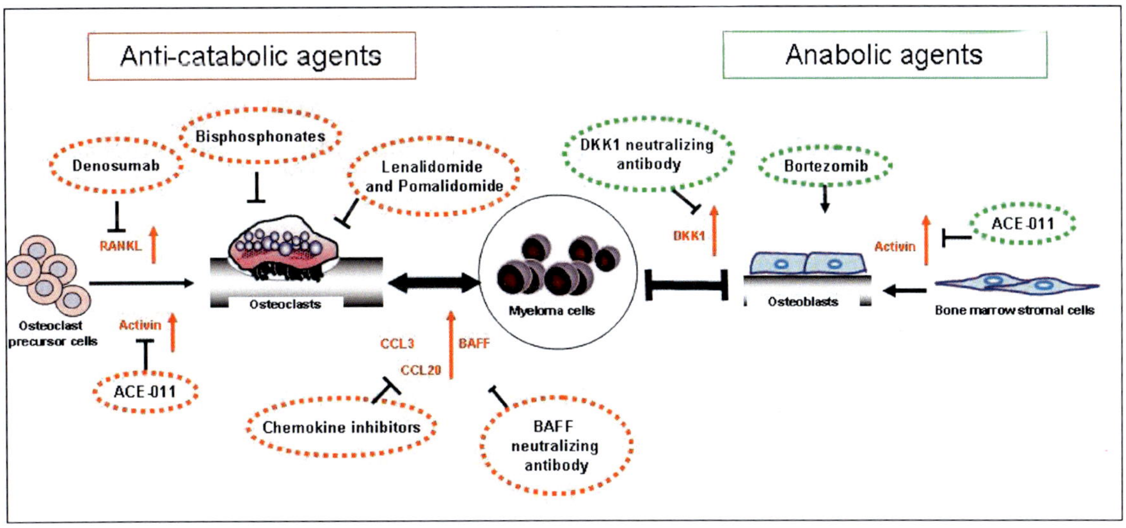

Fig. (2). Targeted therapies to overcome bone disease. The recent advances in the understanding of the pathogenesis of bone disease in multiple myeloma (MM) lead to the development of novel agents with anti-catabolic and/or anabolic properties. Among the anti-catabolic agents, bisphosphonates represent the standard of care and denosumab provide a valid alternative. The most promising anabolic agents are DKK1 antagonists, currently undergoing clinical evaluation. Notably, ACE-011 has a promising dual activity promoting osteoblast differentiation and inhibiting osteoclast development. Several anti-MM agents demonstrated also effects on bone metabolism, mainly thalidomide analogues and bortezomib.

4. CONCLUSIONS AND FUTURE DIRECTIONS

Bone disease in MM contributes to significant morbidity. Until recently BPs were the cornerstone of medical therapy for bone disease. The introduction of several novel targeted agents such as denosumab has now broadened this landscape. Recent studies exploring the MM niche as a therapeutic target are critical to long term anti- tumor strategies. Indeed, numerous studies suggest that restoring the balance between OC and OB, results in delayed tumor growth. Effective long term anti-MM strategies require in-depth knowledge of MM- related osteolysis and the role played by the MM niche in disease progression. These will inform the use of rationally designed optimal combination strategies in the future.

REFERENCES

[1] Saad F, Lipton A, Cook R, *et al.* Pathologic fractures correlate with reduced survival in patients with malignant bone disease. Cancer 2007; 110: 1860-1867.

[2] Coleman Re. Skeletal complications of malignancy. Cancer 1997; 80: 1588-1594.

[3] Martin TJ, Seeman E. Bone remodelling: its local regulation and the emergence of bone fragility. Best Pract Res Clin Endocrinol Metab 2008; 22: 701-722.

[4] Sims NA, Gooi JH. Bone remodeling: Multiple cellular interactions required for coupling of bone formation and resorption. Semin Cell Dev Biol 2008; 19: 444-451.

[5] Zhao C, Irie N, Takada Y, *et al.* Bidirectional ephrinB2-EphB4 signaling controls bone homeostasis. Cell Metab 2006; 4: 111-121.

[6] Lentzsch S, Gries M, Janz M, *et al.* Macrophage inflammatory protein 1-alpha (MIP-1 alpha) triggers migration and signaling cascades mediating survival and proliferation in multiple myeloma (MM) cells. Blood 2003; 101: 3568-3573.

[7] Podar K, Anderson KC. The pathophysiologic role of VEGF in hematologic malignancies: therapeutic implications. Blood 2005; 105: 1383-1395.

[8] Alsayed Y, Ngo H, Runnels J, *et al.* Mechanisms of regulation of CXCR4/SDF-1 (CXCL12)-dependent migration and homing in multiple myeloma. Blood 2007; 109: 2708-2717.

[9] Roodman GD. New potential targets for treating myeloma bone disease. Clin Cancer Res 2006; 12: 6270s-6273s.

[10] Yaccoby S, Wezeman MJ, Zangari M, *et al.* Inhibitory effects of osteoblasts and increased bone formation on myeloma in novel culture systems and a myelomatous mouse model. Haematologica 2006; 91: 192-199.

[11] Giuliani N, Rizzoli V, Roodman GD. Multiple myeloma bone disease: Pathophysiology of osteoblast inhibition. Blood 2006; 108: 3992-3996.

[12] Taube T, Beneton MN, Mccloskey EV, *et al.* Abnormal bone remodelling in patients with myelomatosis and normal biochemical indices of bone resorption. Eur J Haematol 1992; 49: 192-198.

[13] Valentin-Opran A, Charhon SA, Meunier PJ, Edouard CM, Arlot ME. Quantitative histology of myeloma-induced bone changes. Br J Haematol 1982; 52: 601-610.

[14] Bataille R, Chappard D, Marcelli C, *et al.* Mechanisms of bone destruction in multiple myeloma: the importance of an unbalanced process in determining the severity of lytic bone disease. J Clin Oncol 1989; 7: 1909-1914.

[15] Pearse RN, Sordillo EM, Yaccoby S, *et al.* Multiple myeloma disrupts the TRANCE/ osteoprotegerin cytokine axis to trigger bone destruction and promote tumor progression. Proc Natl Acad Sci U S A 2001; 98: 11581-11586.

[16] Seidel C, Hjertner O, Abildgaard N, *et al.* Serum osteoprotegerin levels are reduced in patients with multiple myeloma with lytic bone disease. Blood 2001; 98: 2269-2271.

[17] Giuliani N, Bataille R, Mancini C, Lazzaretti M, Barille S. Myeloma cells induce imbalance in the osteoprotegerin/osteoprotegerin ligand system in the human bone marrow environment. Blood 2001; 98: 3527-3533.

[18] Giuliani N, Colla S, Sala R, *et al.* Human myeloma cells stimulate the receptor activator of nuclear factor-kappa B ligand (RANKL) in T lymphocytes: a potential role in multiple myeloma bone disease. Blood 2002; 100: 4615-4621.

[19] Lai FP, Cole-Sinclair M, Cheng WJ, *et al.* Myeloma cells can directly contribute to the pool of RANKL in bone bypassing the classic stromal and osteoblast pathway of osteoclast stimulation. Br J Haematol 2004; 126: 192-201.

[20] Hiruma Y, Kurihara N, Jelinek DF, Roodman D. Increased Signaling through p62 in the marrow microenvironment increases myeloma cell growth and osteoclast formation. Blood 2008; 112: 239.

[21] Standal T, Seidel C, Hjertner O, *et al.* Osteoprotegerin is bound, internalized, and degraded by multiple myeloma cells. Blood 2002; 100: 3002-3007.

[22] Shipman CM, Croucher PI. Osteoprotegerin is a soluble decoy receptor for tumor necrosis factor-related apoptosis-inducing ligand/Apo2 ligand and can function as a paracrine survival factor for human myeloma cells. Cancer Res 2003; 63: 912-916.

[23] Terpos E, Politou M, Szydlo R, *et al.* Autologous stem cell transplantation normalizes abnormal bone remodeling and sRANKL/osteoprotegerin ratio in patients with multiple myeloma. Leukemia 2004; 18: 1420-1426.

[24] Terpos E, Mihou D, Szydlo R, *et al.* The combination of intermediate doses of thalidomide with dexamethasone is an effective treatment for patients with refractory/relapsed multiple myeloma and normalizes abnormal bone remodeling, through the reduction of sRANKL/osteoprotegerin ratio. Leukemia 2005; 19: 1969-1976.

[25] Han JH, Choi SJ, Kurihara N, *et al.* Macrophage inflammatory protein-1alpha is an osteoclastogenic factor in myeloma that is independent of receptor activator of nuclear factor kappaB ligand. Blood 2001; 97: 3349-3353.

[26] Terpos E, Politou M, Szydlo R, *et al.* Serum levels of macrophage inflammatory protein-1 alpha (MIP-1alpha) correlate with the extent of bone disease and survival in patients with multiple myeloma. Br J Haematol 2003; 123: 106-109.

[27] Choi SJ, Oba Y, Gazitt Y, *et al.* Antisense inhibition of macrophage inflammatory protein 1-alpha blocks bone destruction in a model of myeloma bone disease. J Clin Invest 2001; 108: 1833-1841.

[28] Oyajobi BO, Franchin G, Williams PJ, *et al.* Dual effects of macrophage inflammatory protein-1alpha on osteolysis and tumor burden in the murine 5TGM1 model of myeloma bone disease. Blood 2003; 102: 311-319.

[29] Vallet S, Raje N, Ishitsuka K, *et al.* MLN3897, a novel CCR1 inhibitor, impairs osteoclastogenesis and inhibits the interaction of multiple myeloma cells and osteoclasts. Blood 2007; 110: 3744-3752.

[30] Lee JW, Chung HY, Ehrlich LA, *et al.* IL-3 expression by myeloma cells increases both osteoclast formation and growth of myeloma cells. Blood 2004; 103: 2308-2315.

[31] Giuliani N, Morandi F, Tagliaferri S, *et al.* Interleukin-3 (IL-3) is overexpressed by T lymphocytes in multiple myeloma patients. Blood 2006; 107: 841-842.

[32] Giuliani N, Lisignoli G, Colla S, *et al.* CC-Chemokine ligand 20/macrophage inflammatory protein-3alpha and CC-chemokine receptor 6 are overexpressed in myeloma microenvironment related to osteolytic bone lesions. Cancer Res 2008; 68: 6840-6850.

[33] Vallet S, Mukherjee S, Vaghela N, *et al.* Activin A promotes multiple myeloma-induced osteolysis and is a promising target for myeloma bone disease. Proc Natl Acad Sci U S A 2010; 107(11) 5124-9.

[34] Damiano JS, Cress AE, Hazlehurst LA, Shtil AA, Dalton WS. Cell adhesion mediated drug resistance (CAM-DR): role of integrins and resistance to apoptosis in human myeloma cell lines. Blood 1999; 93: 1658-1667.

[35] Abe M, Kido S, Hiasa M, *et al.* BAFF and APRIL as osteoclast-derived survival factors for myeloma cells: a rationale for TACI-Fc treatment in patients with multiple myeloma. Leukemia 2006; 20: 1313-1315.

[36] Neri P, Kumar S, Fulciniti MT, *et al.* Neutralizing B-cell activating factor antibody improves survival and inhibits osteoclastogenesis in a severe combined immunodeficient human multiple myeloma model. Clin Cancer Res 2007; 13: 5903-5909.

[37] Tian E, Zhan F, Walker R, *et al.* The role of the Wnt-signaling antagonist DKK1 in the development of osteolytic lesions in multiple myeloma. N Engl J Med 2003; 349: 2483-2494.

[38] Giuliani N, Morandi F, Tagliaferri S, *et al.* Production of Wnt inhibitors by myeloma cells: potential effects on canonical Wnt pathway in the bone microenvironment. Cancer Res 2007; 67: 7665-7674.

[39] Giuliani N, Colla S, Morandi F, *et al.* Myeloma cells block RUNX2/CBFA1 activity in human bone marrow osteoblast progenitors and inhibit osteoblast formation and differentiation. Blood 2005; 106: 2472-2483.

[40] Edwards CM, Edwards Jr, Lwin ST, *et al.* Increasing Wnt signaling in the bone marrow microenvironment inhibits the development of myeloma bone disease and reduces tumor burden in bone *in vivo*. Blood 2008; 111: 2833-2842.

[41] Li X, Pennisi A, Yaccoby S. Role of decorin in the antimyeloma effects of osteoblasts. Blood 2008; 112: 159-168.

[42] Weinstein RS, Roberson PK, Manolagas SC. Giant osteoclast formation and long-term oral bisphosphonate therapy. N Engl J Med 2009; 360: 53-62.

[43] Berenson Jr, Lichtenstein A, Porter L, *et al.* Efficacy of pamidronate in reducing skeletal events in patients with advanced multiple myeloma. Myeloma Aredia Study Group. N Engl J Med 1996; 334: 488-493.

[44] Aparicio A, Gardner A, Tu Y, *et al.* *In vitro* cytoreductive effects on multiple myeloma cells induced by bisphosphonates. Leukemia 1998; 12: 220-229.

[45] Musto P, Petrucci MT, Bringhen S, *et al.* A multicenter, randomized clinical trial comparing zoledronic acid versus observation in patients with asymptomatic myeloma. Cancer 2008; 113: 1588-1595.

[46] Kyle RA, Yee GC, Somerfield MR, *et al.* American Society of Clinical Oncology 2007 clinical practice guideline update on the role of bisphosphonates in multiple myeloma. J Clin Oncol 2007; 25: 2464-2472.

[47] Khosla S, Burr D, Cauley J, *et al.* Bisphosphonate-associated osteonecrosis of the jaw: report of a task force of the American Society for Bone and Mineral Research. J Bone Miner Res 2007; 22: 1479-1491.

[48] Bone HG, Hosking D, Devogelaer JP, *et al.* Ten years'experience with alendronate for osteoporosis in postmenopausal women. N Engl J Med 2004; 350: 1189-1199.

[49] Pozzi S, Vallet S, Mukherjee S, *et al.* High-dose zoledronic acid impacts bone remodeling with effects on osteoblastic lineage and bone mechanical properties. Clin Cancer Res 2009; 15: 5829-5839.

[50] Raje N, Woo SB, Hande K, *et al.* Clinical, radiographic, and biochemical characterization of multiple myeloma patients with osteonecrosis of the jaw. Clin Cancer Res 2008; 14: 2387-2395.

[51] Berenson Jr, Rosen LS, Howell A, *et al.* Zoledronic acid reduces skeletal-related events in patients with osteolytic metastases. Cancer 2001; 91: 1191-1200.

[52] Vanderkerken K, De Leenheer E, Shipman C, *et al.* Recombinant osteoprotegerin decreases tumor burden and increases survival in a murine model of multiple myeloma. Cancer Res 2003; 63: 287-289.

[53] Body JJ Greipp P, Coleman RE, *et al.* A phase I study of AMGN-0007, a recombinant osteoprotegerin construct, in patients with multiple myeloma or breast carcinoma related bone metastases. Cancer 2003; 97: 887-892.

[54] Fizazi K, Lipton A, Mariette X, *et al.* Randomized phase II trial of denosumab in patients with bone metastases from prostate cancer, breast cancer, or other neoplasms after intravenous bisphosphonates. J Clin Oncol 2009; 27: 1564-71.

[55] Vij R, Horvath N, Spencer A, *et al.* An open-label, phase 2 trial of denosumab in the treatment of relapsed or plateau-phase multiple myeloma. Am J Hematol 2009; 84: 650-6.

[56] Fulciniti M, Tassone P, Hideshima T, *et al.* Anti-DKK1 mAb (BHQ880) as a Potential Therapeutic for Multiple Myeloma. Blood 2007; 114: 371-9.

[57] Yaccoby S, Ling W, Zhan F, *et al.* Antibody-based inhibition of DKK1 suppresses tumor-induced bone resorption and multiple myeloma growth *in vivo*. Blood 2007; 109: 2106-2111.

[58] Heath DJ, Chantry AD, Buckle CH, *et al.* Inhibiting Dickkopf-1 (Dkk1) Removes Suppression of Bone Formation and Prevents the Development of Osteolytic Bone Disease in Multiple Myeloma. J Bone Miner Res 2008; 24: 425-36

[59] Pearsall RS, Canalis E, Cornwall-Brady M, *et al.* A soluble activin type IIA receptor induces bone formation and improves skeletal integrity. Proc Natl Acad Sci U S A 2008; 105: 7082-7087.

[60] Tai YT, Li XF, Breitkreutz I, *et al.* Role of B-cell-activating factor in adhesion and growth of human multiple myeloma cells in the bone marrow microenvironment. Cancer Res 2006; 66: 6675-6682.

[61] Diamond P, Labrinidis A, Martin SK, *et al.* Targeted disruption of the CXCL12/CXCR4 axis inhibits osteolysis in a murine model of myeloma-associated bone loss. J Bone Miner Res 2009; 24: 1150-1161.

[62] Davies FE, Raje N, Hideshima T, *et al.* Thalidomide and immunomodulatory derivatives augment natural killer cell cytotoxicity in multiple myeloma. Blood 2001; 98: 210-216.

[63] Lentzsch S, Leblanc R, Podar K, *et al.* Immunomodulatory analogs of thalidomide inhibit growth of Hs Sultan cells and angiogenesis *in vivo*. Leukemia 2003; 17: 41-44.

[64] Anderson G, Gries M, Kurihara N, *et al.* Thalidomide derivative CC-4047 inhibits osteoclast formation by down-regulation of PU.1. Blood 2006; 107: 3098-3105.

[65] Breitkreutz I, Raab MS, Vallet S, *et al.* Lenalidomide inhibits osteoclastogenesis, survival factors and bone-remodeling markers in multiple myeloma. Leukemia 2008; 22: 1925-1932.

[66] Von Metzler I, Krebbel H, Hecht M, *et al.* Bortezomib inhibits human osteoclastogenesis. Leukemia 2007; 21: 2025-2034.

[67] Giuliani N, Morandi F, Tagliaferri S, *et al.* The proteasome inhibitor bortezomib affects osteoblast differentiation *in vitro* and *in vivo* in multiple myeloma patients. Blood 2007; 110: 334-338.

[68] Mukherjee S, Raje N, Schoonmaker JA, *et al.* Pharmacologic targeting of a stem/progenitor population *in vivo* is associated with enhanced bone regeneration in mice. J Clin Invest 2008; 118: 491-504.

[69] Zangari M, Esseltine D, Lee CK, *et al.* Response to bortezomib is associated to osteoblastic activation in patients with multiple myeloma. Br J Haematol 2005; 131: 71-73.

[70] Terpos E, Heath DJ, Rahemtulla A, *et al.* Bortezomib reduces serum dickkopf-1 and receptor activator of nuclear factor-kappaB ligand concentrations and normalises indices of bone remodelling in patients with relapsed multiple myeloma. Br J Haematol 2006; 135: 688-692.

[71] Terpos E, Kastritis E, Roussou M, *et al.* The combination of bortezomib, Melphalan, dexamethasone and intermittent thalidomide is an effective regimen for relapsed/refractory myeloma and is associated with improvement of abnormal bone metabolism and angiogenesis. Leukemia 2008; 22: 2247-2256.

[72] Ishitsuka K, Hideshima T, Neri P, *et al.* p38 mitogen-activated protein kinase inhibitor LY2228820 enhances bortezomib-induced cytotoxicity and inhibits osteoclastogenesis in multiple myeloma; therapeutic implications. Br J Haematol 2008; 141: 598-606.

[73] Breitkreutz I, Raab MS, Vallet S, *et al.* Targeting MEK1/2 blocks osteoclast differentiation, function and cytokine secretion in multiple myeloma. Br J Haematol 2007; 139: 55-63.

[74] Okawa Y, Hideshima T, Steed P, *et al.* SNX-2112, a selective Hsp90 inhibitor, potently inhibits tumor cell growth, angiogenesis, and osteoclastogenesis in multiple myeloma and other hematologic tumors by abrogating signaling *via* Akt and ERK. Blood 2009; 113: 846-855.

[75] Deleu S, Lemaire M, Arts J, *et al.* Bortezomib alone or in combination with the histone deacetylase inhibitor JNJ-26481585: effect on myeloma bone disease in the 5T2MM murine model of myeloma. Cancer Res 2009; 69: 5307-5311.

[76] Deleu S, Lemaire M, Arts J, *et al.* The effects of JNJ-26481585, a novel hydroxamate-based histone deacetylase inhibitor, on the development of multiple myeloma in the 5T2MM and 5T33MM murine models. Leukemia 2009; 23: 1894-1903.

CHAPTER 7

Management of Complications in Multiple Myeloma

Suzanne Lentzsch*

Division of Hematology/Oncology, University of Pittsburgh Cancer Institute, Pittsburgh, PA

Abstract: Patients with multiple myeloma have a high rate of complications related to their underlying disease. This includes anemia, renal failure, complications related to bone disease such as hypercalcemia, bone pain and fractures, infection and renal insufficiency. Adequate supportive care is therefore an essential part of each anti-myeloma treatment and can significantly improve overall survival and the quality of life of multiple myeloma patients. This review focuses on the management of specific complications associated with advanced multiple myeloma.

Keywords: Bone disease, hypercalcemia, pain, kyphoplasty, vertebroplasty, osteonecrosis of the jaw (ONJ), infections, renal insufficiency, anemia.

1. INTRODUCTION

Patients with multiple myeloma have a high rate of complications related to their underlying disease. This includes anemia, renal failure, complications related to bone disease, such as hypercalcemia, bone pain and fractures, infection, and renal insufficiency. Adequate supportive care is therefore an essential part of each anti-myeloma treatment and can significantly improve overall survival and the quality of life of multiple myeloma patients. This review focuses on the management of specific complications associated with advanced multiple myeloma.

2. MULTIPLE MYELOMA BONE DISEASE

Almost all patients with multiple myeloma develop osteopenia or osteolytic lesions which may result in pathologic fractures or severe bone pain. The development of osteolytic lesions is attributable to increased bone resorption, caused by stimulation of osteoclast formation and activity [1-3]. Increased osteoclast activity is accompanied by decreased osteoblast function resulting in imbalanced bone remodeling with increased bone resorption and decreased bone formation. Patients subsequently experience severe loss of bone mass, diagnosed as osteopenia or lytic bone lesions. Patients with one or more lesions on radiographs and otherwise unexplained osteopenia should be given bisphosphonate therapy. Randomized trials by Berenson *et al.* have shown that pamidronate and zoledronate significantly reduce skeletal-related events (SRE) in multiple myeloma [4, 5]. Recommended pamidronate dosage is 60-90 mg given over at least 2 hours, and zoledronic acid 4 mg given over 15 minutes.

Complications resulting from bone lesions include:

2.1. Hypercalcemia

Over 10% of patients with multiple myeloma present with hypercalcemia at the time of diagnosis and may require emergent treatment [6]. Hypercalcemia may have no symptoms or present as a variety of symptoms such as nausea, vomiting, polyuria, polydipsia, anorexia, increased constipation, weakness, confusion or stupor. Calcium is bound to proteins, especially albumin. Therefore, abnormal serum albumin levels may not reflect the physiologically important ionized calcium. In myeloma patients with hypoalbuminemia, total serum calcium might be normal when ionized calcium is elevated. In contrast, patients rarely have a calcium binding paraprotein resulting in increased binding of calcium. This causes an elevation of the total calcium concentration without rise in the serum ionized calcium concentration [6]. This phenomenon is

***Address correspondence to Suzanne Lentzsch:** Division of Hematology/Oncology, University of Pittsburgh Cancer Institute, 5150 Centre Ave, #568, Pittsburgh, PA 15232; E-mail: lentzschs@upmc.edu.

Klaus Podar and Kenneth C. Anderson (Eds)

called pseudo-hypercalcemia. Most patients with multiple myeloma with a diagnosis of hypercalcemia do not require the measurement of ionized calcium since the monoclonal protein rarely binds to calcium [7]. The management of hypercalcemia depends upon the level of calcium, the patient's symptoms and rapidity with which the symptoms developed. Treatment should reflect the acuity and degree of symptoms.

- Mild hypercalcemia, serum calcium below 12 mg/dL: Patients with mild asymptomatic hypercalcemia do not require immediate treatment. Treatment should include hydration with isotonic saline. Addition of dexamethasone (40 mg for 4 days) as part of the myeloma therapy, or prednisone (1 mg/kg per day) is effective in most cases.
- Moderate to severe hypercalcemia, serum calcium above 14 mg/dL: Treatment should include hydration, preferably with isotonic saline, corticosteroids such as dexamethasone as part of the myeloma therapy (40 mg for 4 days) or prednisone (1 mg/kg per day), and bisphosphonate such as zoledronic acid or pamidronate. Calcitonin is used if rapid reduction of calcium levels is needed or if patients are refractory to bisphosphonates alone.
- Extremely severe hypercalcemia, serum calcium above 18 mg/dL: In addition to the measures outlined above, patients should undergo hemodialysis.

2.1.1. Saline Hydration in Hypercalcemia

Initial therapy for acute or symptomatic hypercalcemia includes isotonic saline to treat possible volume depletion due to hypercalcemia-induced urinary salt wasting and, in a few cases, vomiting. The infusion rate depends on the severity of hypercalcemia and comorbidities, especially underlying cardiac or renal disease and the age of the patient. A reasonable regimen in the absence of edema is the administration of isotonic saline at an initial rate of 200-300 mL/hour, and then adjusting to maintain urine output of 100-150 mL/hour. Infusion therapy should be carefully monitored to avoid any fluid overload.

2.1.2. Bisphosphonates in Hypercalcemia

The maximum effect of bisphosphonates occurs in 2-4 days. In cases requiring rapid reduction of calcium, bisphosphonates should be administered in conjunction with hydration and calcitonin. Bisphosphonates such as pamidronate and zoledronic acid are given with caution in patients with impaired renal function. Adequate hydration with normal saline and treatment with a reduced dosage and/or slower infusion rate, *e.g.* 4 mg zoledronic acid over 30 minutes or 30-45 mg pamidronate over 4 hours, minimizes the risk of worsening renal failure.

2.1.3. Calcitonin

Calcitonin provides a rapid reduction in serum calcium concentrations by increasing the renal calcium excretion, and decreasing bone reabsorption [8, 9]. Salmon calcitonin (4 IU/kg) is administered intramuscularly or subcutaneously every 12 hours. The dosage can be increased up to 6-8 IU/kg every 6 hours. Nasal application of calcitonin is not recommended for the treatment of hypercalcemia [10]. The efficacy of calcitonin is limited to the first 48 hours, even with repeated doses, suggesting the development of tachyphylaxis. Therefore calcitonin is most beneficial for patients with acute hypercalcemia and a calcium over 14 mg/L (3.5 mmol/L), when combined with hydration and bisphosphonates.

2.2. Bone Pain

Many multiple myeloma patients suffer from moderate to severe skeletal pain, particularly in the spine, which can substantially decrease the quality of life. Pain is frequently the first symptom of multiple myeloma at diagnosis, but also very often is an indicator of relapsed or disease progression. In addition to micro-fractures or pathological fractures of the vertebral bodies, pelvis or the long bones, pain also results from nerve compression or extramedullary multiple myeloma.

Analgesics in combination with chemotherapy usually control the bone pain, especially in cases of response. Pharmacological therapy of lytic lesions includes non-opioids, mild opioids and strong opioids.

Non-opiate analgesics, such as non-steroidal anti-inflammatory drugs (NSAIDs) should be used judiciously since those drugs can contribute to renal failure. Acetaminophen is routinely used for the treatment of myeloma bone pain. A three step treatment plan, also called World Health Organization (WHO) Pain Treatment Ladder is often used for the management of myeloma-related pain [11].

WHO Pain Ladder [11]

Level 1	**Level 2**	**Level 3**
NSAIDs	*Weak opioids*	*Strong opioids*
Aspirin	Codein	Morphine
Ibuprofen	Dihydrocodein	Buprenorphin
Naproxen	Levomethadone	Tramodol
COX-2 inhibitors	Tilidine	Fentanyl

Adjuvant medication (corticosteroid, antiemetics, neuroleptics, anti-depressants, stool softener, benzodiazepines) should be given as required.

Abbreviations: WHO, World Health Organization; NSAIDs, nonsteroidal anti-inflammatory drugs; COX-2, cyclooxygenase-2.

To maintain freedom from pain it is important that the patient should take pain medication according to a strict schedule. Adherence to the pain medication schedule usually results in a higher quality of life with a lower need of high dosage of medication for breakthrough pain.

2.3. Treatment of Fractures

Fracture of long bones occurs most frequently in the proximal parts of the humerus and femur. Pathologic fractures and impending fractures of long bones need stabilization with an intramedullary rod. Close collaboration with an orthopedic surgeon is mandatory in order to recognize impending fractures early and to undertake appropriate actions. If 50% or more destruction of cortical bone is observed, surgical intervention is required [12]. Radiotherapy can be used in selected cases as sole therapy, but should be applied to all impending fractures. Single treatment with 8-10 Gy fraction is recommended [13].

2.3.1. Kyphoplasty and Vertebroplasty

Kyphoplasty and vertebroplasty are indicated to achieve fast pain relief. Dudeney, *et al.* reported a study analyzing kyphoplasty in multiple myeloma patients with osteolytic vertebral compression fractures. Significant improvement in pain and physical function was noted in 80% of the patients. In addition, 34% of the vertebral height lost at the time of fracture was restored with the procedure without major complications [14]. Another study by Fourney *et al.* achieved significant or complete pain relief in 84% of the patients, while no patients experienced worsening of the pain or procedure related complications [15]. Interestingly, reduction of pain scores remained significant up to one year following the procedures. The choice between kyphoplasty and vertebroplasty depends on the expertise of the physician performing the procedure. Possible complications include extrusion of cement, increased pain from heat, or damage to the spinal cord or nerve roots.

2.3.2. Radiation

Radiation should be used judiciously since extensive radiation can reduce the bone marrow reserve, subsequently compromise future chemotherapy, and especially prevent future autologous stem cell procedures. Nevertheless, up to 40% of the patients with multiple myeloma might require radiation to control the disease or pain at some point of the disease course [16]. The most common reasons for radiation therapy include:

- Pain control of lytic lesions which are refractory to systemic therapy
- Impending fractures
- Spinal cord compression from a plasmacytoma
- Primary treatment of a solitary plasmacytoma

Post surgical radiation after stabilization of an impending fracture is not recommended and only needed in circumstances such as scattered fractures [17]. Besides rapid pain relief, radiation can also reduce tumor mass accompanied by a reduction in the monoclonal protein. This should be taken into account especially if systemic chemotherapy is given parallel with radiation. Dosage of radiation varies according to the clinical situation and usually between 20-30 Gy in 5-10 fractions is recommended [18]. Solitary plasmacytoma with a curative treatment approach requires higher dosages up to 50 Gy. In contrast, radiation given for pain management is very effective at a dosage of 8-10 Gy given in a single fraction [18].

2.4. Cord Compression

Epidural spinal cord compression (ESCC) should be suspected in patients with severe back pain, lower extremity weakness, bladder or bowel disfunction, incontinence, or paresthesias of lower extremities. MRI of the entire spine should be initiated immediately if cord compression is suspected. Spinal cord compression is caused either by extramedullary plasmacytoma or retropulsed bone due to vertebral fractures. In order to preserve the neurological function in patients with spinal cord compression, immediate treatment is critical. Rades *et al.* reported that up to 60% of patients with cord compression have improvement of motor function with radiotherapy [19]. For patients who are not surgical candidates, dexamethasone and radiation therapy are usually helpful.

2.4.1. Surgery

Decompression using laminectomy for patients with epidural spinal cord compression (ESCC) is the initial approach in neurologically compromised patients diagnosed very early. Retrospective studies comparing laminectomy with or without radiotherapy vs. radiotherapy alone revealed no advantage to surgical approach [20, 21]. Improvements in surgical therapy led to the use of more aggressive tumor resections combined with postoperative radiotherapy. The benefit of an aggressive tumor debulking with combined radiotherapy (30 Gy over ten days starting within 14 days of surgery) was shown, when patients who were not paraplegic for more than 48 hours showed a significantly higher ambulatory rate if treated with surgery followed by radiotherapy (84% vs. 57% with radiotherapy alone). The patients retained the ability to walk significantly longer than those treated with radiotherapy alone (median 122 vs. 13 days) [22]. In summary, the randomized trials indicate that radical resection followed by radiotherapy increases the likelihood of regaining the ability to walk if cord compression was diagnosed very early (within 24 hours of presentation). Therefore, each patient should be carefully considered. Patients with adequate life expectancy and good medical status who are candidates for an aggressive approach should be identified.

2.4.2. Radiation Therapy

Radiation therapy is still the choice of treatment for patients with ESCC who are not considered surgical candidates or for patients who have already undergone surgical decompression. The dose schedule may vary between 30 and 40 Gy divided into 10-20 fractions [19,23-28]. Glucocorticoids are an integral component of initial management of cord compression and should be initiated as soon as possible.

For all patients with ESCC and either neurologic symptoms or substantial thecal sac compression by imaging, glucocorticoids are recommended. For patients with severe neurologic deficits, such as paraparesis or paraplegia, dexamethasone 96 mg IV followed by 24 mg 4 times daily for three days and then tapered over 10 days is recommended (Grade 2C) [29]. For patients with minimal neurologic symptoms, we suggest moderate doses of dexamethasone as a bolus of 10 mg IV followed by 16 mg daily orally in divided doses (Grade 2C) [29].

3. OSTEONECROSIS OF THE JAW

3.1. Osteonecrosis of the Jaw and Bisphosphonate Therapy

Bisphosphonates have been shown in clinical trials to reduce skeletal-related events such as bone pain, hypercalcemia, fractures, need for radiation, and surgery [4, 5, 30]. Unfortunately, treatment with bisphosphonates is also associated with the development of osteonecrosis of the jaw (ONJ) that has the potential to severely influence the quality of life and might lead to other clinical complications.

The oral bioavailability of bisphosphonates is less than 2% [31]. Intravenous infusion of bisphosphonates results in 50% rapidly binding to the bone surface [32]. Once the drug is bound to the bone, bisphosphonates remain in a pharmacologically inactive form until released from hydroxyapatite by the action of osteoclasts [31-33].

ONJ induced by bisphosphonates often present as a persisting non-healing wound. ONJ might occur after tooth extraction or dental surgery, but it can also occur spontaneously and present initially as oral mucosal ulceration [34]. Interestingly, the mandibular involvement is 2 to 5 times more common than involvement of the maxilla, especially posterior to the canines [34-36]. Symptoms of ONJ include tooth, jaw or facial pain, but also might be completely painless. Patients might have difficulties with eating, speaking or carrying out dental hygiene. Exposed bone on inspection of the oral cavity is a hallmark of ONJ, but cutaneous or mucosal fistulas, draining fluids and loose teeth are also signs of ONJ. The differential diagnosis of ONJ includes myeloma deposits, radio-osteonecrosis, and dental infections unrelated to bisphosphonates.

3.2. Pathogenesis of ONJ

The pathogenesis of ONJ is also not completely understood. The constant bone remodeling, continuous mechanical stress, and consequent microfractures along with the flora of the oral cavity contributes to the mandible being the preferred site of ONJ. Due to decreased osteoclast activity, resorption of decayed or infected bone is inhibited and supports the development of necrosis. ONJ also appears to be a phenomenon of poor wound healing and avascular necrosis [34]. Damage to the mucosal surface and poor dental hygiene may be sufficient to initiate the process [37, 38]. It is very well known that the risk of development of ONJ is closely related to the length and the potency of bisphosphonates [39-43]. It has been shown in several trials that the increased potency of zoledronic acid increases the relative risk of ONJ from 3.4 to 9.5 times in comparison to pamidronate [39-43]. The incidence of ONJ is not exactly known. Multiple trials estimate a range from 1.2 to 15% [40, 44]. In addition, Durie showed that the mean time of onset to ONJ was 18 months for zoledronic acid and 6 years for pamidronate [41]. A retrospective study by Mavrokokki showed a mean time to onset of 12 months for zoledronic acid and 24 months for pamidronate [42]. A prospective study by Bamias *et al.* showed that the rate of ONJ in patients on IV bisphosphonates was 1.5% before 12 months of therapy and 7.7% at 48 months of therapy [39]. Taken together, these reports suggest that the risk of ONJ significantly increases after the first 24 months of IV bisphosphonate therapy with a higher risk with zoledronic acid. Risk factors for ONJ other than type of bisphosphonate and length of use of bisphosphonates are tooth extraction or other oral trauma, poor dentition with bad dental hygiene, age, smoking, diabetes mellitus, and poor-fitting oral appliances [45].

3.3. Prevention of ONJ

According to the recommendations of the American Association of Oral and Maxillofacial Surgeons and the American Society of Clinical Oncology, patients should have an appropriate education about oral hygiene practices and should be informed about the risk of ONJ. The oral cavity should be examined for periodontitis and major dental work should be finished before commencing of bisphosphonate therapy. Evaluation of the patient by a dentist is strongly recommended before initiating bisphosphonates. Further followup should include 6-month dental reviews while on bisphosphonates and tooth extraction should be avoided unless absolutely required [37, 38, 46, 47].

There are no clear guidelines for planning dental surgery. According to Mayo Clinic guidelines, bisphosphonate therapy should be stopped a month before tooth extraction is scheduled and until after healing is complete [48]. The Canadian consensus guidelines recommend a 3-6 month break in treatment [49]. The American Association of Oral and Maxillofacial Surgeons recommends stopping bisphosphonate until wound healing is complete [47]. The Myeloma Scientific Advisory Group of the Myeloma Foundation of Australia (MFA) along with various medical experts published their recommendations in the Internal Medicine Journal in 2009 and recommended patients with low or intermediate risk of skeletal-related events to discontinue bisphosphonates three months before and after dental extractions, and where possible, until complete healing of the extraction site occurs [45, 50].

Based on the experiences from several researchers concerning antibiotic prophylaxis for a planned dental procedure, the prophylaxis should include an appropriate anti-streptococcal/anti-anaerobic agent and should start before the dental procedure. Suggested regimens include amoxicillin-clavulanate 825 mg/125 mg twice a day for 1-7 days before and for 3 days following the procedure [51, 52]. Alternatively clindamycin 300 mg initially followed by 150 mg 4 times per day for 5 days before the procedure and 5-11 days after the procedure can be given [53].

3.4. Management of Established ONJ

Treatment of ONJ can be very problematic since the patients very often do not have complete healing resulting in a severe impairment of the quality of life. It is common sense that after the occurrence of ONJ, bisphosphonate therapy should be suspended. The Medical and Scientific Advisory Group of the Myeloma Foundation of Australia recommended at least three months suspension of bisphosphonates after occurrence of ONJ except in the setting of difficult-to-control hypercalcemia [45]. Reinstitution of bisphosphonates in intermediate or high- risk skeletal-related event groups preferably should occur after the resolution of ONJ. Nevertheless, in some cases the risk of skeletal-related events becomes the overriding concern and use of bisphosphonate before healing is unavoidable [54]. Except for treatment-resistant hypercalcemia, the frequency of bisphosphonates after reinstitution should be less frequent, *e.g.* 3-monthly, or less potent bisphosphonates such as clodronate should be considered.

Dental management of established osteonecrosis of the jaw should include the following [45].

1) Antibiotics (should include treatment of Actinomyces) (penicillin 500 mg daily or amoxicillin 500 mg three times a day remain the treatments of choice), addition of metronidazole for refractory infections; regular Chlorhexidine mouthwash (0.2% BD) [49, 55, 56].
2) Regular dental checks to reinforce preventive care, maintain integrity of dentition and avoid tooth removal.
3) Avoidance of debridement of necrotic bone (debridement will worsen the necrosis, and is only recommended if the bone is causing trauma to surrounding mucosa). Sequestrating fragments should be removed only when mobile and preferably after a drug holiday.
4) Analgesics.

4. INFECTIONS

Patients with multiple myeloma have an increased risk for infections. Factors that contribute to the increased risk include: hypogammaglobulinemia due to the depression of the normal plasma cell clone and function, chemotherapy-induced neutropenia, and impaired lymphocyte function. Urinary tract infections and pneumonias account for the majority of infections. The most common organisms are Streptococcus pneumoniae, Haemophilus influenza, and Escherichia coli. A study of 3,107 newly diagnosed patients showed that the majority of patients acquired infections within the first 60 days of diagnosis or at the time of relapse [57].

Prophylaxis for infection aims at a decreased rate of infection, and includes the use of antibiotics, antivirals, antifungals, vaccines, and intravenous immunoglobulin. Patients with multiple myeloma should have yearly influenza vaccine and a single pneumococcal vaccine at the time of diagnosis. Despite the fact that patients with multiple myeloma most likely have a reduced antibody response, patients may still benefit from obtaining pneumococcal vaccines. There is no evidence that influenza or pneumococcal vaccination is associated with a higher risk of reaction compared to the normal population [12].

Since the antibody response to pneumococcal vaccination may be sub-optimal, patients with frequent pneumococcal infections should be considered to receive penicillin prophylaxis for pneumococcus. But routine prophylaxis for pneumococcal infections is not recommended in general in adults.

4.1. Prophylactic Antibiotics

The use of prophylactic antibiotics in multiple myeloma patients is controversial. There are no prospective studies showing the value of antimicrobial prophylaxis in patients with multiple myeloma. In patients with a high risk of infection, *e.g.* relapsed/refractory multiple myeloma with long term use of high dose steroids, antibiotic prophylaxis with either fluoroquinolone (*e.g.* levofloxacin 500 mg daily), or trimethoprim-sulfamethoxazole (*e.g.* 80/400 mg once daily or 160/800 mg every other day) during the first three or four months of chemotherapy should be considered [12]. Patients receiving thalidomide, lenalidomide or pomalidomide should not receive trimethoprim-sulfamethoxazole prophylaxis since this combination increases the risk of serious skin toxicity. In those patients, fluoroquinolone is preferable.

It is clinically standard for patients treated with bortezomib to receive antiviral prophylaxis with either Acyclovir 400 mg twice daily or valacyclovir 500 mg once daily) because of increased risk of Herpa Zoster or Varicella Zoster reactivation [58-60].

The analysis of 663 patients treated in the APEX trial, a prospective randomized phase II trial comparing bortezomib vs. dexamethasone, found that patients treated with bortezomib had a significantly higher incidence of Herpa Zoster when compared with patients treated with high dose dexamethasone (13 vs. 5 percent respectively) [58]. Based on those findings, antiviral prophylaxis was suggested. Dasanu and Alexandrescu discussed the data critically and raised concerns regarding the safety of routine antiviral drug prophylaxis in patients with relapsed or refractory multiple myeloma [61]. This is especially critical in light of using bortezomib as maintenance therapy which might be given over several years.

A study by Oken *et al.* randomized 54 patients who were about to begin chemotherapy to prophylaxis for two months or no prophylaxis. Antibiotic prophylaxis consisted of trimethoprim-sulfamethoxazole (TMP-SMX 160/800 mg orally every 12 hours) given for the first two months of initial chemotherapy. Patients in the treatment arm had significantly fewer bacterial infections than those in the control arm (11 vs. 2 respectively), and significantly fewer severe infections (8 vs. 1) in the first three months [62]. It is important to point out that patients in both arms received high dose dexamethasone and also induction therapy. The role of prophylactic antibiotics in the setting of myeloma therapy such as thalidomide, lenalidomide, pomalidomide, and bortezomib is less clear. Therefore, the decision to administer prophylactic antibiotics at least in the first few months or in heavily pretreated patients at the time of relapse should be based on the risk of infections and the chemotherapy given to the patient.

4.2. Intravenous Immunoglobulin (IVIG)

In selected patients with recurrent serious infections despite prophylactic antibiotics, IVIG is recommended. Results from prophylactic IVIG are very promising. In a controlled randomized trial, multiple myeloma patients in plateau phase were treated with either monthly IVIG (0.4 g/kg) or placebo. In the IVIG group, significantly fewer serious infections (19 in 449 patient months vs. 38 in 472 patient months) were observed [63]. IVIG should be considered for all patients who have severe hypogammaglobulinemia or increased incidence of infection caused by encapsulated bacteria or common viral pathogens.

5. RENAL INSUFFICIENCY

Around 20% of all multiple myeloma patients experience renal insufficiency presenting as either acute or chronic onset [64]. The mechanisms involved in the development of renal failure vary from an excess production of monoclonal light chains (light chain cast nephrology), deposition of intact light chains causing nephrotic syndrome (light chain deposition disease), light chain amyloidosis, hypercalcemia, radio contrast media-induced acute renal failure, dehydration, and hyperuricemia [12]. The frequency with which renal insufficiency occurs varies by definition. A study by Winearls defines renal insufficiency as a creatinine above 1.5 mg/dL [65]. In a study by Blade *et al.* in which renal failure was defined as a creatinine concentration equal to or over 2 mg/dL, 22% of 423 patients had renal failure [64]. There also is general correlation between the presence and severity of the renal disease and worse patients'survival [65].

All patients with multiple myeloma, especially patients with high levels of urinary free light chain multiple myeloma, should take several precautions to minimize renal damage. All patients should be instructed: 1) to avoid any nonsteroidal antiinflammatory drugs; 2) maintain hydration by drinking enough fluids to produce at least three liters of urine per day; 3) avoiding nephrotoxins such as aminoglycosides.

5.1. Management of Acute Renal Failure

Patients with multiple myeloma and acute renal failure consistent with myeloma cast nephropathy should start chemotherapy as soon as possible, preferably with chemotherapy inducing fast remission, *e.g.* a combination of bortezomib, thalidomide and dexamethasone.

- Intravenous fluids should be given to treat volume depletion. This is especially necessary in the setting of hypercalcemia or hyperuricemia. Hydration of patients with acute renal failure and multiple myeloma is critical and should be provided to all patients unless it is a contraindication in situations such as heart failure or oliguric/anuric acute renal failure. Goals of hydration are to decrease the light chain concentration within the tubular lumen in order to minimize light chain precipitation and induce a high urine flow rate. Reasonable infusion rate for patients who have no volume depletion is the administration of isotonic or half isotonic saline with a rate of 150 mL/hour in order to achieve a urine output of 100-150 mL/hour (approximately 3 L/day) [66]. This needs to be carefully monitored and may require modification to avoid accumulation of fluid due to renal or heart failure. For patients with oliguria or acute renal failure, fluid administration is still recommended. If reversal of oliguria does not occur within 24 hours, fluid administration should be modified to prevent volume overload. Loop diuretics should be used judiciously since there is some concern that they promote cast formation [67].

- Other reasons for acute renal failure such as hypercalcemia should be excluded or treated with bisphosphonates (discussed in Chapter: Bisphosphonates). If the corrected calcium concentration is elevated above 14 mg/dL, the initiation of bisphosphonates is recommended. If the serum calcium concentration is below 14 mg/dL, initial treatment with only fluids is recommended. If the hypercalcemia persists despite 6 to 12 hours of fluids, bisphosphonates should be given.

- If present, hyperuricemia should be treated. Nonsteroidal antiinflammatory drugs, ACE inhibitors or angiotensin receptor blockers should be stopped. In this situation, radiocontrast dye should be avoided if possible to prevent further kidney injury.

5.2. Plasmapheresis in Acute Renal Failure

Results of a clinical trial evaluating the effectiveness of plasmapheresis in patients with multiple myeloma in acute renal failure are conflicting. Zucchelli showed a significantly higher recovery of renal function in patients with Bence Jones proteinuria after receiving plasmapheresis [68]. The Consensus Report from the Scientific Advisors of the International Myeloma Foundation reviewed available studies and concluded that plasmapheresis might be an important adjunct in the management of multiple myeloma cast nephropathy [69]. Due to the possible reduction in dialysis dependency, plasmapheresis should be considered for individuals in acute renal failure suspected to be due to cast nephropathy including the following settings: 1) patients with cast nephropathy on kidney biopsy; and 2) patients with clinical symptoms suggesting that acute renal failure is due to high levels of free monoclonal light chains in the serum or urine, even in the absence of a renal biopsy [66].

The usual plasmapheresis regimen includes five to seven exchanges within seven to ten days. The duration of plasma exchange is to be guided by serum free light chain levels. Plasmapheresis should be started in conjunction with a dexamethasone containing chemotherapy to reduce the rate of light chain production. Free light chain assays should be repeated in order to monitor the success of the plasma exchange, even after completing the plasma cell exchange [66].

5.3. Chronic Renal Failure

The goal of management of chronic renal failure is to slow the progression and subsequent dialysis dependency. Chronic renal failure appears to be due to myeloma cast nephropathy. The most effective therapy to further prevent the progression of chronic renal failure is to minimize risk factors that promote light chain aggregation and subsequent tubular obstruction by casts [70]. As mentioned above, intravenous fluid to prevent volume depletion and maintain high urine output of approximately 3 L/day is indicated in order to decrease the light chain concentration within the tubular lumen and produce a high urine flow rate to minimize light chain precipitation [66]. Chemotherapy should be initiated in order to reduce the free light chain burden. As mentioned already, nonsteroidal antiinflammatory drugs and intravenous radiocontrast should be avoided. Other therapies remain to be proven in humans, such as the following.

- Alkalinization of the urine, raising the urine pH above 6.0 to 6.5 (toward or above the isoelectric point of the light chain) in order to prevent the formation of Tamm- Horsfall mucoprotein [67, 71].

- Loop diuretics should be avoided unless the patient is hypercalcemic. Loop diuretics can raise the tubular fluid sodium chloride concentration, and might contribute to the co-aggregation of light chains with Tamm Horsfall mucoprotein [67]. In addition, diuretics may also contribute to volume depletion, leading to a lower urine flow.

6. ANEMIA

6.1. Indication for Red Blood Cell Transfusion

This review focuses only on anemia associated with multiple myeloma. The grade of anemia associated with multiple myeloma depends upon the severity of multiple myeloma cell infiltration of the bone marrow. It should be evaluated for the presence or absence of symptoms related to anemia and whether the patient is undergoing active treatment. According to the guidelines of the British Committee for Standards in Hematology, patients with a hemoglobin <7 g/dL should receive 2 units of packed red blood cells (PRBC). That will result in an increment of 1-2 g/dL of hemoglobin. Patients > 65 and/or those with cardiovascular or respiratory disease may not tolerate anemia well. Those patients should be transfused when hemoglobin is ≤ 8 g/dL. If hemoglobin is between 7-10 g/dL, there are no exact guidelines, but patients with significant symptoms should receive 2 units of PRBC. If hemoglobin is above 10 g/dL, transfusion is not indicated [72]. If a transfusion is needed, irradiated leukoreduced cross-matched red cells are preferred.

6.2. Use of Erythropoiesis-Stimulating Agents

The use of erythropoiesis-stimulating agents (ESAs) has been the standard of care since the early 1990s, providing high response rates and improving the quality of life for patients [73]. Three randomized trials showed that symptomatic anemia during the plateau phase of multiple myeloma responded to administration of erythropoietin [74-76]. The trial by Dammacco included 145 patients with multiple myeloma and a hemoglobin concentration less than 11 g/dL receiving 150 U/kg of erythropoietin or a matching volume of placebo subcutaneously three times a week for 12 weeks. Patients receiving erythropoietin had a significantly lower incidence of transfusion (28% vs. 47%) and larger increase in hemoglobin concentration (1.8 vs. 0 g/dL) [74]. However, the role of ESAs in the treatment of myeloma-related anemia should be reconsidered due to growing evidence that ESAs might be associated with increased risk of thrombosis and disease progression [77-79]. Therefore, the decision to use ESAs for anemia in multiple myeloma is based upon a number of factors including stage of disease, response to anti-myeloma therapy, serum erythropoietin levels, and reimbursement policies. Newly diagnosed multiple myeloma patients with a good bone marrow capacity usually show improvement of the hemoglobin after responding to anti-myeloma therapy. Very often ESAs are not necessary. In patients with more advanced multiple myeloma, hemoglobin levels below 10 g/dL receiving chemotherapy and/or having additional chronic or acute renal failure, ESAs might be indicated. Those patients usually receive erythropoietin 40,000 units once a week or darbepoetin 200 micrograms every two to three weeks [12].

Even with an increased risk of venous thromboembolism and disease progression in association with ESAs, in selected patients, especially relapsed or refractory after multiple therapies, patients who are on chemotherapy and/or have acute or chronic renal failure might benefit from administration of erythropoietin.

REFERENCES

[1] Barille-Nion S, Bataille R. New insights in myeloma-induced osteolysis. Leuk Lymphoma 2003; 44(9): 1463-7.

[2] Giuliani N, Colla S, Rizzoli V. New insight in the mechanism of osteoclast activation and formation in multiple myeloma: focus on the receptor activator of NF-kappaB ligand (RANKL). Exp Hematol 2004; 32(8): 685-91.

[3] Roodman GD. Pathogenesis of myeloma bone disease. Blood Cells Mol Dis 2004; 32(2): 290-2.

[4] Berenson JR, Lichtenstein A, Porter L, Dimopoulos MA, Bordoni R, George S, *et al.* Long-term pamidronate treatment of advanced multiple myeloma patients reduces skeletal events. J Clin Oncol 1998; 16(2): 593-602.

[5] Berenson JR, Rosen LS, Howell A, Porter L, Coleman RE, Morley W, *et al.* Zoledronic acid reduces skeletal-related events in patients with osteolytic metastases. Cancer 2001; 1; 91(7): 1191-200.

[6] Agus ZS, Berenson JR. Treatment of hypercalcemia. In: Rosen CJ, ed. *UpToDate*. Waltham, MA 2009.

[7] Annesley TM, Burritt MF, Kyle RA. Artifactual hypercalcemia in multiple myeloma. Mayo Clin Proc 1982; 57(9): 572-5.

[8] Austin LA, Heath H, 3rd. Calcitonin: physiology and pathophysiology. N Engl J Med 1981;304(5):269-78.

[9] Deftos LJ, First BP. Calcitonin as a drug. Ann Intern Med 1981; 95(2): 192-7.

[10] Dumon JC, Magritte A, Body JJ. Nasal human calcitonin for tumor-induced hypercalcemia. Calcified Tissue Interna 1992; 51(1): 18-9.

[11] World Health Organization. Cancer pain relief and palliative care: report of a WHO expert panel. WHO Technical Report 804. Geneva; 1990.

[12] Rajkumar SV. Treatment of the Complications of Multiple Myeloma. In: Kyle RA, ed. *UpToDate*. Waltham, MA: UpToDate 2009.

[13] Terpos E, Dimopoulos MA. Myeloma bone disease: pathophysiology and management. Ann Oncol 2005; 16(8): 1223-31.

[14] Dudeney S, Lieberman IH, Reinhardt MK, Hussein M. Kyphoplasty in the treatment of osteolytic vertebral compression fractures as a result of multiple myeloma. J Clin Oncol 2002; 20(9): 2382-7.

[15] Fourney DR, Schomer DF, Nader R, Chlan-Fourney J, Suki D, Ahrar K, *et al.* Percutaneous vertebroplasty and kyphoplasty for painful vertebral body fractures in cancer patients. J Neurosurg 2003; 98(1 Suppl): 21-30.

[16] Featherstone C, Delaney G, Jacob S, Barton M. Estimating the optimal utilization rates of radiotherapy for hematologic malignancies from a review of the evidence: part II-leukemia and myeloma. Cancer 2005; 103(2): 393-401.

[17] Lecouvet F, Richard F, Vande Berg B, Malghem J, Maldague B, Jamart J, *et al.* Long-term effects of localized spinal radiation therapy on vertebral fractures and focal lesions appearance in patients with multiple myeloma. Br J Haematol 1997; 96(4): 743-5.

[18] Leigh BR, Kurtts TA, Mack CF, Matzner MB, Shimm DS. Radiation therapy for the palliation of multiple myeloma. Int J Radiat Oncol Biol Phys 1993; 25(5): 801-4.

[19] Rades D, Hoskin PJ, Stalpers LJ, Schulte R, Poortmans P, Veninga T, *et al.* Short-course radiotherapy is not optimal for spinal cord compression due to myeloma. Int J Radiat Oncol Biol Phys 2006; 64(5): 1452-7.

[20] Findlay GF. Adverse effects of the management of malignant spinal cord compression. Journal Neurol Neurosurg Psychiatry 1984; 47(8): 761-8.

[21] Young RF, Post EM, King GA. Treatment of spinal epidural metastases. Randomized prospective comparison of laminectomy and radiotherapy. J Neurosurg 1980; 53(6): 741-8.

[22] Chi JH, Gokaslan Z, McCormick P, Tibbs PA, Kryscio RJ, Patchell RA. Selecting treatment for patients with malignant epidural spinal cord compression-does age matter? results from a randomized clinical trial. Spine 2009; 34(5): 431-5.

[23] Maranzano E, Bellavita R, Rossi R, De Angelis V, Frattegiani A, Bagnoli R, *et al.* Short-course vs. split-course radiotherapy in metastatic spinal cord compression: results of a phase III, randomized, multicenter trial. J Clin Oncol 2005; 23(15): 3358-65.

[24] Rades D, Karstens JH, Hoskin PJ, Rudat V, Veninga T, Schild SE, *et al.* Escalation of radiation dose beyond 30 Gy in 10 fractions for metastatic spinal cord compression. Int J Radiat Oncol Biol Phys 2007; 67(2): 525-31.

[25] Rades D, Lange M, Veninga T, Rudat V, Bajrovic A, Stalpers LJ, *et al.* Preliminary results of spinal cord compression recurrence evaluation (score-1) study comparing short-course vs. long-course radiotherapy for local control of malignant epidural spinal cord compression. Int J Radiat Oncol Biol Phys 2009; 73(1): 228-34.

[26] Rades D, Stalpers LJ, Schulte R, Veninga T, Basic H, Engenhart-Cabilic R, *et al.* Defining the appropriate radiotherapy regimen for metastatic spinal cord compression in non-small cell lung cancer patients. Eur J Cancer 2006; 42(8): 1052-6.

[27] Rades D, Stalpers LJ, Veninga T, Schulte R, Hoskin PJ, Obralic N, *et al.* Evaluation of five radiation schedules and prognostic factors for metastatic spinal cord compression. J Clin Oncol 2005; 23(15): 3366-75.

[28] Rades D, Walz J, Stalpers LJ, Veninga T, Schulte R, Obralic N, *et al.* Short-course radiotherapy (RT) for metastatic spinal cord compression (MSCC) due to renal cell carcinoma: results of a retrospective multi-center study. Eur Urol 2006; 49(5): 846-52; discussion 52.

[29] Schiff D. Treatment and prognosis of neoplastic epidural spinal cord copression, including cauda equina syndrome. In: Posner JB, ed. *UPToDate*. Waltham, MA 2009.

[30] Rosen LS, Gordon D, Kaminski M, Howell A, Belch A, Mackey J, *et al.* Zoledronic acid vs. pamidronate in the treatment of skeletal metastases in patients with breast cancer or osteolytic lesions of multiple myeloma: a phase III, double-blind, comparative trial. Cancer J 2001; 7(5): 377-87.

[31] Licata AA. Discovery, clinical development, and therapeutic uses of bisphosphonates. Ann Pharmacother 2005 Apr; 9(4): 668-77.

[32] Fleisch H. Bisphosphonates: mechanisms of action. Endocr Rev 1998; 19(1): 80-100.

[33] Roelofs AJ, Thompson K, Gordon S, Robers JJ. Molecular mechanisms of action of bisphosphonates: current status. Clin Cancer Res 2006; 12: 6222s-30s.

[34] Marx RE, Sawatari Y, Fortin M, Broumand V. Bisphosphonate-induced exposed bone (osteonecrosis/ osteopetrosis) of the jaws: risk factors, recognition, prevention, and treatment. J Oral Maxillofac Surg 2005; 63(11): 1567-75.

[35] Badros A, Weikel D, Salama A, Goloubeva O, Schneider A, Rapoport A, *et al.* Osteonecrosis of the jaw in multiple myeloma patients: clinical features and risk factors. J Clin Oncol 2006; 24(6): 945-52.

[36] Woo SB, Hande K, Richardson PG. Osteonecrosis of the jaw and bisphosphonates. N Engl J Med 2005; 353(1): 99-102; discussion 99.

[37] Migliorati CA, Casiglia J, Epstein J, Jacobsen PL, Siegel MA, Woo SB. Managing the care of patients with bisphosphonate- associated osteonecrosis: an American Academy of Oral Medicine position paper. J Am Dent Assoc 2005; 136(12): 658-68.

[38] Woo SB, Hellstein JW, Kalmar JR. Narrative[corrected] review: bisphosphonates and osteonecrosis of the jaws. Ann Intern Med 2006; 144(10): 753-61.

[39] Bamias A, Kastritis E, Bamia C, Moulopoulos LA, Melakopoulos I, Bozas G, *et al.* Osteonecrosis of the jaw in cancer after treatment with bisphosphonates: incidence and risk factors. J Clin Oncol 2005; 23(34): 8580-7.

[40] Dimopoulos MA, Kastritis E, Anagnostopoulos A, Melakopoulos I, Gika D, Moulopoulos LA, *et al.* Osteonecrosis of the jaw in patients with multiple myeloma treated with bisphosphonates: evidence of increased risk after treatment with zoledronic acid. Haematologica 2006; 91(7): 968-71.

[41] Durie BG, Katz M, Crowley J. Osteonecrosis of the jaw and bisphosphonates. N Engl J Med 2005; 353(1): 99-102; discussion 99.

[42] Mavrokokki T, Cheng A, Stein B, Goss A. Nature and frequency of bisphosphonate-associated osteonecrosis of the jaws in Australia. J Oral Maxillofac Surg 2007 Mar; 65(3): 415-23.

[43] Zervas K, Verrou E, Teleioudis Z, Vahtsevanos K, Banti A, Mihou D, *et al.* Incidence, risk factors and management of osteonecrosis of the jaw in patients with multiple myeloma: a single-centre experience in 303 patients. Br J Haematol 2006; 134(6): 620-3.

[44] Hoff A, Toth B, Altundag K, Guarneri V, Adamus A, Nooka AK. Osteonecrosis of the jaw in patients receiving intravenous bisphosphonate therapy. J Clin Oncol 2006; 24: Abstract 8528a.

[45] Dickinson M, Prince HM, Kirsa S, Zannettino A, Gibbs SD, Mileshkin L, *et al.* Osteonecrosis of the jaw complicating bisphosphonate treatment for bone disease in multiple myeloma: an overview with recommendations for prevention and treatment. Intern Med J 2009; 39(5): 304-16.

[46] Kyle RA, Yee GC, Somerfield MR, Flynn PJ, Halabi S, Jagannath S, *et al.* American Society of Clinical Oncology 2007 clinical practice guideline update on the role of bisphosphonates in multiple myeloma. J Clin Oncol 2007; 25(17): 2464-72.

[47] American association of oral and maxillofacial surgeons position paper on bisphosphonate-related osteonecrosis of the jaws. J Oral Maxillofac Surg 2007; 65(3): 369-76.

[48] Lacy MQ, Dispenzieri A, Gertz MA, Greipp PR, Gollbach KL, Hayman SR, *et al.* Mayo clinic consensus statement for the use of bisphosphonates in multiple myeloma. Mayo Clin Proc 2006; 81(8): 1047-53.

[49] Khan AA, Sandor GK, Dore E, Morrison AD, Alsahli M, Amin F, *et al.* Canadian consensus practice guidelines for bisphosphonate associated osteonecrosis of the jaw. J Rheumatol 2008; 35(7): 1391-7.

[50] Dimopoulos MA, Kastritis E, Bamia C, Melakopoulos I, Gika D, Roussou M, *et al.* Reduction of osteonecrosis of the jaw (ONJ) after implementation of preventive measures in patients with multiple myeloma treated with zoledronic acid. Ann Oncol 2009; 20(1): 117-20.

[51] Montefusco V, Gay F, Spina F, Ambrosini MT, Maniezzo M, Farina L. Antibiotic prophylaxis before dental procedures can reduce ONJ incidence. Blood 2007; 110: 3613a.

[52] Ripamonti CI, Maniezzo M, Campa T, Fagnoni E, Brunelli C, Saibene G, *et al.* Decreased occurrence of osteonecrosis of the jaw after implementation of dental preventive measures in solid tumour patients with bone metastases treated with bisphosphonates. The experience of the National Cancer Institute of Milan. Ann Oncol 2009; 20(1): 137-45.

[53] Clinical Practice Guideline: Prevention of Bisphosphonate-Related Osteonecrosis of the Jaw (BRONJ). NSW Health 2008.

[54] Badros A, Goloubeva O, Weikel D, Rapoport P, Akpek G, Yanovich S, *et al.* Interruption of Bisphosphonates (BP) Therapy in Multiple Myeloma (MM) Patients and Osteonecrosis of the Jaw (ONJ). Blood 2006; 108: abstract 5026.

[55] Dental management of patients receiving oral bisphosphonate therapy: expert panel recommendations. J Am Dent Assoc 2006; 137(8): 1144-50.

[56] Ruggiero SL, Mehrotra B, Rosenberg TJ, Engroff SL. Osteonecrosis of the jaws associated with the use of bisphosphonates: a review of 63 cases. J Oral Maxillofac Surg 2004; 62(5): 527-34.

[57] Augustson BM, Begum G, Dunn JA, Barth NJ, Davies F, Morgan G, *et al.* Early mortality after diagnosis of multiple myeloma: analysis of patients entered onto the United kingdom Medical Research Council trials between 1980 and 2002--Medical Research Council Adult Leukaemia Working Party. J Clin Oncol 2005; 23(36): 9219-26.

[58] Chanan-Khan A, Sonneveld P, Schuster MW, Stadtmauer EA, Facon T, Harousseau JL, *et al.* Analysis of herpes zoster events among bortezomib-treated patients in the phase III APEX study. J Clin Oncol 2008; 26(29): 4784-90.

[59] Kim SJ, Kim K, Kim BS, Lee HJ, Kim H, Lee NR, *et al.* Bortezomib and the increased incidence of herpes zoster in patients with multiple myeloma. Clin Lymphoma Myeloma. 2008 Aug; 8(4): 237-40.

[60] Rajkumar SV. Treatment of relapsed or refractory multiple myeloma. In: Kyle RA, ed. *UpToDate*. Waltham, MA 2009.

[61] Dasanu CA, Alexandrescu DT. Prophylactic antivirals may be helpful in prevention of varicella-zoster virus reactivation in myeloma, but are they safe? J Oncol Pharm Pract 2009.

[62] Oken MM, Pomeroy C, Weisdorf D, Bennet JM. Prophylactic antibiotics for the prevention of early infection in multiple myeloma. Am J Med 1996; 100: 624-8.

[63] Chapel HM, Lee M, Hargreaves R, Pamphilon DH, Prentice AG. Randomised trial of intravenous immunoglobulin as prophylaxis against infection in plateau-phase multiple myeloma. The UK Group for Immunoglobulin Replacement Therapy in Multiple Myeloma. Lancet 1994; 343(8905): 1059-63.

[64] Blade J, Fernandez-Llama P, Bosch F, Montoliu J, Lens XM, Montoto S, *et al.* Renal failure in multiple myeloma: presenting features and predictors of outcome in 94 patients from a single institution. Arch Intern Med 1998; 158(17): 1889-93.

[65] Winearls CG. Acute myeloma kidney. Kidney Int 1995 Oct; 48(4): 1347-61.

[66] Rajkumar SV, Kaplan AA, Leung N. Treatment of renal failure in multiple myeloma. In: Glassock RJaK, R. A., ed. *UpToDate*. Waltham, MA 2009.

[67] Sanders PW, Booker BB. Pathobiology of cast nephropathy from human Bence Jones proteins. J Clin Invest 1992; 89(2): 630-9.

[68] Zucchelli P, Pasquali S, Cagnoli L, Ferrari G. Controlled plasma exchange trial in acute renal failure due to multiple myeloma. Kidney Int 1988; 33(6): 1175-80.

[69] Durie BG, Kyle RA, Belch A, Bensinger W, Blade J, Boccadoro M, *et al.* Myeloma management guidelines: a consensus report from the Scientific Advisors of the International Myeloma Foundation. Hematol J 2003; 4(6): 379-98.

[70] Cohen DJ, Sherman WH, Osserman EF, Appel GB. Acute renal failure in patients with multiple myeloma. Am J Med 1984; 76(2): 247-56.

[71] Holland MD, Galla JH, Sanders PW, Luke RG. Effect of urinary pH and diatrizoate on Bence Jones protein nephrotoxicity in the rat. Kidney Interna 1985; 27(1): 46-50.

[72] Murphy MF, Wallington TB, Kelsey P, Boulton F, Bruce M, Cohen H, *et al.* Guidelines for the clinical use of red cell transfusions. Br J Haematol 2001; 113(1): 24-31.

[73] Katodritou E, Dimopoulos MA, Zervas K, Terpos E. Update on the use of erythropoiesis-stimulating agents (ESAs) for the management of anemia of multiple myeloma and lymphoma. Cancer Treat Rev 2009; 35(8): 738-43.

[74] Dammacco F, Castoldi G, Rodjer S. Efficacy of epoetin alfa in the treatment of anaemia of multiple myeloma. Br J Haematol 2001; 113(1): 172-9.

[75] Garton JP, Gertz MA, Witzig TE, Greipp PR, Lust JA, Schroeder G, *et al.* Epoetin alfa for the treatment of the anemia of multiple myeloma. A prospective, randomized, placebo-controlled, double-blind trial. Arch Intern Med 1995 Oct 23; 155(19): 2069-74.

[76] Osterborg A, Boogaerts MA, Cimino R, Essers U, Holowiecki J, Juliusson G, *et al.* Recombinant human erythropoietin in transfusion-dependent anemic patients with multiple myeloma and non-Hodgkin's lymphoma--a randomized multicenter study. The European Study Group of Erythropoietin (Epoetin Beta) Treatment in Multiple Myeloma and Non-Hodgkin's Lymphoma. Blood 1996; 87(7): 2675-82.

[77] Bohlius J, Wilson J, Seidenfeld J, Piper M, Schwarzer G, Sandercock J, *et al.* Recombinant human erythropoietins and cancer patients: updated meta-analysis of 57 studies including 9353 patients. J Natl Cancer Inst 2006; 98(10): 708-14.

[78] Knight R, DeLap RJ, Zeldis JB. Lenalidomide and venous thrombosis in multiple myeloma. N Engl J Med 2006; 354(19): 2079-80.

[79] Smith RE, Jr., Aapro MS, Ludwig H, Pinter T, Smakal M, Ciuleanu TE, *et al.* Darbepoetin alpha for the treatment of anemia in patients with active cancer not receiving chemotherapy or radiotherapy: results of a phase III, multicenter, randomized, double-blind, placebo-controlled study. J Clin Oncol 2008; 26(7): 1040-50.

CHAPTER 8

Promising Clinical Trials in Multiple Myeloma

Shaji Kumar*

Divisions of Hematology and Internal Medicine, Mayo Clinic, Rochester, MN

Abstract: Treatment of multiple myeloma has undergone a significant change in the past decade due to a combination of better understanding of the disease biology, improved risk stratification models and several very effective therapies. As a result, the survival of patients with myeloma nearly doubled during this time period. However, patients eventually become refractory to current therapies and the disease remains incurable even with aggressive treatment approaches. As a result it is important to continue to develop new therapies for the disease, ideally based on better understanding of the basic disease pathophysiology. In fact several promising drugs are currently undergoing clinical evaluation for myeloma, and these drugs are at various stages of development. In this chapter, we summarize the ongoing clinical trials in the treatment of symptomatic myeloma, many of which likely will lead to effective treatments in the near future. Broadly these trials can be classified into three groups; (i) new drugs from drug classes shown to have efficacy in myeloma, (ii) new classes of drugs and (iii) combinations of new and old drugs. Other trials in myeloma are also examining different aspects of disease, including use of many of these drugs in the setting of smoldering myeloma to reduce risk of progression, use of new and current drugs in maintenance and consolidation therapy setting, as well as new drugs that are being examined as part of supportive care for myeloma.

Keywords: Pomalidomide, carfilzomib, salinosporamidine A (NPI-0052), bendamustin, HDAC inhibitors, vorinostat, panabinostat, HSP90 inhibitors, tanespimycin, AKT inhibitor, perifosin, elotuzumab

NEW DRUGS FROM EXISTING CLASSES OF ANTI-MYELOMA DRUGS

The drug classes currently forming the backbone of myeloma therapy include the IMiDs (thalidomide and lenalidomide), the proteasome inhibitor bortezomib, alkylating agents like Melphalan and cyclophosphamide, the anthracycline doxorubicin and corticosteroids. Ongoing clinical trials are evaluating a new IMiD (pomalidomide, CC4047), several new proteasome inhibitors (Carfilzomib, NPI-0052, MLN9708), and another alkylating agent (Bendamustine).

POMALIDOMIDE (ACTIMID, CC4047)

Pomalidomide is a new drug that belongs to the class of the immunomodulatory drugs (IMiDs) and is structurally related to thalidomide and lenalidomide.

Pomalidomide was first studied by Schey *et al.* in a group of relapsed patients with myeloma [1]. In this phase 1 study, twenty-four relapsed or refractory patients were treated with a escalating doses of pomalidomide. The drug was well tolerated with no serious nonhematologic adverse events. At least a minimal response was seen in two thirds of patients, including 13 (54%) who had a partial response, and four (17%) with complete remission. The maximum tolerated dose (MTD) was determined to be 2 mg/d. Additional studies in this trial suggested improvement in tumor specific immune response, suggesting that atleast part of the efficay is due to immune mechanisms.

Lacy *et al.* conducted a phase 2 trial of pomalidomide in combination with dexamethasone, in patients with relapsed myeloma. Sixty patients with relapsed myeloma were treated with pomalidomide, at a dose of 2 mg daily on days 1 through 28 of a 28-day cycle along with dexamethasone 40 mg weekly. Thirty-eight patients (63%) achieved a partial response or better, including complete response in three patients (5%),

***Address correspondence to Shaji Kumar:** Divisions of Hematology and Internal Medicine, Mayo Clinic, Rochester, MN 55905; Phone: 507-266-0523; Fax: 507-266-4972; E-mail: kumar.shaji@mayo.edu

Klaus Podar and Kenneth C. Anderson (Eds)

and very good partial response in 17 patients (28%). Importantly, responses were seen in 40% of lenalidomide-refractory patients, 37% of thalidomide-refractory patients, and 60% of bortezomib-refractory patients. The most common toxicity was myelosuppression with grade 3 or 4 hematologic toxicities being anemia (5%), thrombocytopenia (3%), and neutropenia (32%). The median progression-free survival was 11.6 months and was not significantly different in patients with high-risk disease compared with patients with standard-risk disease. In a follow up study of lenalidomide refractory patients, defined as relapsing on or within 60 days of stopping lenalidomide, pomalidomide along with dexamethasone at the same doses was highly active [2]. Patients received 2 mg daily pomalidomide along with 40 mg dexamethasone weekly in 4-week cycles. The group included nearly half of the patients with high-risk myeloma, with a median of 4 prior therapies and two thirds having received a prior autologous stem cell transplant. Grade 3 and 4 toxicities seen were primarily hematological and three patients had fatigue. The overall response rate was 32% and another 18% had a minimal response. The dose was increased to 4 mg daily in 8 patients, one of who responded. Another follow up trial evaluating the same doses in a bortezomib and lenalidomide refractory population is ongoing and a second trial examining the combination of pomalidomide and bortezomib is currently planned.

Richardson and colleagues conducted a phase 1 study of pomalidomide with dexamethasone added at progression in patients with relapsed myeloma. Thirty-two patients with a median of 7 prior therapies, including lenalidomide and bortezomib in all patients, were enrolled in this dose escalation study. The doses evaluated included 2, 3, 4 and 5 mg daily days 1-21 of a 28-day cycle. Dose limiting hematological toxicity was encountered at 5 mg and the selected dose for phase 2 evaluations was 4 mg given 3 weeks out of 4 weeks. The overall response rate (PR or better) was 28%, however nearly half of the entire group had an MR or better, similar to the previous studies. A randomized phase 2 trial evaluating pomalidomide with or without dexamethasone with dexamethasone added at progression in the latter group is underway.

CARFILZOMIB

Carfilzomib is a new proteasome inhibitor that is in phase 2 and 3 clinical trials currently. It is made up of two key elements: a peptide portion that selectively binds to the substrate binding pocket of the proteasome with high affinity and an epoxyketone pharmacophore thatspecifically interacts with the catalytic threonine residue to irreversibly inhibit enzyme activity resulting in sustained proteasome inhibition[3,4]. The irreversible mechanism, as well as its selectivity for the proteasome relative to the active sites of other protease classes results in high degree of activity. At doses of 15mg/m^2 or greater, more than 80% proteasome inhibition is achieved in PBMCs in humans. In *in vitro* studies, it had significant activity against myeloma cell lines and in animal models [3].

Two phase 1 studies initially evaluated its activity in the setting of myeloma. The 001 study explored five days of continuous dosing very 2 weeks treated 29 patients at doses ranging from 1.2 to 20 mg/m2. The MTD was determined to be 15 mg/m^2 for this dosing schedule [5]. The DLTs were thrombocytopenia and febrile neutropenia. Another phase 1 study (002 study) examined 2 consecutive days of dosing every week for 3/4 weeks and found that doses of up to 20 mg/m^2 for the first cycle followed by an increase of the dose to 27 mg/m^2 thereafter can be safely administered [6].

Jagannath *et al.* studied 46 patients with relapsed multiple myeloma with a median of 5 previous therapies, all of who had received prior lenalidomide and bortezomib. Over 80% of the group also had previous transplants. Patients received 2 daily doses every week for 3 weeks with one week off. 20 mg/m^2 PR or better was seen in 18% of patients, with another 8% obtaining a minimal response. Stable disease was seen ion 41% of the patients and the median time to progression was 5.1 months. Grade 3 and 4 toxicities were mainly hematologic in nature. In the follow up phase of this trial an additional 223 patients (total 269) were enrolled with the dose escalating to 27 mg/m^2 after first cycle and the results are awaited. Interestingly, neuropathy was not a major toxicity distinguishing this drug from bortezomib in terms of toxicity.

The PX171-004 trial evaluated the activity of single agent carfilzomib in patient with relapsed myeloma who had received 1-3 prior therapies, and included patients who were bortezomib naïve as well as those who had previously received the drug [7]. Patients received 2 consecutive doses of the drug at 20 mg/m^2 daily every week for 3 weeks with a week off. MR or better was seen in 30% of the 34 patients with previous treatment with bortezomib, including 18% PR or better. The median time to progression was 5.3 months for this group of patients. In contrast, the MR or better response rate was 61% including 46% PR or better among the 54 patients who were bortezomib naïve [7,8]. The median time to progression was 7.6 months for this cohort. Given the clinical activity of bortezomib-lenalidomide combinations in newly diagnosed and relapsed myeloma, carfilzomib has also been combined with lenalidomide in phase 1 studies. In a dose escalation study, the MTD was not reached at full dose (25 mg days 1-21) of lenalidomide and 20 mg/m2 of carfilzomib at standard dosing along with dexamethasone weekly. The overall response rate was 55% (PR or better) and an additional 21% patients had an MR. A larger randomized phase 3 trial is currently planned for this combination in the setting of relapsed disease.

NPI-0052

NPI-0052 is a novel second-generation 20S proteasome inhibitor (non-peptide based) with a rapid and prolonged inhibition of all 3 proteolytic activities. It has shown significant preclinical activity in myeloma as a single agent and in combination with lenalidomide, which formed the rational for its clinical investigation [9,10]. In a phase 1 study of NPI-0052 in patients with relapsed myeloma, the drug was administered at escalating doses on days 1, 8 and 15 of a three-week cycl [11]. Paraprotein reductions were seen and the best response included stable disease in nearly half of the patients, many of which lasted over 6 months. It has also been combined with lenalidomide with some preliminary evidence of clinical activity [12].

BENDAMUSTINE

Bendamustine hydrochloride (Treanda; Cephalon), is a DNA alkylating anticancer agent, approved by the US FDA for the treatment of chronic lymphocytic leukemia [13]. Bendamustine causes DNA damage that is thought to lead to cell death via several pathways, including apoptosis and mitotic catastrophe. A recent study suggests that bendamustine has mechanistic features that differentiate it from other alkylating agents, which might contribute to its efficacy in patients with disease refractory to these drugs [14,15].

In a Phase I study of bendamustine, Knoop *et al.* enrolled 31 patients with multiple myeloma that had progressed after high-dose chemotherapy. Bendamustine 100 mg/m^2 on days 1 and 2 per cycle was found to be the maximal tolerated dose. The overall response rate was 55% with a median progression- free survival of 26 (0 - 61) weeks. Toxicity was mild and mainly hematologic [16]. A randomized phase III study compared bendamustine and prednisone (BP) to standard Melphalan and prednisone (MP) in previously untreated patients with multiple Myeloma Patients were randomly assigned to receive BP (n=68) or MP (n=63). The overall response rate was 75% in the BP and 70% in the MP group. A significantly higher number of patients treated with BP achieved a complete remission than did patients receiving MP (32 vs. 13%; P=0.007), and the maximum response was achieved more rapidly in patients treated with BP compared to those receiving MP (6.8 vs. 8.7 cycles; P<0.02) [17].

Other trials have examined the activity of bendamustine in combination with bortezomib or IMiDs. In a phase 1 study, 28 patients with refractory or relapsed multiple myeloma were treated with fixed doses of bendamustine (60 mg/m^2) and prednisolone (100 mg), and escalating doses of thalidomide (50, 100, 200 mg) [18]. Treatment cycles were repeated every 28 d until maximum response, DLT, or disease progression. The overall response was 85% (PR or better) including a third of patients with VGPR or better. Median progression-free and overall survival for all patients was 11 and 19 months respectively. No dose limiting toxicity was seen at doses of thalidomide of up to 200 mg and the non-hematological side effects were mild to moderate. Transient grade 3-4 neutropenia was reported in 12 patients, and grade 3-4 thrombocytopenia occurred in two patients.

Lentzsch and colleagues studied the combination of bendamustine and lenalidomide in relapsed and or refractory MM [19]. Bendamustine was given on days 1 and 2, lenalidomide on days 1-21, and oral dexamethasone on days 1, 8, 15, and 22 of each 28-day cycle. At the last report, 12 patients had been treated and an MTD of bendamustine and lenalidomide had not been reached with 100mg/m2 bendamustine and 10 mg lenalidomide. An objective response was observed in 70% of patients, including 3 very good partial responses and 4 partial responses. Two patients experienced stable disease. One previous study examined the activity of benadamustine added to bortezomib and dexamethasone, in patients not responding to the doublet, demonstrating the feasibility of this combination [20]. Other larger studies are ongoing that are testing this combination.

NEW DRUG CLASSES

HDAC Inhibitors

Inhibition of histone deacetylase (HDAC) provides a novel approach for cancer treatment. Histones are part of the core proteins of nucleosomes, and acetylation and deacetylation of these proteins is involved in the regulation of gene expression. Deacetylated histones bind tightly to the phosphate backbone of DNA, inhibiting transcription by limiting access to transcription factors and RNA polymerases. Acetylation neutralizes the charge of histones resulting in a more open DNA conformation and allows transcription factors access to the DNA, resulting in expression of corresponding genes. The opposing activities of histone acetyltransferase (HAT) and HDAC control the amount of acetylation on the DNA and a balance exists between HAT and HDAC activity in normal cells, that leads to cell specific patterns of gene expression. Alteration of gene expression such as silencing of tumor suppressor genes can be brought about by altered activity of the HDAC [21]. HDAC inhibitors (HDACi) have been shown to induce differentiation, cell cycle arrest or apoptosis in cultured tumor cells, and to inhibit the growth of tumors in animal models. In addition, HDAC inhibitor treatment may also be mediated through changes in acetylation of non-histone proteins (*e.g.* HSP90, p53). Recent studies suggest that there is activity in a variety of solid and hematological tumors with suberoylanilide hydroxamic acid (SAHA), an orally administered, HDACi. SAHA has been reported to have single-agent activity in cutaneous T-cell lymphoma (CTCL), diffuse large cell lymphoma, and head and neck cancer. Similar activity has been reported in preclinical studies with valproic acid, PXD101 and MGCD0103 and in clinical studies with other HDACi, including intravenous (IV) depsipeptide and oral MS-275 [22].

SAHA: SAHA (vorinostat, Zolinza) is an oral histone deacetylase inhibitor that is currently in clinical trials. Vorinostat was approved by the United States FDA in October 2006 for the treatment of cutaneous manifestations in patients with cutaneous T-cell lymphoma who have progressive, persistent or recurrent disease on or following 2 systemic therapies. Vorinostat has also demonstrated promising preclinical activity in multiple myeloma. In a phase 1 trial of 13 patients with relapsed or refractory myeloma, oral vorinostat was generally well tolerated at 250 mg bid for 5 days each week of a 4 week cycle or 200 mg bid for 14 days/3 week cycle [23]. Modest activity was demonstrated in relapsed and/or refractory multiple myeloma.

In vitro, SAHA shows synergistic cytotoxicity with bortezomib in MM cells by disrupting aggregates of the ubiquitin conjugated aggresomes. Twenty-one patients were enrolled into a phase 1 study evaluating the combination of SAHA with bortezomib [24]. The MTD for SAHA plus Bort was 400 mg daily x 8 days plus 1.3 mg/m2 days 1, 4, 8 and 11. Myelosuppression was a commonly seen toxicity and non-hematological toxicities grade 2 and higher included fatigue, diarrhea, atrial fibrillation, shingles, and pneumonia. The overall response rate of 50% among the 16 evaluable patients. Long term results of this phase 1 trial among 9 patients receiving at least 12 cycles, showed 5 PR, 2 MR and 2 stable diseases as the best response to therapy. [25] The most common drug-related toxicities of any grade were diarrhea, nausea, and fatigue. The median time to progression was 294 days among these 9 patients. In an ongoing Phase IIb, international, multicenter, open-label study of vorinostat in combination with bortezomib in advanced MM, patients with two prior treatment regimens, including at least one bortezomib-containing regimen are being enrolled [26]. Patients will receive intravenous bortezomib 1.3 mg/m2 on Days 1, 4, 8, and 11 and oral vorinostat 400 mg once daily on Days 1-14 of each 21-day cycle. The addition of oral dexamethasone (20 mg on the day of and day after each bortezomib dose) is permitted for patients who experience disease progression after two treatment cycles or no change (stable disease) after four cycles, until further disease progression.

In another phase I clinical trial, vorinostat was combined with pegylated liposomal doxorubicin (PLD) and bortezomib in patients with relapsed/refractory MM [27]. Treatment consisted of bortezomib at 1.3mg/m^2

on days 1, 4, 8, and 11; PLD at 30mg/m2 on day 4, and escalating doses of vorinostat (200 to 400mg once daily) on days 4 through 11 of a 3-week cycle. As of last report, 6 out of 7 evaluable patients have responded to treatment, including 1 CR, 1 VGPR, and 4 PR.

Vorinostat has also been combined with lenalidomide and dexamethasone in a phase 1 trial of relapsed myeloma [28]. Patients received vorinostat daily, administered orally for 14 days with 7 days on (Days 1-7 and 15-21), combined with oral lenalidomide daily for 21 days, and oral dexamethasone 40 mg/day (Days 1, 8, 15, and 22; cycles were repeated every 28 days). Early data shows partial response in 1 patient, and minimal response in 1 patient among the 6 evaluable patients.

LBH589: LBH589 (Panabinostat) is a new chemical entity that is a potent inhibitor of DAC and HSP90 belonging to a structurally novel class of the cinnamic hydroxamic acid class of compounds, and is formulated as an oral capsule. LBH589 was devised through iterative design and combinatorial approach using *in vitro* histone deacetylase inhibition assays, activation of the p21 promoter and inhibition of the proliferation of tumor cell lines in monolayer as selection criteria. LBH589 exhibits potent antiproliferative activity against a broad range of tumor cell lines and its antiproliferative activity in the tumor cell lines is accompanied by increased histone acetylation, suggesting that LBH589 modulates the intended target.

In a Phase II, single arm, multicenter study of panobinostat in patients with relapsed MM, 20 mg/day of oral panobinostat was given on a Monday/Wednesday/Friday (MWF) dosing schedule [29]. Thirty eight patients were enrolled. Mild or moderate level of nausea, as well as fatigue or asthenia, occurred in half of the patients. The most common Grade 3/4 adverse events were cytopenias, with neutropenia, thrombocytopenia, and anemia in 32%, 26%, and 16% of patients, respectively. One patient obtained a VGPR and an MR was seen in another patient.

Panobinostat has been combined with bortezomib in a phase 1 study that had enrolled 29 patients at the time of last report [30]. Patients were treated with escalating doses of bortezomib and panobinostat up to 30 mg panobinostat given three times weekly + 1.3 mg/m2 bortezomib given on days 1, 4, 8, 11 of a three week cycle. Clinical efficacy observed includes 50% patients with a PR or better including 4 with immunofixation (IF) negative complete response (CR). Four additional patients achieved minor responses, resulting in 64% overall response rate. Responses were also seen in patients refractory to prior bortezomib, suggesting synergistic activiity. Ongoing trials are evaluating this combination further. Ongoing clinical trials are also examining the activity of panobinostat in combination with lenalidomide, Melphalan [31], and everolimus.

Hsp90 Inhibitors

Heat shock protein 90 (Hsp90) is part of a chaperone complex that interacts with a variety of intracellular client proteins to facilitate their proper folding, prevent misfolding or aggregation, and preserve their 3-dimensional conformation to a functionally competent state [32]. *In vitro* studies have suggested significant antimyeloma activity of this molecule, suppressing proliferation and survival of MM cells both *in vitro* and *in vivo* by a variety of mechanisms [33]. Hsp90 inhibition was able to negate resistance to conventional myeloma therapies as well as block the protective effects of their interaction with BMSCs.

Tanespimycin (KOS-953) is an hsp90 inhibitor that is currently in clinical evaluation. In a phase 1/2 study of tanespimycin + bortezomib in patients with relapsed/refractory MM, increasing doses of bortezomib (0.7, 1.0, or 1.3 mg/m^2) was combined with escalating doses of tanespimycin (100, 150, 220, 275, or 340 mg/m^2) given as IV infusion on days 1, 4, 8, and 11 in each 21-day cycle [34]. The MTD was highest dose tested (340 mg/m^2 tanespimycin, 1.3 mg/m2 bortezomib) and seventy-two patients were enrolled with 42 patients treated at MTD. The median number of prior regimens was 5 (range 1-15) including stem cell transplant (69%), thalidomide (74%), bortezomib (69%), and lenalidomide (28%). The overall response rates (MR or better) were 48% in the 21 bortezomib-naive patients, 22% in the 23 bortezomib-pretreated patients, and 13% in the 23 bortezomib-refractory patients. Grade 3 or 4 thrombocytopenia and neutropenia were seen in 25% and 3% of patients respectively. Another randomized phase 2 study of this combination examined three different doses of the drug with standard bortezomib dose and found similar results [35]. An ongoing phase 3 trial is evaluating this combination.

Akt Inhibitor

Perifosine is an oral, novel synthetic alkylphospholipid, with multiple effects on signal transduction pathways, including inhibition of Akt and activation of JNK. Preclinical *in vitro* studies showed that perifosine induces significant cytotoxicity in both multiple myeloma (MM) cell lines and patient MM cells resistant to conventional therapies, and augments dexamethasone (dex), doxorubicin, Melphalan and bortezomib-induced MM cell cytotoxicity [36]. *In vivo* studies showed significant antitumor activity in a human plasmacytoma mouse model. Phase I studies in solid tumors have shown that perifosine is well tolerated at a dose of up to 150mg daily, with responses also seen.

In the initial Phase II trial of perifosine, alone or in combination with dexamethasone, in relapsed or relapsed/refractory MM, patients were treated with 150mg of perifosine daily [37]. Among 25 patients evaluable for response, best response to single agent perifosine after 2 cycles was stable disease (<25% reduction in M-protein) in 6 patients (24%). Dexamethaosne was added in 15 of 25 pts with progression 3 patients with MR among the 9 evaluable for response. The most common adverse events included nausea, vomiting, diarrhea, fatigue, and increased creatinine.

Richardson *et al.* presented results of a phase 1/2 study of perifosine combined with bortezomib. The phase I stage of the study enrolled a total of 18 patients and the MTD was determined to be perifosine 50 mg qd + Vel 1.3 mg/m^2 (d 1, 4, 8, 11) in 21-day cycles. The phase II portion enrolled 66 patients with a median of 5 lines of prior treatment including bortezomib in all and lenalidomide in 75%. Most common grade 1/2 events included nausea, diarrhea, vomiting, fatigue and anorexia and grade 3/4 adverse events included thrombocytopenia, neutropenia, anemia, hyponatremia and diarrhea. The median OS for all evaluable patients was not reached with 55% patients still alive. The ORR of the combination was 38% and median OS was 16 months.

Anti-CS1 Antibody (Elotuzumab)

The cell surface glycoprotein CS1 (CD2 subset 1, CRACC, SLAMF7, CD319, or 19A24), is a member of the immunoglobulin gene superfamily and is highly and uniformly expressed on multiple myeloma cells, with restricted expression on NK cells and little to no expression on normal tissues. A humanized monoclonal IgG1 targeting CS1, a cell surface glycoprotein (Elouzumab, HuLuc63) is currently undergoing clinical trials, having shown significant *in vitro* activity in myeloma, alone and in combination with bortezomib [38,39]. Pre-clinical data indicates mechanism of action is mainly through NK-mediated ADCC.

Twenty-eight patients were enrolled into a phase 1/2 study in relapsed myeloma patients, where increasing does of the antibody was combined with lenalidomide given in the standard doses along with weekly dexamethasone. The combination was well tolerated and no DLTs were seen. The most common grade 3/4 events were myelosuppression and fatigue. The overall response (PR or better) was 82% and was 95% among the 22 patients who were lenalidomide naïve. Additional studies are ongoing.

REFERENCES

[1] Schey SA, Fields P, Bartlett JB, *et al.* Phase I study of an immunomodulatory thalidomide analog, CC-4047, in relapsed or refractory multiple myeloma. J Clin Oncol 2004; 22: 3269-3276.

[2] Lacy MQ, Gertz MA, Hayman SR, *et al.* Pomalidomide (CC4047) Plus Low Dose Dexamethasone (Pom/dex) Is Active and Well Tolerated in Lenalidomide Refractory Multiple Myeloma (MM). Blood 2009; 114: 429.

[3] Kuhn DJ, Chen Q, Voorhees PM, *et al.* Potent activity of carfilzomib, a novel, irreversible inhibitor of the ubiquitin-proteasome pathway, against preclinical models of multiple myeloma. Blood 2007; 110: 3281-3290.

[4] Parlati F, Lee SJ, Aujay M, *et al.* Carfilzomib can induce tumor cell death through selective inhibition of the chymotrypsin-like activity of the proteasome. Blood 2009; 114: 3439-3447.

[5] Orlowski RZ, Stewart K, Vallone M, *et al.* Safety and Antitumor Efficacy of the Proteasome Inhibitor Carfilzomib (PR-171) Dosed for Five Consecutive Days in Hematologic Malignancies: Phase 1 Results. ASH Annual Meeting Abstracts 2007; 110: 409.

[6] Stewart KA, O'Connor OA, Alsina M, *et al.* Phase I evaluation of carfilzomib (PR-171) in hematological malignancies: Responses in multiple myeloma and Waldenstrom's macroglobulinemia at well-tolerated doses. ASCO Meeting Abstracts 2007; 25: 8003.

[7] Siegel D, Wang L, Orlowski RZ, *et al.* PX-171-004, An Ongoing Open-Label, Phase II Study of Single-Agent Carfilzomib (CFZ) in Patients with Relapsed or Refractory Myeloma (MM); Updated Results From the Bortezomib-Treated Cohort. Blood 2009; 114: 303.

[8] Wang L, Siegel D, Kaufman JL, *et al.* Updated Results of Bortezomib-Naive Patients in PX-171-004, An Ongoing Open-Label, Phase II Study of Single-Agent Carfilzomib (CFZ) in Patients with Relapsed or Refractory Myeloma (MM). Blood 2009; 114: 302.

[9] Chauhan D, Singh AV, Ciccarelli B, *et al.* Combination of novel proteasome inhibitor NPI-0052 and lenalidomide trigger *in vitro* and *in vivo* synergistic cytotoxicity in multiple myeloma. Blood 2010; 115: 834-845.

[10] Chauhan D, Catley L, Li G, *et al.* A novel orally active proteasome inhibitor induces apoptosis in multiple myeloma cells with mechanisms distinct from Bortezomib. Cancer Cell 2005; 8: 407-419.

[11] Richardson P, Wolf JL, Jakubowiak A, *et al.* Perifosine in Combination with Bortezomib and Dexamethasone Extends Progression-Free Survival and Overall Survival in Relapsed/Refractory Multiple Myeloma Patients Previously Treated with Bortezombib: Updated Phase I/II Trial Results. Blood 2009; 114: 1869-.

[12] Jakubowiak A, Richardson P, Zimmerman TM, *et al.* Phase I Results of Perifosine (KRX-0401) in Combination with Lenalidomide and Dexamethasone in Patients with Relapsed or Refractory Multiple Myeloma (MM). Blood 2008; 112: 3691.

[13] Cheson BD. Bendamustine: a new therapeutic option for hematologic malignancies. Clin Adv Hematol Oncol 2008; 6: 631-633.

[14] Leoni LM, Bailey B, Reifert J, *et al.* Bendamustine (Treanda) displays a distinct pattern of cytotoxicity and unique mechanistic features compared with other alkylating agents. Clin Cancer Res 2008; 14: 309-317.

[15] Gaul L, Mandl-Weber S, Baumann P, Emmerich B, Schmidmaier R. Bendamustine induces G2 cell cycle arrest and apoptosis in myeloma cells: the role of ATM-Chk2-Cdc25A and ATM-p53-p21-pathways. J Cancer Res Clin Oncol 2008; 134: 245-253.

[16] Knop S, Straka C, Haen M, *et al.* The efficacy and toxicity of bendamustine in recurrent multiple myeloma after high-dose chemotherapy. Haematologica 2005; 90: 1287-1288.

[17] Ponisch W, Mitrou PS, Merkle K, *et al.* Treatment of bendamustine and prednisone in patients with newly diagnosed multiple myeloma results in superior complete response rate, prolonged time to treatment failure and improved quality of life compared to treatment with Melphalan and prednisone--a randomized phase III study of the East German Study Group of Hematology and Oncology (OSHO). J Cancer Res Clin Oncol 2006; 132: 205-212.

[18] Ponisch W, Rozanski M, Goldschmidt H, *et al.* Combined bendamustine, prednisolone and thalidomide for refractory or relapsed multiple myeloma after autologous stem-cell transplantation or conventional chemotherapy: results of a Phase I clinical trial. Br J Haematol 2008; 143: 191-200.

[19] Lentzsch S, O'Sullivan A, Lalo S, *et al.* A Phase I Study of Bendamustine Combined with Lenalidomide and Dexamethasone in Patients with Refractory or Relapsed Multiple Myeloma. Blood 2009; 114: 1856.

[20] Fenk R, Michael M, Zohren F, *et al.* Escalation therapy with bortezomib, dexamethasone and bendamustine for patients with relapsed or refractory multiple myeloma. Leuk Lymphoma 2007; 48: 2345-2351.

[21] Szyf M. DNA methylation properties: consequences for pharmacology. Trends Pharmacol Sci 1994; 15: 233-238.

[22] Saito A, Yamashita T, Mariko Y, *et al.* A synthetic inhibitor of histone deacetylase, MS-27-275, with marked *in vivo* antitumor activity against human tumors. Proc Natl Acad Sci U S A 1999; 96: 4592-4597.

[23] Richardson PG, Mitsiades CS, Colson K, *et al.* Final Results of a Phase I Trial of Oral Vorinostat (Suberoylanilide Hydroxamic Acid, SAHA) in Patients with Advanced Multiple Myeloma. Blood 2007; 110: 1179.

[24] Badros A, Philip S, Niesvizky R, *et al.* Phase I Trial of Suberoylanilide Hydroxamic Acid (SAHA) plus Bortezomib (Bort) in Relapsed Multiple Myeloma (MM) Patients (pts). ASH Annual Meeting Abstracts 2007; 110: 1168-.

[25] Jagannath S, Weber D, Sobecks R, *et al.* The Combination of Vorinostat and Bortezomib Provides Long-Term Responses in Patients with Relapsed or Refractory Multiple Myeloma. Blood 2009; 114: 3886.

[26] Siegel D, Jagannath S, Lonial S, *et al.* Update On the Phase IIb, Open-Label Study of Vorinostat in Combination with Bortezomib in Patients with Relapsed and Refractory Multiple Myeloma. Blood 2009; 114: 3890.

[27] Voorhees PM, Gasparetto C, Richards KL, *et al.* Vorinostat in Combination with Pegylated Liposomal Doxorubicin and Bortezomib for Patients with Relapsed/Refractory Multiple Myeloma: Results of a phase I study. Blood 2009; 114: 306.

[28] Siegel D, Weber D, Mitsiades CS, *et al.* A phase I study of vorinostat in combination with lenalidomide and dexamethasone in patients with relapsed or refractory multiple myeloma. Blood 2008; 112: 3705-.

[29] Wolf JL, Siegel D, Matous J, *et al.* A phase II study of oral panobinostat (LBH589) in adult patients with advanced refractory multiple myeloma. Blood 2008; 112: 2774.

[30] San-Miguel JF, Sezer O, Siegel D, *et al.* A phase IB, multi-center, open-label dose-escalation study of oral panobinostat (LBH589) and i.v. bortezomib in patients with relapsed multiple myeloma. Blood 2009; 114: 3852.

[31] Berenson JR, Yellin O, Boccia RV, *et al.* A Phase I Study of Oral Melphalan Combined with LBH589 for Patients with Relapsed or Refractory Multiple Myeloma (MM). Blood 2009; 114: 1855-.

[32] Isaacs JS, Xu W, Neckers L. Heat shock protein 90 as a molecular target for cancer therapeutics. Cancer Cell 2003; 3: 213-217.

[33] Mitsiades CS, Mitsiades NS, McMullan CJ, *et al.* Antimyeloma activity of heat shock protein-90 inhibition. Blood 2006; 107: 1092-1100.

[34] Richardson PG, Chanan-Khan AA, Lonial S, *et al.* Tanespimycin plus bortezomib demonstrates safety, activity, and effective target inhibition in relapsed/refractory myeloma patients: updated results of a phase 1/2 study. Blood 2009; 114: 2890.

[35] Badros AZ, Richardson PG, Albitar M, *et al.* Tanespimycin plus bortezomib in relapsed/refractory myeloma patients: results from the time-2 study. Blood 2009; 114: 1871.

[36] Hideshima T, Catley L, Yasui H, *et al.* Perifosine, an oral bioactive novel alkylphospholipid, inhibits Akt and induces *in vitro* and *in vivo* cytotoxicity in human multiple myeloma cells. Blood 2006; 107: 4053-4062.

[37] Richardson P, Lonial S, Jakubowiak A, *et al.* A multicenter phase II study of perifosine (KRX-0401) alone and in combination with dexamethasone (Dex) for patients with relapsed or relapsed/refractory multiple myeloma (MM). Blood 2006; 108: 3582.

[38] van Rhee F, Szmania SM, Dillon M, *et al.* Combinatorial efficacy of anti-CS1 monoclonal antibody elotuzumab (HuLuc63) and bortezomib against multiple myeloma. Mol Cancer Ther 2009; 8: 2616-2624.

[39] Tai YT, Dillon M, Song W, *et al.* Anti-CS1 humanized monoclonal antibody HuLuc63 inhibits myeloma cell adhesion and induces antibody-dependent cellular cytotoxicity in the bone marrow milieu. Blood 2008; 112: 1329-1337.

CHAPTER 9

The Multiple Myeloma Bone Marrow Microenvironment

Aldo M. Roccaro[1,2*], Angelo Vacca[3], Giuseppe Rossi[2] and Irene Ghobrial[1]

[1]Dana-Farber Cancer Institute, Harvard Medical School, Boston, MA, USA; [2]Dept. of Hematology, Spedali Civili di Brescia, Brescia, BS, Italy and [3]Dept. of Internal Medicine and Clinical Oncology, University of Bari Medical School, Bari, BA Italy

Abstract: Multiple myeloma (MM) is a plasma cell malignancy that characteristically involves extensive infiltration of bone marrow (BM), with the formation of plasmacytomas, as clusters of malignant plasma cells inside or outside the BM milieu. Despite limits to our understanding of the molecular events of neoplastic transformation in MM, substantial advances have been made in understanding the biology of the disease through the study of the BM microenvironment, which appears to be fundamental for the proliferation, survival, and resistance of myeloma; providing the preclinical evidences for targeting MM cells and BMSCs as an anti-tumor strategy in this disease.

Keywords: Bone marrow stromal cells (BMSCs), cell adhesion mediated drug resistance (CAM-DR), extracellular matrix (ECM), adhesion molecules, interleukin-6, insulin-like-growth-factor 1, vascular endothelial growth factor (VEGF), bone marrow niches, B-cell activating factor (BAFF), a proliferation-inducing ligand (APRIL), stromal derived factor-1 (SDF-1), hypoxia, BM endothelial cells (BMECs), angiogenesis.

1. INTRODUCTION

Substantial advances have been made in understanding the biology of multiple myeloma (MM) through the study of the bone marrow (BM) microenvironment, which appears to be fundamental for the proliferation, survival, and resistance of MM cells [1]. The cellular components of the bone marrow milieu include BM stromal cells or mesenchymal cells, osteoclasts (OCLs), osteoblasts (OBLs), and vascular endothelial cells (BMEC). Cytokines, such as interleukin 6 (IL-6), play important roles in the pathogenesis and progression of the disease and its pathophysiologic manifestations (Fig. **1**) [2]. BM stromal cells (BMSCs) are a major source of IL-6, which acts to promote myeloma cell survival by inhibiting apoptosis. IL-6 also contributes to bone loss in myeloma by stimulating osteoclast formation and inhibiting bone formation [2]. It has been demonstrated that malignant plasma cells interact with extracellular matrix (ECM) proteins and that these interactions protect the cells from chemotherapy- and radiation therapy-induced cell death.

MM cells home to the BM and adhere to ECM proteins and to BMSCs, a process which not only localizes tumor cells in the BM milieu but also has important functional sequelae. Specifically, adhesion of MM cells to ECM proteins confers cell adhesion mediated drug resistance (CAM-DR), and binding of MM cells to BMSCs triggers transcription and secretion of cytokines (ie, IL-6, IGF-1, or vascular endothelial growth factor [VEGF]) from BMSCs, which not only promotes growth, survival, and migration of MM cells but also further confers resistance to conventional chemotherapy [3-5]. Therefore, delineation of mechanisms mediating MM cell growth, survival and drug resistance in the BM milieu provides the framework to develop and validate novel therapeutic agents to improve the outcomes of patients with MM.

The present chapter will focus on the liquid and solid BM milieu components in order to better delineate how BM may support MM cell growth and disease progression (Fig. **1**).

2. ROLE OF ADHESION MOLECULES

Adhesion molecules mediate both homotypic and heterotypic adhesion of MM cells to either ECM proteins

***Address correspondence to Aldo M. Roccaro:** Dana-Farber Cancer Institute, 44 Binney Street, Harvard Medical School, 02115 Boston, MA, USA; E-mail: aldo_roccaro@dfci.harvard.edu

Klaus Podar and Kenneth C. Anderson (Eds)

or BMSCs [6,7]. Adhesion molecules CD44, very late antigen 4 (VLA-4, CD49d), VLA-5 (CD49e), leukocyte function-associated antigen 1 (LFA-1, CD11a), neuronal adhesion molecule (NCAM, CD56), intercellular adhesion molecule (ICAM-1, CD54), syndecan 1 (CD138), and MPC-1 mediate homing of MM cells to the BM. Subsequently, tumor cells bind to ECM proteins, ie, *via* syndecan 1 and VLA-4 on MM cells to type I collagen and fibronectin, respectively, and to BMSCs, *i.e.*, *via* VLA-4 on MM cells to VCAM-1 (CD106) on BMSCs. This MM cell adherence to BMSCs not only localizes tumor cells in the BM microenvironment but also has important functional and clinical sequelae [8]. Elevated level of serum syndecan 1 correlates with increased tumor cell mass, decreased metalloproteinase 9 activity, and poor prognosis. Furthermore, adhesion of MM cells *via* syndecan 1 to collagen induces matrix metalloproteinase 1, thereby promoting bone resorption and tumor invasion. Moreover, binding *via* VLA-4 on MM cells to fibronectin up-regulates p27Kip1 and other genetic changes, which confer CAM-DR [9,10]. Importantly, serum IL-6 and IL-6 receptors are prognostic factors in MM and reflect the proliferative fraction of MM cells within patients. CRP, an acute phase reactant synthesized in the liver in response to IL-6, can serve as a surrogate prognostic factor. IL-6 or CRP, either alone or coupled with $b_2$microglobulin as a measure of MM cell mass, provides the framework for a biologically based staging system in MM. As adhesion molecules play a crucial role in the pathogenesis of MM, targeting these molecules has provided an important platform for novel therapeutic strategies [11].

3. ROLE OF CYTOKINES IN MULTIPLE MYELOMA

Interleukin-6

Although some MM cells secrete IL-6 and grow in an autocrine fashion, IL-6 is primarily produced in BMSCs and mediates paracrine MM cell growth [2,12]. IL-6 secretion from BMSCs is up- regulated by many molecules/cytokines (*i.e.* CD40, tumor necrosis factor α [TNF-α], VEGF, IL-1ß, TGF-β) and MM cell adherence. Importantly, nuclear factor (NF)-*k*B plays a central role in cytokine- and adhesion-mediated IL-6 up-regulation, and specific inhibition of NF-*k*B blocks IL-6 secretion [13]. Many of MM cell lines and patient tumor cells respond to IL-6. Interestingly, CD45+ MM cells have recently been identified as those MM cells responsive to IL-6.

Clinically, serum IL-6 and IL-6 receptors are prognostic factors in MM and reflect the proliferative fraction of MM cells within patients. CRP, an acute phase reactant synthesized in the liver in response to IL-6, can serve as a surrogate prognostic factor [14]. IL-6 or CRP, either alone or coupled with $b_2$microglobulin as a measure of MM cell mass, provides the framework for a biologically based staging system in MM. Attempts to target IL-6 in treatment strategies to date have included antibodies to IL-6 and IL-6 receptor, as well as IL-6 superantagonists that bind to IL-6R but do not trigger downstream signaling. To date, however, only transient responses have been observed [15].

Insulin-Like Growth Factor 1

Insulin-like growth factor 1 (IGF-1) is a multifunctional peptide that regulates cell proliferation, differentiation, and apoptosis [16]. In the circulation, IGF-I binds primarily to the main IGF binding protein, IGFBP-3. Several studies of risk in malignancies including lung, breast, prostate, and colorectal cancer suggest that high concentrations of circulating IGF-1 are associated with an increased risk of cancer, whereas high IGFBP-3 concentrations are associated with a decreased risk. However, the direct relationship of serum IGF-1 level and prognosis in MM has not yet been clarified. Indeed mean IGF-1 level does not differ between myeloma patients and controls. However, IGF-1 was a strong indicator of prognosis53. Therapies targeting IGF-1, such as inhibitors of IGF-1 receptor, have already have shown preclinical anti-MM activity and will undergo clinical evaluation [17].

Vascular Endothelial Growth Factor (VEGF)

VEGF is a known angiogenic factor in both solid tumor and hematologic malignancies [18]. In MM, it is produced both by MM cells and BMSCs and may account, at least in part, for the increased angiogenesis observed in MM patients's BM [19]. It has been shown that increased microvessel density (MVD) in MM patients'BM specimens is associated with poor prognosis, and BM MVD at diagnosis is an important prognostic factor for survival of patients who undergo autologous transplantation as frontline therapy [14,20].

BAFF and APRIL

B-cell activating factor (BAFF) and a proliferation-inducing ligand (APRIL) have also been shown to promote MM cell growth [21-24]. Previous studies have shown that the production for BAFF and APRIL is the BM environment, and that production is mainly by monocytes and neutrophils [25]. In addition, osteoclasts produce very high levels of APRIL, unlike BM stromal cells. MM cells express TACI (transmembrane activator and calcium modulator and cyclophilin ligand interactor), the receptor of BAFF/APRIL, at varying levels64. These factors also activate nuclear factor (NF)-*k*B, phosphatidylinositol-3 (PI-3) kinase/AKT, and mitogen-activated protein kinase (MAPK) kinase pathways, and protect MM cells from dexamethasone-induced apoptosis [23].

4. BM MILIEU AND ITS ABILITY TO MODULATE TRAFFICKING OF MM CELLS

MM is characterized by the presence of multiple lytic lesions in most patients indicating continuous spread of MM cells into and out of the BM [26]. Indeed, studies have demonstrated the presence of a small number of circulating plasma cells in over 70% of patients with MM [27], indicating that progression of MM occurs through the continuous trafficking of malignant cells to new sites of the BM. Therefore, adhesion of MM cells to the bone marrow niches is not a static process, but an active dynamic process that involves migration of the malignant cells to the specific bone marrow niches, adhesion to the microenvironment, and egress or mobilization of some of these cells into the peripheral circulation to home to other new sites in the bone marrow.

Migration of cells through the blood to the bone marrow niches requires active navigation, a process termed homing. Homing is thought to be a coordinated, multistep process, which involves signaling by stromal derived factor-1 (SDF-1), and its chemokine receptor CXCR4, activation of adhesion receptors such as lymphocyte function–associated antigen 1 (LFA-1), very late antigen (VLA-4/5), cytoskeleton rearrangement, and activation of metalloproteases MMP2/9 [28-30]. Other cytokines that also regulate migration of MM cells include VEGF and IGF-1. Studies of chemokine receptors in multiple myeloma have demonstrated that MM cell lines express high levels of CXCR3, CXCR4, CCR1 and CCR6. The ligands of these receptors are MIP-1α, MIP-1β, SDF-1, CXC, and RANTES. Of these, the CXCR4/SDF-1 axis plays a critical role in regulating migration and adhesion of MM cells. Studies to identify expression of chemokine receptors in MM have shown large variations in CXCR4 expression ranging from 10 to 100% [31]. SDF-1 induces migration of MM cells *in vitro* and homing into the bone marrow *in vivo*. In addition, SDF-1 induces modest proliferation of MM cells, as well phosphorylation of MEK1/2, p42/44 MAPK, and AKT in a time-dependent fashion in MM cell lines and primary MM cells [32]. CXCR4 is essential for the migration of MM cells *in vitro* and their homing *in vivo* [33]. CXCR4 knockdown led to significant inhibition of migration to SDF-1 in MM cell lines and primary CD138+ cells [33].

Mobilization or egress of cells out of the bone marrow could be enhanced by disrupting the SDF-1/CXCR4 axis. This may occur by decreasing the concentration of endogenous SDF-1 (*e.g.*, after infusion of G-CSF or cyclophosphamide) in BM as performed for stem cell transplant in MM [34], or by the cleavage and inactivation of SDF-1 by proteases in the BM [35]; or by upregulation of CXCR4 expression by hypoxia. Mobilization of stem cells from the BM may also occur if CXCR4 is inhibited [36]. Inhibitors of CXCR4 such as plerixafor have been shown to induce mobilization of stem cells [37,38]. Plerixafor (Genzyme, MA) is a bicyclam molecule that reversibly blocks the binding of CXCR4 with SDF-1 [39]. A recent report showed that the CXCR4 inhibitor plerixafor induced disruption of the interaction of MM cells with the bone marrow reflected by mobilization of MM cells into the circulation *in vivo*, with kinetics that differed from that of hematopoeitic stem cells [40]. Plerixafor enhanced sensitivity to bortezomib *in vitro* by disrupting adhesion of MM cells to stromal cells, with the combination of plerixafor and bortezomib induces significant tumor reduction in this experiment [40].

5. HYPOXIC BM MAY SUPPORT DISSEMINATION OF MM CELLS

MM is characterized by the disseminated involvement of the BM, and its progression involves a continuous circulation of the MM cells in the peripheral blood and homing back to the BM. Several reports have described the mechanism involved in homing of MM cells to the BM. However, the driving force to metastasize from one site of the BM to another is not yet understood. Hypoxia has been shown to be associated with poor patient prognosis in solid tumors, and several studies have shown that BM has a hypoxic nature. Therefore, Azab and Coll. have hyothesized that the hypoxic nature of the BM and the rapid development of MM may cause induction of hypoxia in the tumor microenvironment, induce stress in the MM cells, and drive them to disseminate to new BM niches with normal oxygen levels [41]. Authors have tested the level of oxygenation of MM cells and cells from its BM microenvironment by injection of pimonidazole (PIM) to mice with MM and determined the levels of PIM binding in MM cells and stromal cells in the microenvironment by flow cytometry. The whole cells population in the BM was hypoxic, while the MM cells were more hypoxic compared to cells in the microenvironment. These results *in vitro* by incubation of MM cells in hypoxic conditions. Induction of hypoxia was also verified by detection of increased binding of PIM by flow cytometry, and increased levels of HIF1 and HIF2 in MM cells by immunoblotting. MTT assay showed that hypoxia significantly decreased the survival of MM cells. Immunoblotting showed a downregulation of proliferative signaling pathway, including PI3K, AKT, mTOR and ERK; and induction of stress pathways including MKK-3 and 6, and p38. While hypoxia did not induce apoptosis, G1-phase cell cycle arrest was observed under hypoxic conditions. Importantly, hypoxic MM cells were 50% less adherent to BMSCs compared to normoxic MM cells. Also, hypoxic BMSCs induced 30% less adhesion of MM cells compared to normoxic BMSCs. Mechanistically, immunoblotting showed a significant decrease in the expression of cadherins in both hypoxic MM cells and hypoxic BMSCs. The chemokine stromal-cell derived factor-1-alpha (SDF1) is known to increase adhesive properties of MM cells, and to induce MM retention in the BM. Testing the levels of SDF1 revealed that hypoxia decreased SDF1 secretion (40%) from BMSCs. As a result, media from hypoxic BMSCs induce significantly decreased MM cell chemotaxis (20%) compared to media from normoxic BMSCs. These findings suggest that hypoxic BM will retain less MM cells in the BM and allow more egression. Comparison of the ability of hypoxic and normoxic MM cells to migrate towards normoxic BMSCs or SDF1 revealed that hypoxic MM cells had increased chemotactic properties compared to normoxic MM cells. These findings correlated with the increased expression of CXCR4 on hypoxic MM cells. These results suggest that hypoxic MM cells will home to normoxic BM niches more efficiently than normoxic MM cells. These findings suggest that hypoxia inhibited the proliferation of MM cells and decreased their adhesion to BMSCs, as a first step of egress and metastasize to new normoxic BM niches.

6. ENDOTHELIAL CELLS AND ANGIOGENSIS IN MM

BM angiogenesis represents a constant hallmark of MM progression, partly driven by release of pro-angiogenic cytokines from the tumor plasmacells, fibroblasts and osteoclasts, such as vascular endothelial growth factor (VEGF), basic-fibroblast growth factor (bFGF) and metalloproteinases (MMPs).

BM endothelial cells (BMEC) are also involved in the initial homing of myeloma cells to the BM stromal compartment, and medullary angiogenesis in active MM is driven by the paracrine activation of BMEC by angiogenic cytokines and proteases secreted by myeloma cells, fibroblasts, and osteoclasts. The adhesion between MM cells and BMSCs up-regulates many cytokines with angiogenic activity, most notably VEGF and basic fibroblast growth factor (bFGF) [18]. In myeloma cells, these angiogenic factors may also be produced constitutively as a result of oncogene activation and/or genetic mutations [42].

Evidence for the importance of angiogenesis in the pathogenesis of MM was obtained from BM samples from MM patients [20]. The level of BM angiogenesis, as assessed by grading and/or MVD, is consistently increased in patients with active MM as compared to those with inactive disease or MGUS, a less advanced plasma cell disorder [20]. Among patients with active MM, MVD has been directly correlated with the degree of plasma cell proliferation and infiltration, revealing MVD to be an adverse prognostic marker [43].

BMSC from MM patients were found to express VEGF and bFGF in addition to several other proangiogenic molecules, including angiopoietin 1 (Ang-1), TGF-β, PDGF, HGF, IL-1, and others [44]. An analysis in newly diagnosed MM found a correlation between MVD, syndecan 1 (in blood and BM), and level of serum HGF [45].

Therefore, role of primary BMECs has been investigated and have been shown to directly support MM cell growth. DNA array has been performed on BMECs derived from 10 patients with MM and showed enhanced expression of tumor vascular phase-inducers, suah as bFGF, several VEGF isoforms, Tie2/Tek, TGF-b receptor 1, fibronectin, osteopontin and many others. [46], in contrast with normal human umbilical vein endothelial cells (HUVECs) that expressed lower amount of growth factors genes. BMECs are therefore indicative of both a vasculogenic and an angiogenic state in patients with MM and may form an organized vascular network on matrigel more rapidly and efficiently than HUVECs, showing a growth advantage over HUVECs together with a high intrinsic ability to form vessels, perhaps due to the autocrine loops of wroth (*i.e.* VEGF/VEGF-R; bFGF-bFGF-R). Interestingly these data have been further confirmed and validated in the *in vivo* chorio-allantoic membrane assay [46].

To determine a "gene/molecular fingerprint" of multiple myeloma endothelial cells; and to identify vascular mechanisms governing the malignant progression from quiescent monoclonal gammopathy of undetermined significance, comparative gene expression profiling of multiple myeloma endothelial cells and monoclonal gammopathy of undetermined significance endothelial cells has been recently performed [47]. Twenty-two genes were found differentially expressed at relatively high stringency in multiple myeloma endothelial cells compared with monoclonal gammopathy of undetermined significance endothelial cells. Functional annotation revealed a role of these genes in the regulation of extracellular matrix formation and bone remodeling, cell adhesion, chemotaxis, angiogenesis, resistance to apoptosis, and cell-cycle regulation. The small interfering RNA knockdown of BNIP3, IER3, and SEPW1 genes affected critical multiple myeloma endothelial cell functions correlated with the overangiogenic phenotype. The distinct endothelial cell gene expression profiles and vascular phenotypes detected in this study may influence remodeling of the bone marrow microenvironment in patients with active multiple myeloma. Among extracellular matrix-related proteins, COL6A1 and COL6A3, responsible for cell anchorage to the extracellular matrix [48], were down-regulated in multiple myeloma endothelial cells, which may account for the increased migration of multiple myeloma endothelial cells and fast sprouting of neovessels in active multiple myeloma patients [49]. In contrast, COL4A1, a major component of the vascular basement membranc, was up-regulated and probably provides a track support for the assembly and maturation of newly formed multiple myeloma microvessels. COL4A1 is closely involved in angiogenesis, one reason being that it is a substrate of metalloproteinase-2 and matrix metalloproteinase-9 secreted by multiple myeloma plasma cells and multiple myeloma endothelial cells [49].

In addition, genes involved in cell proliferation, such as serglycin (SRGN) and epidermal growth factor receptor (EGFR) [50], were respectively up-and down-regulated in multiple myeloma endothelial cells. The LIM domain binding 2 (LDB2), involved in the maintenance of cell homeostasis [51], and SEPW1, a gene with antioxidant function [52], were espectively down-and up-regulated in multiple myeloma endothelial cells. SEPW1-mediated homeostasis seems to be crucial for angiogenesis in multiple myeloma because small interfering RNA–silenced expression of the gene inhibited multiple myeloma endothelial cell adhesion and angiogenic activity.

Overall, these evidences suggest that BMECs present with functional, genetic and morphologic features indicating their ability to induce BM-neovacsularization; resulting in MM cells growth; and disease progression; providing preclinical evidences for using anti-angiogenic compounds in the treatment of MM.

7. OSTEOCLAST IN MULTIPLE MYELOMA

Osteolytic bone lesions develop in over 70-80% of patients throughout the axial skeleton and are one of the major sources of morbidity and mortality for patients with MM [53]. These lesions are frequently associated with severe and debilitating bone pain, and pathologic fractures [54]. The usual balance between bone resorption and new bone formation is lost in many cases of MM, resulting in bone destruction and the development of osteolytic lesions [55]. Bone destruction develops adjacent to MM cells, yet not in areas of normal bone marrow. Furthermore, new bone formation, which would normally develop at sites of prior bone destruction, is absent and there is evidence, at these sites of apoptotic osteoblasts [56]. The lack of osteoblasts explains why nuclear medicine bone scans underestimate the degree of bone destruction in patients with MM. The bone lesions that develop rarely heal, even when patients are in a complete remission. As a consequence of increased bone resorption, nearly 15% of MM patients develop hypercalcemia. The combination of hypercalcemia, pathologic fractures, nerve compression and severe bone pain lead to significant morbidity and mortality for patients with MM [57].

There are several factors implicated in osteoclast activation, including receptor activator of NF-κB ligand (RANKL), macrophage inflammatory protein-1a (MIP-1a), interleukin-3 (IL-3), and interleukin-6 (IL-6) [58]. RANK ligand is a member of the tumor necrosis factor (TNF) family and plays a major role in the increased osteoclastogenesis implicated in MM bone disease [58]. MM cell binding to neighboring stromal cells within the bone marrow of patients with MM results in increased RANKL expression. This leads to an increase in osteoclast activity through the binding of RANKL to its receptor, on osteoclast precursor cells, which further promotes their differentiation [59]. RANKL is also involved in inhibition of osteoclast apoptosis.

8. OSTEOBLAST IN MULTIPLE MYELOMA

There are reports indicating that osteoblasts may contribute to MM pathogenesis by supporting MM cells growth and survival [60]. This could potentially result from the ability of osteoblasts secrete IL-6 in cocolture system with MM cells, thus increasing IL-6 levels within the BM milieu and therefore inducing MM plasmacells growth. Other mechanisms include the possible role of osteoblast in stimulating MM cells survival by blocking TRAIL-mediated programmed MM cell death, by secreting osteoprotegerin, a decoy receptor for either RANKL and TRAIL. Further *in vitro* evidences have been demonstrated that osteoblasts could reduce the stimulatory effect of osteoclasts on MM cells survival [61]. Interestingly, these *in vitro* data have been validated *in vivo*, where MM cell growth was inhibited by stimulating bone formation in SCID-hu MM model [60].

Several factors are felt to be responsible for suppression of osteoblast activity in MM and the precise mechanisms through which they execute their effect is currently under investigation. Some of these markers include: IL-3, dickkopf 1 (DKK1), secreted frizzled-related protein-2 and IL-7 [62-65]. Certain factors (DKK1 and sFRP-2) appear to affect the Wnt signaling pathway, critical for osteoblast differentiation [66], while others (IL-3 and IL-7) do not appear to directly affect this signaling pathway. These are soluble inhibitors of signaling pathways which affect osteoblast differentiation and not osteoblast survival, suggesting that their inhibitory effects should be reversible when MM cells are no longer present [67]. DKK1 plays an important role in osteoblast suppression in myeloma [65]. DKK1 is secreted by MM cells and it inhibits osteoblast differentiation. A high correlation of DKK1 gene expression levels with the extent of bone disease was demonstrated in MM patients. A soluble inhibitor of the Wnt signaling pathway, it is produced by osteoblasts and plays a critical role in osteoblast differentiation [64,65]. In contrast, other investigators have found DKK1 not to be expressed by MM cells [64,65], no evidence of upregulation following MM cell binding to preosteoblasts, and an absence of blockade on the inhibitory effects of MM cell lines on human osteoblast differentiation when treated with antibody to DKK1. A more recent study showed that levels of DKK1 were elevated in patients with MM as compared to either those with MGUS or normal controls. A sustained decrease in levels following autologous stem cell transplantation correlated with a normalization of markers of bone turnover, suggesting a return of osteoblast activity [68]. Another study demonstrated that treating severe combined immunodeficiency (SCID) mice implanted with rabbit bone rudiments containing primary myeloma cells with an antibody to DKK1 decreased bone destruction, increased bone formation, and decreased tumor growth [69].

CONCLUSIONS

Based on the understanding of interaction between BMSCs and MM cells, new therapeutical approaches have been established, in order to better target not only the MM cell clone, but also the BM milieu which has been clearly shown to support MM cell growth and disease progression. These new small molecules, used either alone or in combination with steroids or conventional agents, offer promising results to improve patient outcome. Further research will be required to better define genetic and epigenetic modification of the BM milieu component, thereby providing the framework for developing more selective; more potent; and less toxic targeted MM therapies.

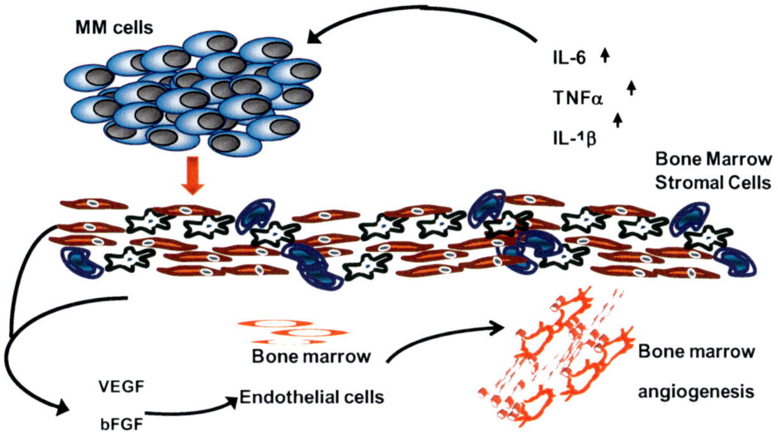

Fig. (1). Crosstalk between bone marrow stromal cells and myeloma cells.

REFERENCES

[1] Roodman GD. Role of the bone marrow microenvironment in multiple myeloma. J Bone Miner Res 2002; 17: 1921-5.

[2] Hideshima T, Nakamura N, Chauhan D, Anderson KC. Biologic sequelae of interleukin-6 induced PI3-K/Akt signaling in multiple myeloma. Oncogene 2001; 20: 5991-6000.

[3] Damiano JS, Dalton WS. Integrin-mediated drug resistance in multiple myeloma. Leuk Lymphoma. 2000; 38: 71-81.

[4] Damiano JS. Integrins as novel drug targets for overcoming innate drug resistance. Curr Cancer Drug Targets 2002; 2: 37-43.

[5] Damiano JS, Cress AE, Hazlehurst LA, Shtil AA, and Dalton WS. Cell adhesion mediated drug resistance (CAM-DR): Role of integrins and resistance to apoptosis in human myeloma cell lines. Blood 1999; 93: 1658-67.

[6] Uchiyama H, Barut BA, Chauhan D, Cannistra SA, Anderson KC. Characterization of adhesion molecules on human myeloma cell lines. Blood 1992; 80: 2306-14.

[7] Podar K, Richardson PG, Hideshima T, Chauhan D, Anderson KC. The malignant clone and the bone-marrow environment. Best Pract Res Clin Haematol 2007; 20: 597-612.

[8] Uchiyama H, Barut BA, Mohrbacher AF, Chauhan D, Anderson KC. Adhesion of human myeloma-derived cell lines to bone marrow stromal cells stimulates interleukin-6 secretion. Blood 1993; 82: 3712-20.

[9] Chauhan D, Uchiyama H, Akbarali Y, *et al.* Multiple myeloma cell adhesion-induced interleukin-6 expression in bone marrow stromal cells involves activation of NF-kappa B. Blood 1996; 87: 1104-12.

[10] Shain KH, Yarde DN, Meads MB, *et al.* Beta1 integrin adhesion enhances IL-6-mediated STAT3 signaling in myeloma cells: implications for microenvironment influence on tumor survival and proliferation. Cancer Res 2009; 69: 1009-15.

[11] Schmidmaier R, Baumann P. ANTI-ADHESION evolves to a promising therapeutic concept in oncology. Curr Med Chem 2008; 15: 978-90.

[12] Hideshima T, Podar K, Chauhan D, Anderson KC. Cytokines and signal transduction. Best Pract Res Clin Haematol 2005; 18: 509-24.

[13] Chauhan D, Kharbanda S, Ogata A, *et al.* Interleukin-6 inhibits Fas-induced apoptosis and stress-activated protein kinase activation in multiple myeloma cells. Blood 1997; 89: 227-34.

[14] Guo YQ, Chen SL.[The significance of IGF-1, VEGF, IL-6 in multiple myeloma progression]. Zhonghua Xue Ye Xue Za Zhi 2006; 27: 231-234.

[15] Richardson P, Mitsiades C, Schlossman R, *et al.* The treatment of relapsed and refractory multiple myeloma. Hematology. Am Soc Hematol Educ Prog 2007; 2007: 317-323.

[16] Pene F, Claessens YE, Muller O, *et al.* Role of the phosphatidylinositol 3-kinase/Akt and mTOR/P70S6-kinase pathways in the proliferation and apoptosis in multiple myeloma. Oncogene 2002; 21: 6587-97.

[17] Mitsiades CS, Mitsiades NS, McMullan CJ, *et al.* Inhibition of the insulin-like growth factor receptor-1 tyrosine kinase activity as a therapeutic strategy for multiple myeloma, other hematologic malignancies, and solid tumors. Cancer Cell 2004; 5: 221-30.

[18] Podar K, Anderson KC. The pathophysiologic role of VEGF in hematologic malignancies: therapeutic implications. Blood 2005; 105: 1383-95.

[19] Le Gouill S, Podar K, Amiot M, *et al.* VEGF induces Mcl-1 up-regulation and protects multiple myeloma cells against apoptosis. Blood 2004; 104: 2886-92.

[20] Kumar S, Gertz MA, Dispenzieri A, *et al.* Prognostic value of bone marrow angiogenesis in patients with multiple myeloma undergoing high-dose therapy. Bone Marrow Transplant 2004; 34: 235-9.

[21] Rossi J, Moreaux J, Rose M, *et al.* Phase I/II study of atacicept (TACI-Ig) to neutralize APRIL and BLyS in patients with refractory or relapsed multiple myeloma (MM) or active previously treated Waldenstrom's macroglobulinemia (WM). Blood 2006; 108: abstract 3578.

[22] Moreaux J, Sprynski AC, Dillon SR, *et al.* APRIL and TACI interact with syndecan-1 on the surface of multiple myeloma cells to form an essential survival loop. Eur J Haematol 2009; 83: 119-29.

[23] Moreaux J, Legouffe E, Jourdan E, *et al.* BAFF and APRIL protect myeloma cells from apoptosis induced by interleukin 6 deprivation and dexamethasone. Blood 2004; 103: 3148-57.

[24] Moreaux J, Hose D, Jourdan M, *et al.* TACI expression is associated with a mature bone marrow plasma cell signature and C-MAF overexpression in human myeloma cell lines. Haematologica 2007; 92: 803-11.

[25] Moreaux J, Cremer FW, Reme T, *et al.* The level of TACI gene expression in myeloma cells is associated with a signature of microenvironment dependence versus a plasmablastic signature. Blood 2005; 106: 1021-30.

[26] Kyle RA, Rajkumar SV. Multiple myeloma. N Engl J Med 2004; 351: 1860-73.

[27] Nowakowski GS, Witzig TE, Dingli D, *et al.* Circulating plasma cells detected by flow cytometry as a predictor of survival in 302 patients with newly diagnosed multiple myeloma. Blood 2005; 106: 2276-9.

[28] Lapidot T, Dar A, Kollet O. How do stem cells find their way home? Blood 2005; 106: 1901-10.

[29] Avecilla ST, Hattori K, Heissig B, *et al.* Chemokine-mediated interaction of hematopoietic progenitors with the bone marrow vascular niche is required for thrombopoiesis. Nat Med 2004; 10: 64-71.

[30] Kollet O, Shivtiel S, Chen YQ, *et al.* HGF, SDF-1, and MMP-9 are involved in stress-induced human CD34+ stem cell recruitment to the liver. J Clin Invest 2003; 112: 160-69.

[31] Moller C, Stromberg T, Juremalm M, Nilsson K, Nilsson G. Expression and function of chemokine receptors in human multiple myeloma. Leukemia 2003; 17: 203-10.

[32] Hideshima T, Chauhan D, Hayashi T, *et al.* The biological sequelae of stromal cell-derived factor-1alpha in multiple myeloma. Mol Cancer Ther 2002; 1: 539-44.

[33] Alsayed Y, Ngo H, Runnels J, *et al.* Mechanisms of regulation of CXCR4/SDF-1 (CXCL12)-dependent migration and homing in multiple myeloma. Blood 2007; 109: 2708-17.

[34] Petit I, Szyper-Kravitz M, Nagler A, *et al.* G-CSF induces stem cell mobilization by decreasing bone marrow SDF-1 and up-regulating CXCR4. Nat Immunol 2002; 3: 687-94.

[35] Lapidot T. Mechanism of human stem cell migration and repopulation of NOD/SCID and B2mnull NOD/SCID mice. The role of SDF-1/CXCR4 interactions. Ann N Y Acad Sci 2001; 938: 83-95.

[36] Flomenberg N, Devine SM, Dipersio JF, *et al.* The use of AMD3100 plus G-CSF for autologous hematopoietic progenitor cell mobilization is superior to G-CSF alone. Blood 2005; 106: 1867-74.

[37] Broxmeyer HE, Orschell CM, Clapp DW, *et al.* Rapid mobilization of murine and human hematopoietic stem and progenitor cells with AMD3100, a CXCR4 antagonist. J Exp Med 2005; 201: 1307-18.

[38] Grignani G, Perissinotto E, Cavalloni G, Carnevale Schianca F, Aglietta M. Clinical use of AMD3100 to mobilize CD34+ cells in patients affected by non-Hodgkin's lymphoma or multiple myeloma. J Clin Oncol 2005; 23: 3871-3872; author reply 3872-3.

[39] De Clercq E. Potential clinical applications of the CXCR4 antagonist bicyclam AMD3100. Mini Rev Med Chem 2005; 5: 805-24.

[40] Azab AK, Runnels JM, Pitsillides C, *et al.* The CXCR4 inhibitor AMD3100 disrupts the interaction of multiple myeloma cells with the bone marrow microenvironment and enhances their sensitivity to therapy. Blood 2009; 113: 4341-51.

[41] Azab AK, Quang P, Azab F, *et al.* Role of hypoxia in the progression and dissemination of multiple myeloma. Blood 2009; abstract
[42] Rajkumar SV, Witzig TE. A review of angiogenesis and antiangiogenic therapy with thalidomide in multiple myeloma. Cancer Treat Rev 2000; 26: 351-62.
[43] Rajkumar SV, Kyle RA. Angiogenesis in multiple myeloma. Semin Oncol 2001; 28: 560-4.
[44] Alexandrakis MG, Passam FJ, Ganotakis E, *et al.* Bone marrow microvascular density and angiogenic growth factors in multiple myeloma. Clin Chem Lab Med 2004; 42: 1122-6.
[45] Scudla V, Budikova M, Pika T, *et al.* Comparison of serum levels of selected biological parameters in monoclonal gammopathy of undetermined significance and multiple myeloma. Vnitr Lek 2006; 52: 232-40.
[46] Vacca A, Ria R, Semeraro F, *et al.* Endothelial cells in the bone marrow of patients with multiple myeloma. Blood 2003; 102: 3340-8.
[47] Ria R, Todoerti K, Berardi S, *et al.* Gene expression profiling of bone marrow endothelial cells in patients with multiple myeloma. Clin Cancer Res 2009; 15: 5369-78.
[48] Aumailley M, Mann K, von der Mark H, Timpl R. Cell attachment properties of collagen type VI and Arg-Gly-Asp dependent binding to its α2 (VI) and α3 (VI) chains. Exp Cell Res 1989; 181: 463–74.
[49] Vacca A, Ria R, Semeraro F, *et al.* Endothelial cells in the bone marrow of patients with multiple myeloma. Blood 2003; 102: 3340–8.
[50] Schäfer H, Diebel J, Arlt A, Trauzold A, Schmidt WE. The promoter of human p22/PACAP response gene 1 (PRG1) contains functional binding sites for the p53 tumor suppressor and for NFκB. FEBS Lett 1998; 436: 139–43.
[51] Ueki N, Seki N, Yano K, *et al.* Isolation and chromosomal assignment of human genes encoding cofactor of LIM homeodomain proteins, CLIM1 and CLIM2. J Hum Genet 1999; 44: 112–5.
[52] Loflin J, Lopez N, Whanger PD, Kioussi C. Selenoprotein W during development and oxidative stress. J Inorg Biochem 2006; 100: 1679–84.
[53] Callander NS, Roodman GD. Myeloma bone disease. Semin Hematol 2001; 38: 276-285.
[54] Melton LJ, 3rd, Kyle RA, Achenbach SJ, Oberg AL, Rajkumar SV. Fracture risk with multiple myeloma: a population-based study. J Bone Miner Res 2005; 20: 487-93.
[55] Bataille R, Chappard D, Marcelli C, *et al.* Mechanisms of bone destruction in multiple myeloma: the importance of an unbalanced process in determining the severity of lytic bone disease. J Clin Oncol 1989; 7: 1909-14.
[56] Taube T, Beneton MN, McCloskey EV, Rogers S, Greaves M, Kanis JA. Abnormal bone remodelling in patients with myelomatosis and normal biochemical indices of bone resorption. Eur J Haematol 1992; 49: 192-8.
[57] Roodman GD. Pathogenesis of myeloma bone disease. Blood Cells Mol Dis 2004; 32:290-2.
[58] Roodman GD. Pathogenesis of myeloma bone disease. Leukemia 2009; 23:435-41.
[59] Ehrlich LA, Roodman GD. The role of immune cells and inflammatory cytokines in Paget's disease and multiple myeloma. Immunol Rev 2005; 208: 252-66.
[60] Karadag A, Oyajobi BO, Apperley JF, *et al.* Human myeloma cells promote the production of interleukin-6 by primary human osteoblasts. Br J Haematol 2000; 108: 383-90.
[61] Yacobby S, Wezeman MJ, Zangari M, *et al.* Inhibitory effects of osteoblasts and increased bone formation on myeloma in novel culture systems and a myelomatous mouse model. Haematologica 2006; 91: 192-9.
[62] Ehrlich LA, Chung HY, Ghobrial I, *et al.* IL-3 is a potential inhibitor of osteoblast differentiation in multiple myeloma. Blood 2005; 106: 1407-14.
[63] Giuliani N, Colla S, Morandi F, *et al.* Myeloma cells block RUNX2/CBFA1 activity in human bone marrow osteoblast progenitors and inhibit osteoblast formation and differentiation. Blood 2005; 106: 2472-83.
[64] Oshima T, Abe M, Asano J, *et al.* Myeloma cells suppress bone formation by secreting a soluble Wnt inhibitor, sFRP-2. Blood 2005; 106: 3160-5.
[65] Tian E, Zhan F, Walker R, *et al.* The role of the Wnt-signaling antagonist DKK1 in the development of osteolytic lesions in multiple myeloma. N Engl J Med 2003; 349: 2483-94.
[66] Canalis E, Deregowski V, Pereira RC, Gazzerro E. Signals that determine the fate of osteoblastic cells. J Endocrinol Invest 2005; 28: 3-7.
[67] Huston A, Roodman GD. Role of the microenvironment in multiple myeloma bone disease. Future Oncol 2006; 2: 371-8.
[68] Politou MC, Heath DJ, Rahemtulla A, *et al.* Serum concentrations of Dickkopf-1 protein are increased in patients with multiple myeloma and reduced after autologous stem cell transplantation. Int J Cancer 2006; 119: 1728-31.

[69] Yaccoby S, Ling W, Zhan F, Walker R, Barlogie B, Shaughnessy Jr JD. Antibody-based inhibition of DKK1 suppresses tumor- induced bone resorption and multiple myeloma growth in- vivo. Blood 2007; 109: 2106-11.

CHAPTER 10

Multiple Myeloma Bone Marrow Angiogenesis

Domenico Ribatti[1*] and Angelo Vacca[2]

[1]Department of Human Anatomy and Histology, [2]Department of Biomedical Sciences and Human Oncology, University of Bari Medical School, Bari, Italy

Abstract: Angiogenesis is a constant hallmark of multiple myeloma (MM) progression and has prognostic potential. It is induced by plasma cells *via* angiogenic factors with the transition from monoclonal gammopathy of undetermined significance (MGUS) to MM, and probably with loss of angiostatic activity on the part of MGUS. Soluble angiogenic factors are elevated in the bone marrow and peripheral blood samples form MM patients. The pathophysiology of MM-induced angiogenesis involves both direct production of angiogenic cytokines by plasma cells and their induction within the bone marrow microenvironment cells. The latter are secreted by stromal cells and promote plasma cell growth, survival and migration, as well as paracrine cytokine secretion and angiogenesis in the bone marrow milieu. More recently, a direct involvement of bone marrow macrophages and mast cells in vasculogenic mimicry has been demonstrated, thus contributing together with circulating endothelial cells and endothelial precursor cells (EPCs) to the MM neovascularization. Finally, controversial data are available concerning the correlation between angiogenesis and disease stage and prognosis.

Keywords: Angiogenesis, VEGF, FGF-2, HGF, Ang-1, Ang-2, IGF-1, IL-8, OPN, ADM, TNF, MMP-2/9, CXCL8/IL8, CXCL11/I-TAC, CXCL12/ SDF-1, bone marrow endothelial cells, circulating endothelial cells, endothelial precursor cells, macrophages, mast cells, vascular mimicry.

1. FIRST EVIDENCE OF AN INCREASED ANGIOGENESIS IN BONE MARROW OF MULTIPLE MYELOMA PATIENTS

Multiple myeloma (MM) is a B-cell neoplasm characterized by clonal expansion of malignant plasma cells in the bone marrow, where they proliferate and become resistant to apoptosis and eventually lead to osteolysis, renal dysfunction and anemia. It is still incurable with a median survival of approximately 4 years. In 1994, Vacca and colleagues demonstrated for the first time that bone marrow microvascular density was significantly increased in MM compared to monoclonal gammoapthy of undetermined significance (MGUS) and moreover in active (diagnosis, relapse, leukemic phase) vs. non-active (complete/ objective response, plateau) MM. The authors first hypothesized that progression from MGUS to MM is accompanied by an increase in bone marrow microvascular density [1]. As progression from *in situ* to invasive and metastatic solid tumors is accompained and enhanced by the switch from the perivascular to the vascular phase, these findings suggest that active MM may represent the'vascular phase'of plasma cell tumors, and non-active MM and MGUS their'perivascular phase'. Subsequent studies by other groups confirmed the observation of increased angiogenesis in active MM compared to healthy individuals or MGUS patients [2-5].

2. ANGIOGENIC FACTORS INVOLVED IN THE ANGIOGENIC SWITCH

The cause of induction of the vascular phase is the subject of current investigation [6] (Fig. **1**, Table **1**). Several studies show overexpression and secretion of vascular endothelial growth factor (VEGF) by the clonal plasma cells. VEGF stimulates proliferation and chemotaxis in both endothelial cells *via* VEGF receptor-2 (VEGFR-2) and stromal cells *via* VEGFR-1. These cells are rapidly phosphorylated by the interaction with VEGF, and signal *via* extracellular signal-related kinase-2 (ERK-2) [7]. Plasma cell derived

***Address correspondence to Domenico Ribatti:** Department of Human Anatomy and Histology, Piazza Giulio Cesare, 11 Policlinico, I-70124 Bari, Italy; Tel: +39.080.5478240; Fax: + 39.080.5478310; E-mail: ribatti@anatomia.uniba.it and **Prof. Angelo Vacca:** Department of Internal Medicine and Clinical Oncology, Piazza Giulio Cesare, 11 Policlinico I-70124 Bari, Italy; Tel: +39.080.5593444; Fax:+39.080.5592189; E-mail: a.vacca@dimo.uniba.it

Klaus Podar and Kenneth C. Anderson (Eds)

VEGF stimulates interleukin-6 (IL-6) and VEGF secretion in bone marrow stromal cells (BMSCs), whereas BMSC-derived IL-6 promotes proliferation, survival and VEGF production in plasma cells [8]. The most successful therapeutic approach to target VEGF in cancer is the use of a humanized monoclonal antibody against VEGF, bevacizumab (Avastin®) [9] (Fig. **2**, Table **2**). Several ongoing clinical trials in MM are testing the effects of bevacizumab used in conjunction with other agents including lenalinomide, dexamethasone or bortezomib. In addition to bevacizumab, other VEGF-targeting compounds are under investigation in MM including, dasatinib, pazopanib, sorafenib and sunitinib.

Fibroblast growth factor-2 (FGF-2) is also secreted directly by MM cells [10]. Levels of FGF-2 are significantly higher in the plasma cell lysates of patients with active MM compared with non-active MM and MGUS patients. Inhibition of FGF-2 by means of a polyclonal anti-FGF-2 antibody suppresses the angiogenic potential of plasma cells from patients with active MM, as reflected by inhibition of human umbilical vein endothelial cell (HUVECs) proliferation and chemotaxis, monocyte chemotaxis and *in vivo* chorioallantoic membrane (CAM) angiogenesis [10]. Moreover, FGF-2 triggers paracrine MM-stromal cell interactions in an IL-6/FGF-2 paracrine loop [11]. Syndecan-1 (CD138), a low affinity receptor of FGF-2, is also expressed by MM cells [12]. Hepatocyte growth factor (HGF) and its receptors c-Met and angiopoietin-1 (Ang-1) have been described as additional angiogenic factors in MM [13-15] (Fig. **1**, Table **1**). HGF has been identified in human MM cell lines [13] and in freshly isolated MM plasma cells [14]. Serum levels of this factor are high in approximately 40% of patients at diagnosis and decline to normal levels as they respond to induction therapy. There is no decline if the therapy is ineffective, and the levels become high again upon relapse [16]. Giuliani and colleagues [15] found that Ang-1 expression is up-regulated in MM cell lines or in plasma cells obtained from MM patients and that the Ang-1 expression in the patient samples correlate with the bone marrow microvascular density. Furthermore, they demonstrated that the angiopoietin receptor Tie-2 is up-regulated in the bone marrow endothelial cells in the presence of MM cells and that anti-Tie-2 antibodies blocked the *in vitro* angiogenic activity of MM cells.

Insulin like growth factor-1 (IGF-1) plays a role in the angiogenic process by stimulating MM cells to secrete VEGF [17]. Plasma IL-8 has been reported to increase in MM [18]. Osteopontin (OPN) was found to contribute to angiogenesis in MM [19] and OPN expression correlated with bone marrow microvascular density [20].

Table 1. Main angiogenic factors in active myeloma

Angiogenic Factor	Origin	Receptors	Experimental Observations
• **VEGF** (Vascular endothelial growth factor)	-Multiple myeloma (MM) plasma cells (MMPCs) - MM endothelial cells (MMECs)	1. **VEGFR-2** on endothelial cells (ECs) 2. **VEGFR-1** on bone marrow stromal cells (BMSCs) 3. **VEGFR-3** on MMPCs	Promotes MMECs and BMSCs proliferation, growth and chemotaxis. Promotes IL-6 and VEGF secretion by BMSCs. Up-regulated in active MM. Its expression correlates with bone marrow microvascular density.
• **FGF-2** (Fibroblast growth factor-2)	MMPCs	**FGF-2R-2**	Promotes MMECs and BMSCs proliferation, growth and chemotaxis. Promotes IL-6 and VEGF secretion by BMSCs. Up-regulated in active MM. Its expression correlates with bone marrow microvascular density.
• **HGF** (Hepatocyte growth factor)	MMPCs	**c-Met**	Identified in MM cell lines. Up-regulated in active MM.
• **Ang-1** (Angiopoietin-1)	MMPCs	**Tie-2/Tek**	Up-regulated in active MM. Its expression correlates with bone marrow microvascular density. Stabilises nascent vessels by tightening endo-periendothelial cell interactions.
• **Ang-2** (Angiopoietin-2)	MMPCs	**Tie-2/Tek**	Angiogenic in the presence of VEGF *via* loosening of periendothelial cells.
• **IGF-1** (Insulin-like growth factor-1)	MMPCs (BMSCs) MMECs	**IGF-1R**	Stimulates MMPCs to secrete VEGF. Up-regulated in active MM. Promotes MMECs and BMSCs proliferation, growth and chemotaxis.

Table 1. cont….

• **IL-8** (Interleukin-8)	BMSCs MMECs	**IL-8R**	Up-regulated in active MM.
• **OPN** (Osteopontin)	MMPCs BMSCs MMECs	**CD44**	Its expression correlates with bone marrow microvascular density.
• **MMP-2/9** (Matrix metalloproteinases-2/9)	MMPCs BMSCs MMECs	**Collagen isoforms**	Up-regulated in active MM. MMP-2 expression is stronger.
• **PDGF-BB** (Platelet-derived growth factor-BB)	MMPCs	**PDGFRβ**	This pathway was selectively induced by VEGF. Recruits smooth muscle cells around nascent endothelial channels.
• **ADM** (Adrenomedullin)	MMPCs	**ADMR**	Induces *in vitro* angiogenesis.
• **TNF-alpha** (Tumor necrosis factor-α)	MMPCs BMSCs MMECs	**TNF-αR**	Stimulation of IL-6 secretion, bone resorption and expression of adhesion molecules.
• **TGF-beta 1** (Transforming growth factor-β1)	MMPCs BMSCs MMECs	**TGF-β1R**	Stabilises nascent vessels by stimulating ECM production.
• **CXCL8/IL8** (CXC-chemokine CXCl8/IL8)	MMECs	**CXCR2**	Takes part in a paracrine loop between MMECs and MMPCs to mediate MMPCs proliferation and chemotaxis.
• **CXCL11/I-TAC** (CXCL11-interferon-inducible T-cell α chemoattractant)	MMECs	**CXCR3**	Takes part in a paracrine loop between MMECs and MMPCs to mediate MMPCs proliferation and chemotaxis.
• **CXCL12/SDF-1alpha** (CXCL12/stromal cell-derived factor-1α)	MMECs	**CXCR4**	Takes part in a paracrine loop between MMECs and MMPCs to mediate MMPCs proliferation and chemotaxis.

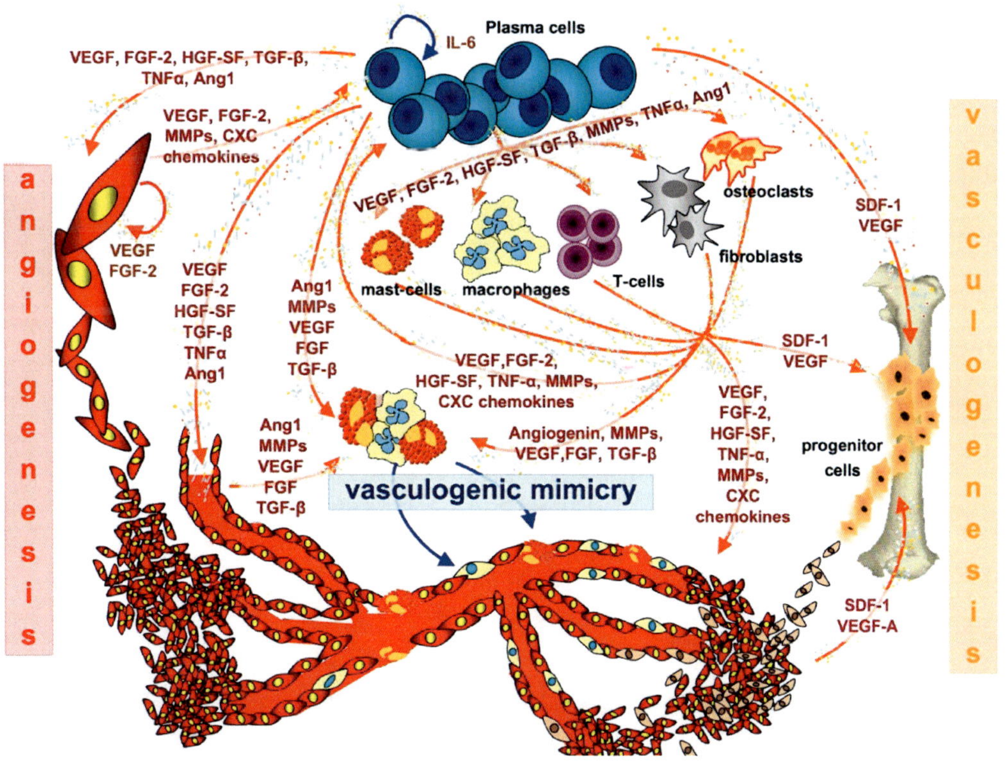

Fig. (1). Interrelationships between plasma cells and various microenvironmental cells and factors promoting angiogenesis and vasculogenesis in the bone marrow of patients with multiple myeloma.

A number of MM cell lines and freshly isolated bone marrow plasma cells of MM patients produce MMP-9, although correlation with disease activity has not been assessed [21]. MMP secretion of MM cells is triggered by BMSCs or bone marrow endothelial cells [22]. We have demonstrated that platelet-derived growth factor (PDGF)-receptor beta (PDGF-Rβ) and pp60-Src as shared constitutively activated tyrosine kinases (TKs) are expressed in plasma cells of MM patients [23]. PDGF-BB/PDGF-Rβ kinase axis promote MM tumor growth by activating ERK-1/2, and AKT. This activity was selectively induced by VEGF and the use of small interfering (si)RNAs validated pp60c-Src as a key signaling effector of the VEGF loop required for MMEC survival, migration and angiogenesis. Finally, we have assessed the antitumor activity of dasatinib, a novel orally bioactive PDGF-Rβ/Src TK-inhibitor that significantly delays MM tumor growth. Airoldi *et al.* [24] demonstrated that IL-12 receptor B2 (IL-12Rβ2) was expressed in primary MM cells but down-regulated compared with normal polyclonal plasmablastic cells and plasma cells. Moreover, IL-12 reduced the pro- angiogenic activity of primary MM cells *in vitro* and decreased significantly the tumorigenicity of NCI-H929 cell line in SCID/NOD mice by inhibiting cell proliferation and angiogenesis. More recently, Hose *et al.* [25] have reported that normal bone marrow plasma cells express several proangiogenic genes, including VEGF-A, IGF-1 and adrenomedullin (ADM) and their culture supernatants significantly induce angiogenesis *in vitro*. Malignant plasma cells show a various pattern of aberrant expression of several pro-angiogenic factors, and culture supernatants of primary MM cells and human MM cell lines induce angiogenesis *in vitro*. However, none of these factors is expressed in all of the MM patient samples, and no significant correlation with microvascular density could be found.

3. THE ROLE OF BONE MARROW MICROENVIRONMENT

The pathogenesis of most cancers includes complex and mutual interactions that affect the number and phenotype of the tumor cells and host stromal cells. Since MM mainly progresses in the bone marrow, signals from this microenvironment play a critical role in maintaining plasma cell growth, migration and survival. The MM microenvironment is formed by clonal plasma cells, extracellular matrix proteins, and BMSCs, which are intimately involved in all biological stages of intramedullary growth [26].

Reciprocal positive and negative interactions between plasma cells and BMSCs, namely hematopoietic stem cells, hematopoietic and mesenchymal progenitor and precursor cells, fibroblasts, osteoblasts, osteoclasts, chondroclasts, endothelial cells, endothelial cell progenitor cells, B lymphocytes, T lymphocytes, NK cells, erythrocytes, megakaryocytes, platelets, macrophages and mast cells, are mediated by any array of cytokines, receptors, and adhesion molecules.

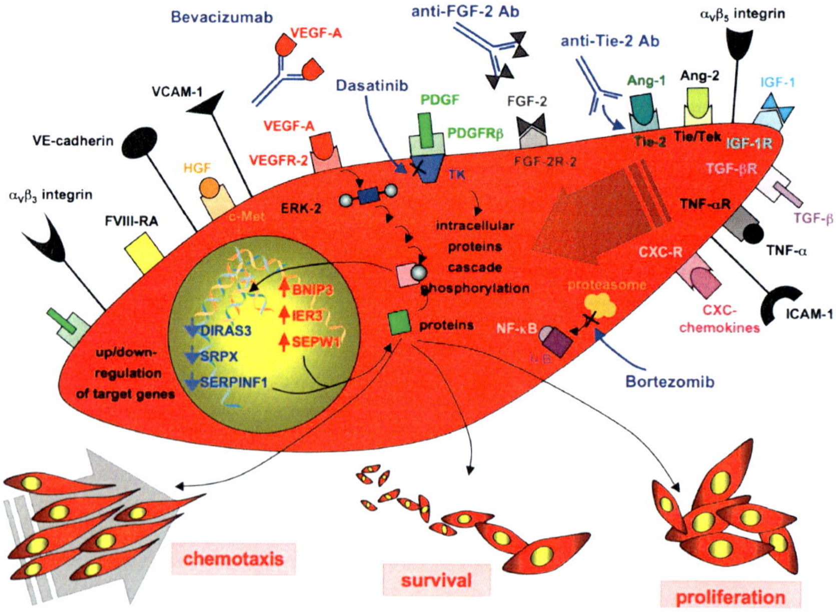

Fig. (2). Schematic representation of pathways of myeloma endothelial cells which can serve as targets for antiangiogenic therapy.

Interactions between these components determine the proliferation, migration and survival of plasma cells, as well as their acquisition of drug resistance and the development of diseases [27-29]. Receptors expressed by plasma cells, such as $\alpha_V\beta_3$ integrin, are crucial for their relationships with each other (homotypic interrelationships) and with extracellular matrix proteins [30] (Table **3**).

Very late activating antigen-4 (VLA-4), leukocyte function-associated antigen (LFA-1), mucin-1 antigen (MUC-1) expressed by plasma cells, and vascular cell adhesion molecule-1 (VCAM-1) and intercellular adhesion molecule-1 (ICAM-1) expressed by BMSCs mediate their heterotypic and homotypic interactions. All these interactions result in enhanced expression and release of cytokines and growth factors needed for the plasma cell survival [31]. Plasma cells in the bone marrow microenvironment secrete cytokines, such as TNF-α [32], TGF-β, VEGF, FGF-2 [10], HGF [13], Ang-1 and MMPs [10, 15].

Moreover, binding of plasma cells to BMSCs triggers transcription and secretion by the latter of cytokines, such as IL-6 [8], IGF-1 [33] and VEGF [34] and CXCL12/stromal cell derived factor-1α (SDF-1α) [35] that mediates cell growth (IL-6, IGF-1, VEGF), survival (IL-6, IGF-1), drug resistance (IL-6, IGF-1, VEGF), migration (IGF-1, VEGF, MMPs, SDF-1α) and angiogenesis (VEGF) in the bone marrow.

4. THE ROLE OF BONE MARROW ENDOTHELIAL CELLS

Vacca and colleagues [36] demonstrated differences in bone marrow endothelial cells isolated from MM patients compared to quiescent HUVECs. MM bone marrow endothelial cells are characterized by an enhanced expression of specific angiogenic factors and their receptors such as VEGF and VEGFR-2, FGF-2 and FGF-2R-2, Ang-2 and Tie-2, by an increased *in vitro* and *in vivo* angiogenic activity. Bone marrow MM endothelial cells (MMECs) express more mRNA and secrete larger amounts of the CXC-chemokines CXCL8/IL-8, CXCL11/interferon-inducible T-cell alpha chemoattractant (I-TAC), CXCL12/SDF-1α and CCL2/monocyte chemotactic protein-1 (MCP-1) than HUVECs, and paired plasma cells express cognate receptors to a variable extent, which suggests that paracrine loops between MMECs and plasma cells involving CXC-chemokines and their receptors are operative in MM patients and mediate plasma cell proliferation and chemotaxis [35].

Attempting a fine characterization of the angiogenic response induced by MM endothelial cells in the CAM assay by using reverse transcriptase-polymerase chain reaction (RT-PCR), we have demonstrated that the expression of endostatin mRNA in MM treated CAMs is significantly lower as compared to control CAMs [37]. These data suggest that angiogenic switch in MM may involve loss of an endogenous angiogenesis inhibitor, namely endostatin. More recently, we have carried out a comparative gene expression profiling of MMECs and MGUS endothelial cells (MGECs) with Affymetrix U133A Arrays [38]. Twenty-two genes were found differentially expressed (14 down-regulated and 8 up-regulated) at relatively high stringency in MMECs compared with MGECs. Deregulated genes are mostly involved in extracellular matrix formation and bone remodeling, cell adhesion, chemotaxis, angiogenesis, resistance to apoptosis, and cell-cycle regulation. Validation was focused on *DIRAS3*, *SERPINF1*, *SRPX*, *BNIP3*, *IER3*, and *SEPW1* genes, which were not previously found to be functionally correlated to the overangiogenic phenotype of MMECs. The siRNA for the up-regulated genes BNIP3, IER3, and SEPW1 affected critical MMEC functions mediating the cell overangiogenic phenotype, that are proliferation, apoptosis, adhesion, and capillary tube formation.

5. THE ROLE OF CIRCULATING ENDOTHELIAL CELLS AND ENDOTHELIAL PRECURSOR CELLS

Zhang *et al.* [39] demonstrated that circulating endothelial cells (CECs) and endothelial precursor cells (EPCs) in peripheral blood were 6-fold higher in MM patients compared to controls and correlated positively with serum M protein and β2-microglobulin. Circulating EPCs displayed late colony formation/outgrowth and capillary-like network formation on Matrigel; these processes were inhibited after thalidomide treatment. Co-expression of VEGFR-2 and CD133 characterized EPC and VEGFR-2 mRNA

Table 2. Targeted antiangiogenic therapy in multiple myeloma

NAME	CLASS	TARGET
• **Bevacizumab**	Humanized monoclonal antibody (HMoAb)	VEGF
• **Anti -FGF-2 Ab**	HMoAb	FGF-2
• **Anti-Tie-2 Ab**	HMoAb	Tie-2
• **Dasatinib, Sorafenib, Sunitinib**	Tyrosine kynases (TK)-inhibitor (TKI)	PDGFRβ/ Src TK

elevations correlated with M protein levels. EPCs are closed associated with hematopoietic stem and progenitor cells (HSPCs) with a typical phenotype including the CD133, CD34 and VEGFR-2 molecules [40, 41]. We have recently demonstrated that in patients with active MM, plasma cells and stromal cells in the bone marrow microenvironment recruit haematopoietic stem precursor cells (HSPCs), and induce their differentiation into mature MMECs [42]. In fact, when HSPCs of MM patients were incubated with VEGF, FGF-2 and IGF, cells differentiated into endothelial cell-like cells expressing typical markers of mature endothelium, such as FVIII-RA, VEGFR-2 and VE-cadherin, and form capillary-like networks *in vitro* [42]. Bone marrow biopsies revealed HPSCs inside the neovessel wall in patients with MM, but not in those with MGUS, suggesting that in the former HSPCs contribute to the new vessel building together with MMECs. Therefore, besides angiogenesis, HSPC-linked vasculogenesis contributes to neovascularization in MM patients.

6. THE INVOLVEMENT OF MACROPHAGES AND MAST CELLS IN THE VASCULAR MIMICRY IN MM

We have shown that when bone marrow macrophages from MM patients are exposed to VEGF and FGF-2, they transform into cells functionally and phenotypically similar to paired MMECs, and generate capillary-like networks mimicking those of MMECs [43]. By contrast, macrophages from non-active MM, MGUS, and benign anemia patients display similar, albeit weaker features. Endothelial cell-like macrophages and apparently typical macrophages contribute sizeably to the formation of the neovessel wall in patients with active MM, whereas their vascular supply is minimal in non-active MM, and absent in MGUS and control patients [43]. In patients with active MM, FACS analysis on freshly isolated bone marrow mononuclear cells revealed higher percentages of CD14/CD68 double-positive cells than in those with non-active disease and MGUS. Furthermore, in active MM patients bone marrow biopsies displayed macrophages with both endothelial cell-like (*i.e.* CD68/FVIII-RA double positive) and apparently typical (*i.e.* CD68 positive/FVIII-RA negative) features located in the microvessel wall and collaborating with MMECs to line the vessel lumen. Figures of this type were rare in non-active MM patients and absent in MGUS. Thus, macrophage involvement in the vasculogenic pathway proceeds in step with MM activity, and with progression of plasma cell tumors as well [43]. Overall, these data suggest that in active MM, macrophages contribute to neovascularization through a vasculogenic pathway, and that in non-active MM and MGUS they are prone to behave accordingly, marching in step with progression, hence with the vascular switch [44].

Chen *et al.* [45] demonstrated that monocytes induces vascular endothelial cell gene expression and develop tube-like structures when they were cultured with bone marrow from patients with MM that express an angiogenic factor, namely pleiotrophin, effect specifically blocked with anti-pleiotrophin antibodies. Moreover, when co-injected with human MM cells into SCID mice, green fluorescent protein-marked human monocytes were found to be incorporated into tumor blood vessels and expressed human vascular endothelial cell protein markers and genes that were blocked by anti-pleiotrophin antibodies. These results suggest that vasculogenesis in human MM may develop from tumoral production of pleiotrophin which induces the transdifferentiation of monocytes into vascular endothelial cells.

We have demonstrated that bone marrow angiogenesis, evaluated as microvessel area, and mast cell density counts are highly correlated in patients with non-active and active MM and in those with MGUS, and that both parameters increased simultaneously in active MM [46]. At the ultrastructural level, the majority of cells displayed semilunar aspects of cytoplasmic granules, suggesting a chronic and slow release of mediators in response to a degranulatory stimulus [46]. More recently, we demonstrated that at the ultrastructural level vessels from MM biopsies are lined by mast cells whose cytoplasm was filled with numerous and irregularly shaped electron dense granules [47]. Moreover, thick endothelial cells, containing endocytotic vesicles, but lacking granules, were connected by a junctional system with the mast cells lining the vessel wall, whereas the vessels from MGUS biopsies were lined with thin endothelial cells, often surrounded by mast cells [47]. These ultrastructural findings have been confirmed by confocal laser microscopy using double anti-tryptase (to mark mast cells) and anti-FVIII-RA (to mark endothelial cells) antibodies. Vessels from MM biopsies displayed regions stained by FVIII-RA alternating with regions stained by both tryptase and FVIII-RA. In the MGUS biopsies, the vessels were uniformly stained by the anti-FVIII-RA antibody only, while tryptase-positive mast cells were only recognizable perivascularly [47]. Overall, these data suggest that in MM mast cells contribute to neovascularization. The bone marrow of MM patients, in fact, displays typical tryptase-positive mast cells in the vessel wall that collaborate with endothelial cell to line the lumina. Since mast cells keep their lineage marker, they can be regarded as cells that do not transdifferentiate into endothelial cells.

Table 3. Main intercellular plasma cell and endothelial cell adhesion molecules.

Plasma cell	
•	**VLA-4** (Very late activating antigen-4)
•	**$\alpha_V\beta_3$, $\alpha_V\beta_5$ integrins**
•	**LFA-1** (Leukocyte function-associated antigen-1)
•	**MUC-1** (Mucin antigen-1)
Endothelial cell	
•	**VCAM-1** (Vascular cell adhesion molecule-1)
•	**ICAM-1** (Intracellular adhesion molecule-1)
•	**$\alpha_V\beta_3$, $\alpha_V\beta_5$ integrins**
•	**VE-cadherin**

During embryo life, blood vessels first appear as the result of vasculogenesis, *i.e.* the formation of capillaries from endothelial cells differentiating *in situ* from groups of mesodermal cells. The primitive heart and primitive vascular plexus form in this way [48]. Remodeling of the primary vascular plexus into a more mature vascular system is thought to occur by angiogenesis, a term applied to the formation of capillaries from existing vessels, *i.e.* capillaries and post-capillary venules, based on endothelial sprouting or intussusceptive (non-sprouting) microvascular growth [48]. In tumors, near angiogenesis, vasculogenesis contributes to the formation of the microvascular plexus that is important for local and systemic diffusion [49].

Experimental data show that in MM, in association with angiogenesis, also vasculogenesis occurs and monocyte-macrophages and mast cells actively participate to this process together with hematopoietic stem and progenitor cells, as we have recently demonstrated [42]. Tumor vessels in MM show an abnormal structure, consisting of endothelial cells, as well as highly proliferating circulating endothelial precursors/angioblasts, hematopoietic stem cells, macrophages, mast cells and tumor cells (vasculogenic mimicry) [39, 43, 47].

Tumor-associated vasculature causes chaotic and variable blood flow as well as vessel leakiness, resulting in lowered drug delivery and further selection of more malignant tumor cells. The ability of the tumor to support continued growth through non angiogenesis-dependent pathways represents an important mechanism of tumor resistance to conventional anti-angiogenic treatment and requires adjustment of these therapies to counter such new pathways.

7. CLINICAL EVIDENCE

In 2000, independently Rajkumar and co-workers and Sezer and co-workers demonstrated that increased bone marrow microvascular density in MM patients is associated with an unfavourable prognosis [50, 51].

In 2001, Munshi and Wilson showed a prognostic significance of pre-treatment microvascular density for progression-free survival and for median duration of complete response in newly diagnosed MM patients who were treated in the total therapy protocol. In 2001, Sezer and colleagues, by comparing pre-versus post-treatment bone marrow microvascular density, demonstrated that this decreases significantly in MM patients achieving remission after therapy, but not in patients who did no respond to therapy.

In 2002, Rajkumar and colleagues demonstrated in a cohort of 400 patients that a progressive increase in bone marrow microvascular density occurs across the whole spectrum of plasma cell disorders, including primary amyloidosis, MGUS, smoldering and active MM [3].

In 2002, Kumar and colleagues investigated the effect of chemotherapy on bone marrow angiogenesis of MM by using immunohistochemistry techniques and microvascular density estimation [52]. They found that the grade of vascularization before initiation of therapy was a predictive factor for survival but they did not find significant changes in the grade of angiogenesis after chemotherapy. Other groups found no significant difference between bone marrow microvascular density in responsive and non-responsive patients [53, 54] while others had found a significant decrease [55, 56]. Persistence of pathological angiogenesis after therapy may reflect a continuous angiogenic stimulation of endothelial cells by residual MM cells and may contribute to relapse and progression.

The prognostic significance of pre-treatment microvascular density for progression-free and overall survival was also confirmed in patients undergoing high-dose chemotherapy [57]. In a further study, Kumar and colleagues [58] reported the effect of thalidomide on the bone marrow vascularization in 81 MM patients treated with thalidomide alone or in association with dexamethasone. They studied bone marrow biopsies at baseline and after 4-6 months of therapy found a significant decrease of microvascular density in responding patients, supporting an antiangiogenic effect of thalidomide. The findings have been confirmed by another study [59], and suggest that angiogenesis and primary resistance to therapy are related features of more aggressive disease, and decrease after therapy; this aspect could partially be mediated by reduction of the release of angiogenic factors from MM cells and by direct toxic effect of the therapy on endothelial cells.

More recently, Seckinger and colleagues [60] demonstrated that bone marrow morphogenetic protein-6 (BMP-6) expression was significantly lower in proliferating MM cells, MM cell lines or plasmablasts. BMP-6 significantly inhibited the proliferation of MM cell lines, survival of primary MM cells and *in vitro* angiogenesis. Finally, a high BMP-6 expression in primary MM cell samples delineated significantly higher survival for patients undergoing high-dose chemotherapy independent of conventional prognostic factors.

Negaard and colleagues [61] demonstrated that patients with hematological malignancies, including MM, had higher pretreatment bone marrow microvascular density than controls, and elevated pretreatment plasma levels of VEGF, IL-6 and IL-8. Moreover, they did not find any association between bone marrow microvascular density and complete response. IL-6 plasma levels did not correlate with treatment response in patients with MM [62] and no significant differences were found according to the MM stage [53].

Pour and colleagues [63] have analyzed 96 patients with secretory MM and demonstrated a significant decrease of VEGF and HGF levels and a significant increase of the endogenous angiogenesis inhibitor thrombospondin-1 (TSP-1) concentrations in the bone marrow plasma of patients who achieved complete or very good partial response in contrast to those who had partial or no response.

8. CONCLUDING REMARKS

Angiogenesis is intimately involved in the pathobiology of MM in both preclinical and clinical models. An improved understanding of the importance of angiogenesis-related signaling in MM has allowed for the rational use of antiangiogenic therapies in patients affected by this malignancy. Considering the complex angiogenesis regulatory network that involves multiple angiogenic factors produced by various cell types, any antiangiogenesis therapy aimed at a single angiogenic factor is not likely to be highly effective.

Further investigation into the complex pathogenic process involved in angiogenesis in MM is important to increase our knowledge of the pathobiology of this malignancy in order to develop more effective therapeutic strategies. Areas of future investigation include identifying factors other than VEGF that are critical in the angiogenesis cascade, elucidating mechanisms of therapeutic resistance, and developing markers for identifying patients most likely to benefit from antiangiogenis treatment.

ACKNOWLEDGEMENTS

Partially supported by MIUR (PRIN 2007), Rome, and Fondazione Cassa di Risparmio di Puglia, Bari, Italy.

REFERENCES

[1] Vacca A, Ribatti D, Roncali L, *et al.* Bone marrow angiogenesis and progression in multiple myeloma. Br J Haematol 1994; 87: 503-8.
[2] Schreiber S, Ackermann J, Obermair A, *et al.* Multiple myeloma with deletion of chromosome 13q is characterized by increased bone marrow neovascularization. Br J Haematol 2000; 110: 605-9.
[3] Rajkumar SV, Mesa RA, Fonseca R, *et al.* Bone marrow angiogenesis in 400 patients with monoclonal gammopathy of undetermined significance, multiple myeloma, and primary amyloidosis. Clin Cancer Res 2002; 8: 2210-6.
[4] Pruneri G, Ponzoni M, Ferreri AJ, *et al.* Microvessel density, a surrogate marker of angiogenesis, is significantly related to survival in multiple myeloma patients. Br J Haematol 2002; 118: 817-20.
[5] Alexandrakis MG, Passam FJ, Ganotakis E, *et al.* Bone marrow microvascular density and angiogenic growth factors in multiple myeloma. Clin Chem Lab Med 2004; 42: 1122-6.
[6] Vacca A, Ribatti D. Bone marrow angiogenesis in multiple myeloma. Leukemia 2006; 20: 193-9.
[7] Vacca A, Ria R, Ribatti D, *et al.* A paracrine loop in the vascular endothelial growth factor pathway triggers tumor angiogenesis and growth in multiple myeloma. Haematologica 2003; 88: 176-85.
[8] Dankbar B, Padro T, Leo R, *et al.* Vascular endothelial growth factor and interleukin-6 in paracrine tumor-stromal cell interactions in multiple myeloma. Blood 2000; 95: 2630-6.
[9] Ferrara N, Hillan KJ, Gerber HP, Novotny W. Discovery and development of bevacizumab, an anti-VEGF antibody for treating cancer. Nat Rev Drug Discov 2004; 3: 391-400.
[10] Vacca A, Ribatti D, Presta M, *et al.* Bone marrow neovascularization, plasma cell angiogenic potential, and matrix metalloproteinase-2 secretion parallel progression of human multiple myeloma. Blood 1999; 93: 3064-73.
[11] Bisping G, Leo R, Wenning D, *et al.* Paracrine interactions of basic fibroblast growth factor and interleukin-6 in multiple myeloma. Blood 2003; 101: 2775-83.
[12] Witzig T, Kimlinger T, Stenson M, Thereneau T. Syndecan-1 expression on malignant cells from the blood and marrow of patients with plasma cell proliferative disorders and B-cell chronic lymphocytic leukemia. Leuk Lymphoma 1998; 31: 167-75.
[13] Borset M, Lien E, Espevik T, Helseth E, Waage A, Sundan A. Concomitant expression of hepatocyte growth factor/scatter factor and the receptor c-MET in human myeloma cell lines. J Biol Chem 1996; 271: 24655-61.
[14] Borset M, Hjorth-Hansen H, Seidel C, Sundan A, Waage A. Hepatocyte growth factor and its receptor c-met in multiple myeloma. Blood 1996; 88: 3998-4004.
[15] Giuliani N, Colla S, Lazzaretti M *et al.* Proangiogenic properties of human myeloma cells: production of angiopoietin-1 and its potential relationship to myeloma-induced angiogenesis. Blood 2003; 102: 638-45.
[16] Seidel C, Børset M, Turesson I, Abildgaard N, Sundan A, Waage A. Elevated serum concentrations of hepatocyte growth factor in patients with multiple myeloma. The Nordic Myeloma Study Group. Blood 1998; 91: 806-12.
[17] Mitsiades CS, Mitsiades NS, McMullan CJ, *et al.* Inhibition of the insulin-like growth factor receptor-1 tyrosine kinase activity as a therapeutic strategy for multiple myeloma, other hematologic malignancies, and solid tumors. Cancer Cell 2004; 5: 221-30.
[18] Kuku I, Bayraktar MR, Kaya E *et al.* Serum proinflammatory mediators at different periods of therapy in patients with multiple myeloma. Mediators Inflamm 2005; 2005: 171-4.

[19] Cheriyath V, Husein MA. Osteopontin, angiogenesis and multiple myeloma. Leukemia 2005; 19: 2203-5.

[20] Colla S, Morandi F, Lazzaretti M, *et al.* Human myeloma cells express the bone regulating gen Runx2/Cbfa1 and produce osteopontin that is involved in angiogenesis in multiple myeloma patients. Leukemia 2005; 19: 2166-76.

[21] Barillé S, Akhoundi C, Collette M, *et al.* Metalloproteinases in multiple myeloma: production of matrix metalloproteinase-9 (MMP-9), activation of proMMP-2, and induction of MMP-1 by myeloma cells. Blood 1997; 90: 1649-55.

[22] Vande Broek I, Asosingh K, Allegaert V, *et al.* Bone marrow endothelial cells increase the invasiveness of human multiple myeloma cells through upregulation of MMP-9: evidence for a role of hepatocyte growth factor. Leukemia 2004; 18: 976-82.

[23] Coluccia AML, Cirulli T, Neri P, *et al.* Validation of PDGFRβ and c-Src tyrosine kinases as tumor/vessel targets in patients with multiple myeloma: preclinical efficacy of the novel, orally available inhibitor dasatinib. Blood 2008; 12: 1346-56.

[24] Airoldi I, Cocco C, Giuliani N, *et al.* Constitutive expression of IL-12Rβ2 on human multiple myeloma cells delineates a novel therapeutic target. Blood 2008; 112: 750-9.

[25] Hose D, Moreaux J, Meissner T, *et al.* Induction of angiogenesis by normal and malignant plasma cells. Blood 2009; 114: 128-43.

[26] Kuehl WM, Bergsagel PL. Multiple myeloma: evolving genetic events and host interactions. Nat Rev Cancer 2002; 2: 175-87.

[27] Damiano JS, Cress AE, Hazlehurst LA, Shtil AA, Dalton WS. Cell adhesion mediated drug resistance (CAM-DR): role of integrins and resistance to apoptosis in human myeloma cell lines. Blood 199; 93: 1658-67.

[28] Hazlehurst LA, Damiano JS, Buyuksal I, Pledger WJ, Dalton WS. Adhesion to fibronectin *via* beta 1 integrin regulates p27kip1 levels and contributes to cell adhesion mediated drug resistance (CAM-DR). Oncogene 2000; 19: 4319-27.

[29] Hazlehurst LA,Enkemann SA, Beam CA, *et al.* Genotypic and phenotypic comparisons of de novo and acquired Melphalan resistance in an isogenic multiple myeloma cell line model. Cancer Res 2003; 63: 7900-6.

[30] Vacca A, Ria R, Presta M, *et al.* Alpha (v) beta (3) integrin engagement modulates cell adhesion, proliferation, and protease secretion in human lymphoid tumor cells. Exp Hematol 2001; 29: 993-1003.

[31] Hideshima T, Podar K, Chauhan D, Anderson KC. Cytokines and signal transduction. Best Pract Res Clin Haematol 2005; 18: 509-24.

[32] Hideshima T, Nakamura N, Chauhan D, Anderson HC. The role of tumor necrosis factor alpha in the pathophysiology of human multiple myeloma: therapeutic applications. Oncogene 2001; 20: 5991-6000.

[33] Ferlin M, Noraz N, Hertogh C, Brochier J, Taylor N, Klein B. Insulin-like growth factor induces the survival and proliferation of myeloma cells through an interleukin-6 independent transduction pathway. Br J Haematol 2000; 111: 626-34.

[34] Gupta D, Treon SP, Shima Y, *et al.* Adherence of multiple myeloma cells to bone marrow stromal cells upregulates vascular endothelial growth factor secretion: therapeutic applications. Leukemia 2001; 15: 1950-61.

[35] Pellegrino A, Ria R, Di Pietro G, *et al.* Bone marrow endothelial cells in multiple myeloma secrete CXC-chemokines that mediates interactions with plasma cells. Br J Haematol 2005; 129: 248-56.

[36] Vacca A, Ria R, Semeraro F, *et al.* Endothelial cells in the bone marrow of patients with multiple myeloma. Blood 2003; 102: 3340-8.

[37] Mangieri D, Nico B, Benagiano V, De Giorgis M, Vacca A, Ribatti D. Angiogenic activity of multiple myeloma endothelial cells *in vivo* in the chick embryo chorioallantoic membrane assay is associated to a down-regulation in the expression of endogenous endostatin. J Cell Mol Med 2008; 12: 1023-8.

[38] Ria R, Todoerti K, Berardi S, *et al.* Gene expression profiling of bone marrow endothelial cells in patients with multiple myeloma. Clin Cancer Res 2009; 15: 5369-78.

[39] Zhang H, Vakil V, Braunstein M, *et al.* Circulating endothelial progenitor cells in multiple myeloma: implications and significance. Blood 2005; 3286-94.

[40] Yin AH, Miraglia S, Zanjani ED, *et al.* AC133, a novel marker for human hematopoietic stem and progenitor cells. Blood 1997; 90: 5002-12.

[41] Peichev M, Naiyer AJ, Pereira D, *et al.* Expression of VEGFR-2 and AC133 by circulating human CD34(+) cells identifies a population of functional endothelial precursors. Blood 2000; sssss95: 952-8.

[42] Ria R, Piccoli C, Cirulli T, *et al.* Endothelial differentiation of hematopoietic stem and prgenitor cells from patients with multiple myeloma. Clin Cancer Res 2008; 14: 1678-85.

[43] Scavelli C, Nico B, Cirulli T, *et al.* Vasculogenic mimicry by bone marrow macrophages in patient with multiple myeloma. Oncogene 2008; 27: 663-74.

[44] Kumar S, Witzig TE, Timm M, *et al.* Bone marrow angiogenic ability and expression of angiogenic cytokines in myeloma: evidence favouring loss of marrow angiogenesis inhibitory activity with disease progression. Blood 2004; 104: 1159-65.

[45] Chen H, Campbell RA, Chang Y, *et al.* Pleiotrophin produced by multiple myeloma induces transdifferentiation of monocytes into vascular endothelial cells: a novel mechanism of tumor-induced vasculogenesis. Blood 2008; 113: 1992-2002.

[46] Ribatti D, Vacca A, Nico B, *et al.* Bone marrow angiogenesis and mast cell density increase simultaneously with progression of human multiple myeloma. Br J Cancer 1999; 79: 451-5.

[47] Nico B, Mangieri D, Crivellato E, Vacca A, Ribatti D. Mast cells contribute to vasculogenic mimicry in multiple myeloma. Stem Cells Dev 2008; 17: 19-22.

[48] Ribatti D, Nico B, Crivellato E. Morphological and molecular aspects of physiological vascular morphogenesis. Angiogenesis 2009; 12: 101-11.

[49] Ribatti D, Vacca A, Nico B, Roncali L, Dammacco F, 2001. Postnatal vasculogenesis. Mech Dev 2001; 100: 157-63.

[50] Rajkumar SV, Leong T, Roche PC, *et al.* Prognostic value of bone marrow angiogenesis in multiple myeloma. Clin Cancer Res 2000; 6: 3111-6.

[51] Sezer O, Niemöller K, Jakob C, *et al.* Bone marrow microvessel density is a prognostic factor for survival in patients with multiple myeloma. Ann Haematol 2000; 79: 574-7.

[52] Kumar S, Fonseca R, Dispenzieri A, *et al.* Bone marrow angiogenesis in multiple myeloma: effect of therapy. Br J Haematol 2002; 119: 665-71.

[53] Sezer O, Jakob C, Eucker J, *et al.* Serum levels of the angiogenic cytokines basic fibroblast growth factor (bFGF), vascular endothelial growth factor (VEGF) and hepatocyte growth factor (HGF) in multiple myeloma. Eur J Haematol 2001; 66: 83-8.

[54] Thompson MA, Witzig TE, Kumar S, *et al.* Plasma levels of tumor necrosis factor alpha and interleukin-6 predict progression-free survival following thalidomide therapy in patients with previously untreated multiple myeloma. Br J Haematol 2003; 123: 305-8.

[55] Oh HS, Choi JH, Park CK, *et al.* Comparison of microvessel desnity before and after peripheral blood stem cell transplantation in multiple myeloma patients and its clinical implications: multicenter trial. Int J Hematol 2002; 76: 465-70.

[56] Alexandrakis MG, Passam FH, Dambaki C, Pappa CA, Stathopoulos EN. The relationship between bone marrow angiogenesis and the proliferation index Ki-67 in multiple myeloma. J Clin Pathol 2004; 57: 856-0.

[57] Kumar S, Gertz MA, Dispenzieri A, *et al.* Prognostic value of bone marrow angiogenesis in patients with multiple myeloma undergoing high-dose therapy. Bone Marrow Transplant 2004; 34: 235-9.

[58] Kumar S, Witzig TE, Dispenzieri A, *et al.* Effect of thalidomide therapy on bone marrow angiogenesis in multiple myeloma. Leukemia 2004; 18: 624-7.

[59] Bhatti SS, Kumar L, Dinda AK, Dawar R. Prognostic value of bone marrow angiogenesis in multiple myeloma: use of light microscopy as well as computerized image analyzer in the assessment of microvessel density and total vascular area in multiple myeloma and its correlation with various clinical, histological and laboratory parameters. Am J Hematol 2006; 81: 649-56.

[60] Seckinger A, Meißner T, Moreaux J, *et al.* Bone morphogenic protein 6: a member of a novel class of prognostic factors expressed by normal and malignant plasma cells inhibiting proliferation and angiogenesis. Oncogene 2009; 28: 3866-79.

[61] Negaard HF, Iversen N, Bowitz-Lothe IM, *et al.* Increased bone marrow microvascular density in haematological malignancies is associated with differential regulation of angiogenic factors. Leukemia 2009; 23: 162-9.

[62] Rosiñol L, Cibeira MT, Segarra M, *et al.* Response to thalidomide in multiple myeloma: impact of angiogenic factors. Cytokine 2004; 26: 145-8.

[63] Pour L, Svachova H, Adam Z, *et al.* Levels of angiogenic factors in patients with multiple myeloma correlate with treatment response. Ann Haematol 2010; 89: 385-9.

CHAPTER 11

Mouse Models of Multiple Myeloma: Advantages and Pitfalls

Mariateresa Fulciniti[1*], Paola Neri[2], Pierosandro Tagliaferri[3] and Pierfrancesco Tassone[3]

[1]Jerome Lipper Multiple Myeloma Center, Dana-Farber Cancer Institute, Boston, MA), 02115, USA; [2]Division of Hematology and Bone Marrow Transplant, University of Calgary, AB, Canada and [3]Medical Oncology Unit, University of Magna Græcia and T. Campanella Cancer Center, Catanzaro, Italy.

Abstract: Multiple myeloma (MM) is a complex disease which strongly relies on a network of humoral and cellular interactions within the human bone marrow milieu. Although outcomes of anti-MM treatments have improved over the past decade, the disease is still incurable. Translational research for the development of novel therapeutic approaches against MM requires experimental preclinical models able to recapitulate the disease microenvironment. Over the last few years, a variety of murine MM models have been developed. These models have significantly improved our understanding of the disease and led to the development of new therapeutics. We here review the most known models of MM and discuss both advantages and pitfalls.

Keywords: Xenograft mouse models, diffuse xenograft mouse models, SCID mouse, SCID-hu mouse, SCID rab mouse, NOD/SCID mouse, 5TMM, VK* myc, LAGλ-1 model.

1. INTRODUCTION

In the recent years, the availability of *in vivo* models of multiple myeloma (MM) has provided a valuable preclinical setting for understanding the pathobiology of the disease, the critical role of the human bone marrow microenvironment (HuBMM) and for evaluating the anti-tumor activity of investigational new drugs. Specifically, the recognition of the role of HuBMM in the growth, survival and drug resistance of MM cells [1] has highlighted the importance of pre-clinical MM models able to recapitulate the complex circuitry of human tumor-bone marrow interactions. While most *in vitro* experimental models are mainly based on cell interactions on a two-dimensional surface, animal models of MM provide the optimal framework to study complex interactions in a three-dimensional support. We here review the most known MM models, as reported in Table **1**, and discuss both advantages and pitfalls. These aspects are important in the selection of the appropriate model for the experimental purpose and should be taken in account for data interpretation.

Theoretically, an experimental animal model of MM must fulfill the following criteria:

- It must reproduce all genotypic and phenotypic features of human MM;
- It must allow the growth of human disease within its natural autologous bone marrow milieu;
- It must recapitulate clinical features and laboratory abnormalities of human MM;
- It must warrant that therapies active against human MM are effective in the animal model and vice versa.

At present, the available mouse models have a variety of features resembling the human disease, but none of them fulfils all the criteria listed above [2-4].

Overall, small-animal models of human cancer include inbred strains that spontaneously develop cancer [5-7], rodents exposed to chemical mutagens [8-10], and mice in which tumors are produced by viral or bacterial infection [11,12]. As expected, animals that spontaneously develop cancer are flawed to predict

***Address correspondence to Mariateresa Fulciniti:** Jerome Lipper Multiple Myeloma Center, Dana-Farber Cancer Institute, Boston, MA 02115, USA; Fax: 617-632-2140; E-mail: mariateresa_fulciniti@dfci.harvard.edu;

Klaus Podar and Kenneth C. Anderson (Eds)

human diseases. In addition, a number of approaches have been applied to develop genetically engineered models of malignancies, in which the tumor arises "naturally" in the host.

Table 1. MM mouse models

Model Name	Description
SCID s.c.	Immunoincompetent model, transplanted s.c. with MM cell lines
SCID-hu	Immunoincompetent model, transplanted with human fetal bone and human MM primary cells or cell lines.
SCID-rab	Xenograft model, transplanted with rabbit bone and human MM primary cells or cell lines. Immunoincompetent.
NOD/SCID	Diffuse xenograft model, transplanted with human MM primary cells or cell lines. Immunoincompetent.
ARH-77	Diffuse xenograft model, transplanted with the human ARH-77 MM cell line. Immunoincompetent.
LAKl-1	Fresh whole core bone marrow biopsies obtained from MM patients engrafted en bloc into hind limb muscle of SCID mice. Immunoincompetent.
5TMM series	Immunocompetent models obtained from serial transplantations of syngeneic recipients with murine MM cells spontaneously arising in C57BL/KaLwRij mice.
Vk*myc	Transgenic mouse model in which c-myc gene is activated in postgerminal B cells of C57B16/J mice by somatic hypermutation.

These models have been used to study the molecular processes critical for the onset, growth and survival of malignancies and to identify potential therapeutic targets.

The development of human tumor xenograft models represented a big step towards more clinically relevant models [4,13,14]. Human MM cell lines have been engrafted in immunocompromised mice to study the disease [15] but most importantly to test novel therapeutics *in vivo* [4]. Over the last few years, different models of MM that recapitulate the pathophysiology of the disease in animals have been developed, including the SCID-hu [16,17] and the 5TMM [18] model. These models provide an effective opportunity to study the relevance of bone marrow stromal cells (BMSCs) – MM cell interactions and to evaluate new treatment approaches targeting the MM cell and/or its HuBMM. Taken together, all these models have contributed to our understanding of MM and to pre-clinical evaluation of novel therapeutics that have been translated to the bedside for clinical treatment of MM patients [19]

2. MM MODELS OF THE 5T SERIES

The 5TMM is a model of murine MM based on serial transplantations of syngeneic recipients with MM cells spontaneously arising in C57BL/KaLwRij aging mice [20,21]. Different 5TMM lines have been established by transplanting primary MM cells into syngeneic recipients and subsequently propagated by intravenous (iv) injection of the tumor cells into young syngeneic mice. The more commonly used 5T cell lines are 5T2MM and 5T33MM models, which share some common features. Mice develop monoclonal gammopathy, renal damage and hypercalcemia. Mice present BM infiltration by MM cells and bone lesions [22] characterized by increased osteoclasts activity [23]. In addition, the 5T2MM and 5T33MM have similar patterns of expression of adhesion molecules and express isoforms of CD44 such as V6, V7, and V10 that appear to be critical for the interaction between the 5T cells and the BM endothelium [24,25]. However, the 5T2MM is the most similar model to the human disease with moderate proliferation activity and consistent development of osteolytic lesions [26, 27], while the 5T33MM discloses more aggressive features similar to advanced MM. In fact, 5T33 cells show early infiltration of the BM as compared to 5T2MM cells (2 weeks vs. 9 weeks, respectively) and home also in the spleen and liver [24].

In the past, these models have provided valuable insights into MM bone disease contributing to elucidate the role of osteoprotegerin and RANK/RANKL interaction in the development of osteolytic lesions [28,29,30] and the activity of bisphosphonates in the treatment of MM-related bone disease [29,31]. Moreover, the use of these models has improved the understanding of MM pathophysiology, including the functional involvement of cell adhesion molecules in MM proliferation or homing to the BM [25,32,33], the influence of chemokines on MM cell homing *in vivo* [34-36], as well as the process of MM-associated neoangiogenesis [27,37,38], the status of normoxia vs. hypoxia in the BM with lesions [39] and the role of matrix metalloproteinases [37]. Finally, these models have been useful for the preclinical development of a variety of novel agents for MM, jncluding erythropoietin, all-trans retinoic acid, IGF-1R kinase inhibitors, HMG-CoA reductase inhibitor and bortezomib alone or in combination with novel histone deacetylase inhibitor [29,35,40-43].

Overall, a key advantage of the 5T models is the syngeneic nature of the interaction between murine MM cells and the murine BMM of the host. Importantly, these mice are immunocompetent and therefore suitable for evaluation of immunotherapeutic strategies, which cannot be readily addressed in models based on immunocompromised rodents. However, the major limitation of the use of 5T models is the difference in the biology of murine vs. human MM. Furthermore, the murine cell lines used for serial transplantation do not reproduce, even in a mouse specular system, the wide spectrum of genetic heterogeneity of human disease in its HuBMM. A further important disadvantage of this model is the low frequency of spontaneous tumorigenesis in these mice [44].

3. ENGINEERED MODELS OF MM

MM is a multistep process involving numerous genetic and epigenetic events [45]. Several mouse MM models have been developed taking in account the genetic background underlying the pathogenesis of the disease. Several strategies based on knock-in or knock-out of certain genes [46,47] have been used to develop genetically engineered models of malignancy. In general, DNA-constructs generated by coupling gene sequences with specific or universal promoters and/or enhancers are microinjected into fertilized 1-2 day old mouse eggs that are then surgically implanted into surrogate mothers. The majority of the offsprings will incorporate the exogenous gene into their germline and can be used to breed mouse transgenic lines. The transgene expression can be directed or restricted to specific cell lineages. In MM significant effort has been directed towards the construction of mice with restricted expression of MM relevant activated oncogenes and mutated tumor suppressor genes in the B cell lineage. Untreated transgenic mice carrying either Eμ-v-abl, Eμ- IL-6 or Eμ-bcl-2 were reported to develop plasma cell malignancies with variable incidences [48-52].

New emerging mouse models of human plasma cell neoplasms are based on the transgenic expression in B-cells of IL-6 [53], or fusion protein of nucleophosmin and anaplastic lymphoma kinase (NPM-ALK) [54] as well as targeted deregulation of c-Myc and Bcl-xl in the B-cell compartment [55,56]. Chesi and colleagues have recently developed a new mouse model where c-myc is activated in postgerminal B-cells of C57Bl6/J mice by somatic hypermutation [57]. These mice (Vk*myc) spontaneously develop monoclonal gammopathies and plasma cell expansion in the BM but not in secondary lymphoid organs. They exhibit monoclonal paraproteinemia, BM infiltration with plasma cells, anemia and decreased bone mineral density. Interestingly, these mice are also responsive to drugs commonly used to treat MM (Melphalan, dexamethasone, and bortezomib) [57].

Another transgenic mouse model in which the spliced form of the plasma cell differentiation factor XBP-1 (XBP-1s) is targeted to the B cell lineage under the control of the IgH promoter and enhancer elements (pEμ) has been recently generated [58]. XBP-1 is a transcription factor that is required for plasma cell differentiation and is expressed at high levels in MM cells vs. normal plasma cells [59]. The pEμXBP-1 transgenic mice develop features closely resembling MGUS and progress to MM. Indeed, by one year of age, a significant proportion of the pEμXBP-1s transgenic mice demonstrates a clinical and histopathologic pictures similar to human MM. They show marked elevation of serum IgM and IgG, expansion of the plasma cell population in the BM (with plasma cells ranging from 5 to 30% of total BM cellularity), development of plasmacytic tumors resembling human MGUS or MM and eventually presence of bone lytic lesions on X-ray examination. The long latency period in the development of MM in this model indicates that additional genetic lesions are required for full malignant transformation. In addition, the transcriptional profiles of the lymphoid and MM cells show deregulation of genes with known dysfunction in human MM including Cyclin D1, IL-6R (gp80), gp130, MAF, MAFB, BAFF and APRIL providing an opportunity to study the biology of human MM and the role of genetic lesions in the evolution and progression of the disease as well as to assess novel therapies *in vivo*.

In conclusion, transgenic mice can been useful for clarifying how specific oncogenes participate in normal cell differentiation and for understanding the oncogenic pathways able to induce malignancy. Moreover, these models offer the opportunity of testing new agent targeting the specific genetic alteration, but they are not representative of the complexity of the genetic scenario of MM in humans. Moreover, in some of models such as knock-in or knock-out mice, tumor arises "naturally" in the host, but in a mutated murine microenvironment which is similar to the hereditary cancer onset scenario. This scenario does not reflect the "natural" microenvironment where the human tumor arises in a context of non-mutated HuBMM. Further limits are represented by obvious differences between murine and human stroma, by the impossibility to reproduce different tumor stages and to follow tumor development, therefore limiting the potential translational value of this model for testing of investigational agents. Moreover, transgenic mouse strains are extremely labor intensive and can be very costly, therefore limiting their use by many institutions.

4. SUBCUTANEOUS XENOGRAFTS OF HUMAN MM

Similarly to subcutaneous (sc) xenograft models of solid tumors, human MM cell lines can be injected in immunocompromised mice. MM cell lines autonomously engraft and generate palpable tumors, providing an *in vivo* setting for the study of MM [60,61]. The severe combined immunodeficiency (SCID) mouse provides an attractive model for the study of a variety of human tumors *in vivo*. In this model, progenitor B- and T-cells consistently fail to develop to a fully functional mature state and eventually undergo apoptosis [62]. Despite the immune deficiencies, the haematopoietic microenvironment of SCID, including the thymic stroma, remains intact [63]. All these properties make these mice unable to reject allogeneic or xenogeneic organ grafts allowing the successful engraftment of normal or neoplastic lymphoid populations in SCID mice [64]. In this model MM cells have been injected sc in a mixture with matrigel to facilitate the engraftment. Tumors grow as solid sc tumors and the tumor growth is measured in three dimensions using a caliper and the following formula. $V = (a^2 \times b)/2$; where a is the width of the tumor (smaller diameter) and b is the length (larger diameter). The primary endpoint for preclinical studies of anti-MM agents is typically the effect on the volume of sc tumors. Mice are euthanized when the tumor reaches a predetermined threshold of size (typically a diameter of 2 cm) or when significant compromise in their quality of life is noted (*e.g.*, significant weight loss, bleeding, infection, and so forth).

So far, the sc xenograft model in immunodeficient mice has allowed the evaluation of a variety of investigational therapeutics against human MM *in vivo* [65-68] and some of these studies have been translated to the bedside in clinical protocols treating patients with refractory relapsed MM, including proteasome inhibitors [69,70], thalidomide and its immunomodulatory analogs [71].

Human sc xenografts have the advantage that MM lesions can be easily monitored and any changes in their size can be quantified easily with caliper measurements. In addition, tumors can be easily excised and evaluated for histological and molecular profiling studies. However, there are some important limitations in the use of these models that should be taken in account by researchers. A key problem is the use of MM cell lines that are used to create xenografts. In fact these cell lines do not recapitulate the wide heterogeneity of MM in humans. Most importantly, since several MM cell lines have been obtained from advanced extramedullary disease (pleural or peritoneal effusions or peripheral blood of plasma cell leukemia patients), these cells are biologically different from primary MM cells which closely adhere to cells of the HuBMM and therefore do not recapitulate the biological features of early disease (*i.e.* they have high rate of cells in S phase, when compared to fresh MM cells that do not usually divide rapidly). These differences are important since therapeutics that target cell division may works well against cell lines *in vitro* or *in vivo* but not in MM patients. Moreover, these cell lines evolve over time and undergo several mutations not present at the time of intramedullay disease. It is interesting to note that nearly half of MM tumors are nonhyperdiploid and usually have one of five recurrent IgH translocations [72]. Furthermore, there are virtually no MM cell lines representing the hyperdiploid D1 group [73]. In addition, many MM cell lines are EBV positive and therefore not representative of human disease since few human MM express EBV. It should be also noted that while exchanged and spread among different research institutions, these cells are manipulated with similar but not identical culture conditions which in turn favour the onset of cell instability and increase the heterogeneity of the parental clones.

Together with above considerations on the genetic nature of MM cell lines, more critical considerations would be taken in account on the use of these models. In fact, in these models, the growth of the disease is not consistent with the diffuse systemic nature of MM and places MM cells in a murine sc microenvironment which is far from the complex scenario of the HuBMM where cells are significantly influenced by the milieu for MM proliferation, survival, and development of drug resistance [74-78]. It is in fact well known that several conventional anti-MM therapeutics (eg, dexamethasone, alkylating agents, anthracyclines) are active *in vitro* against MM cells when they are cultured alone, but considerably less effective when MM cells are cocultured in the presence of BMSCs [1,79]. Since sc xenografts do not allow the interaction between MM cell and human BMSCs, some agents may exhibit anti-MM activity in these models but may be not active in MM patients. It is also conceivable that these models can't assess the effect on MM cell growth of drugs targeting only the BMM, as well as do not lead to the characteristic skeletal complications of MM (eg, bone resorption, spontaneous fractures), which further limits the relevance of these models. Finally, the requirement of immunocompromised animals makes these models unable to characterize the anti-tumor activity of many immunotherapeutic drugs.

5. DIFFUSE XENOGRAFTS MODELS OF HUMAN MM

To address the limitations of the sc xenograft model of MM, models of intravenous (iv) or intra-peritoneal (ip) injections of tumor cells in non-obese diabetic scid (NOD/SCID) mice have been developed. Feo-Zuppardi *et al.* [15] have first showed engraftment of highly purified primary cells from BM of MM patients after intra-peritoneal injections in SCID mice. Secretion of monoclonal human immunoglobulins was described in this model and pathologic studies showed engraftment of MM cells in the peritoneal cavity where cells were injected, and evidence of metastatic spread to lymph nodes and various tissues without metastasis to murine BM. Other investigators [80] have also used the iv route to inject the murine tumor MOPC-315 into Balb/c mice, but mice did not develop the disseminated BM involvement characteristic of MM in humans.

Later, Huang *et al.* [81] have successfully engrafted into SCID mice a human MM cell line ARH-77 derived from peripheral plasma cells of a patient with IgG plasma cell leukemia [82,83], showing tumor engraftment at the inoculation site where ARH-77 cells were injected sc. Disseminated tumor growth in the BM, kidney, brain and liver was detected when mice were irradiated with 150 rads and injected iv with 1 x 10^7 ARH-77 cells. Tumor cells proliferated in the BM of vertebrae and in bones of the skull resulting in osteolytic lesions and spinal cord compression, mimicking the growth pattern observed in human MM. This model has been used to demonstrate the *in vivo* anti-tumor effects of the monoclonal anti-human CD54 antibody in MM [84].

To better understand the mechanisms of bone destruction in MM, Alsina *et al.* [85] have also injected ARH-77 cells iv in SCID mice previous irradiated (400 rads) to develop an *in vivo* model of human MM-related bone disease, able to mimic the clinical scenario of MM patients. All injected mice developed hypercalcemia, hind limb paralysis and osteolytic lesions, as assesses radiographically, 28 to 35 days after MM cells injections. Histologic examination of murine tissues also demonstrated infiltration of MM cells in the liver and spleen, and increased osteoclastic bone resorption in vertebrae and long bones adjacent to MM cell deposit, mimicking the behaviour of MM disease in humans. However, no increase in murine or human cytokines involved in bone resorption, such as IL-6, IL-1, or TNF-α, were observed in this model.

Other studies have also demonstrated the ability of peripheral MM cells, contaminating mobilized blood mononucleated cells or CD34-enriched cell explants, from patients with advanced disease, to produce MM and cause lytic bone disease in irradiated NOD/SCID mice when injected intra-cardically or intraosseous [86,87]. Injection of MM cells into the left cardiac ventricle (IC) or into the murine sternal BM (IO) were used to measure the ability of MM cells to home in the BM, and to migrate to distant BM sites. Phenotypic, pathologic and molecular analyses have shown presence of lytic bone lesions, BM plasma cells, and high frequency of clonotypic cells in the murine BM and in the femoral BM, following IC and IO injections. Overall, these data showed that peripheral cells from MM patients with aggressive disease include malignant clones that are myelomagenic, able to expand and migrate in the murine BM which is a supportive environment for MM cells, highlighting the importance of effective purging strategies before transplant.

Although the systemic nature of MM may be recapitulated by these *in vivo* models of iv/ic injections of MM cells, these experimental *in vivo* systems do not allow for sensitive and effective detection of disease progression and tumor load. Recently, visualization of cancer cells in mice has become possible by improved imaging technologies and the use of cells stably expressing the bioluminescent jellyfish Aequorea Victoria protein, green fluorescent protein (GFP). RPMI-8226 MM cells stably transfected with GFP were injected iv in SCID/NOD mice and the development of diffuse MM lesions was monitored by whole-body fluorescence imaging. This approach allowed the detection of the fluorescence emitted by the GFP+ MM cells when illuminated with near-infrared light, and confirmed histologically or by flow cytometric detection of GFP+ cells [88]. More than 95% of mice injected with GFP+ MM cells developed bone lesions in the spine and in the axial skeleton consistent with the distribution of MM bone diseases observed clinically and showed paralysis secondary to vertebral MM involvement. Extraskeletal tumors were also observed without significant tumor spread to lungs, liver, spleen and kidney. In addition, the murine MM 5TGM1 cells were also engineered to stably express GFP and inoculated into syngeneic C57BL mice to produce fluorescent tumors throughout the mouse skeleton [89]. Whole-body images of tumor-bearing mice revealed that GFP+ MM cells have a predilection for the skeleton in all mice with multifocal lesions in the axial skeleton, consistent with the typical tumor distribution in MM patients.

These models has been successfully used to evaluate the anti-tumor effects of new agents such as Bortezomib [89] and heat shock protein 90 inhibitor [90] showing the utility of this approach for rapid and inexpensive detection of MM engraftment and for the screening of novel anti-MM agents. The weakness of these approaches is mainly the lack of HuBMM which does not allow the recapitulation of human disease and the study of drug targeting also or specifically the non-tumor compartment.

6. SCID-HU MODEL

Primary MM cells from most patients do not grow in SCID mice, due to the dependence of MM cells on BM microenvironment factors that cannot be replaced by the murine microenvironment. To overcome these limitations murine models based on sc implantation of human fetal bone chips, where MM cells are directly injected, have been developed (SCID-hu). The SCID-hu model was initially used to study normal hematopoiesis [63], cytokines [91] and gene therapies [92] and then exploited as model to study the growth of primary leukemic cells [93] and the homing of MM cell lines and primary MM cells. Urashima *et al.* [94] have first shown engraftment and proliferation of human MM cell lines (ARH-77, OCI-My5, U-266, RPMI-8226) in the implanted fetal bone chips, where MM cells are injected in irradiated SCID-hu mice. By histologic examinations they have also demonstrated the ability of MM cells to home and spread to human BM within an additional not injected bone chip, without spread to murine BM, highlighting the importance of the human BM microenvironment to facilitate human MM cell growth. Later, Yaccoby *et al* [95] have successfully engrafted purified primary cells from MM patients in this system, showing the typical MM clinical features in the SCID host, such as the appearance of monotypic human Igs in the serum, high blood calcium levels and changes in the implanted human bone, which often result in osteolysis of the human bone. New formed blood vessels were also detectable in areas infiltrated by MM cells, demonstrating active angiogenesis.

Overall the SCID-hu MM model is the only available model in which primary MM cells can grow *in vivo* in a HuBMM. Using this model it has been possible to demonstrate the activity of several investigational compound targeting MM cells and its HuBMM, such as the antiangiogenic agent thalidomide [96], the IkappaB kinase (IKK) inhibitor MLN120B [97], and others. Although the SCID-hu model remains the most biologically relevant system for the study of interaction of MM cells with the human BM milieu, its use is difficult in experimental settings that require a large number of animals bearing MM, such as drug combinations studies. A limited number of MM cells can be obtained from each patient sample limiting the number of mice that can be injected with the same material and increasing variability in the engraftment of disease in mice. To overcome these limitations, Tassone *et al.* [16] have recently developed a novel SCID-hu model obtained injecting the IL-6 and BMSCs dependent MM cell line INA-6, stably transduced with GFP, into SCID mice previously implanted with human fetal bone chips (Fig. **1**). MM engraftment was observed only in mice implanted with human fetal bone and not in animals injected s.c. or i.v. with INA-6 cells. Serum level of shuIL-6R, released by INA-6 cell in mice sera and external real time fluorescence imaging of SCID-hu mice were used as sensitive indicators of tumor growth. Disseminated growth of MM cells in the BM was also confirmed by histologic examination of human fetal bone chips. Although the use of a single MM cell line limits the reproduction of the natural heterogeneity of MM in humans, the INA-6 SCID-hu model is highly reproducible and useful for preclinical evaluation of novel anti-MM agents. By the use of this model has been possible to demonstrate the anti-MM activity of several drugs such as the anti-inflammatory drug Atiprimod [98], the anti-BAFF mAb [99], the anti-DKK1 mAb (BHQ880) [100], a fully human anti-IL6 mAb [101] the immunoconjugated anti CD138 BB4-DM1 [67], the IL-6 superantagonist SANT-7 [102] and others [103,104].

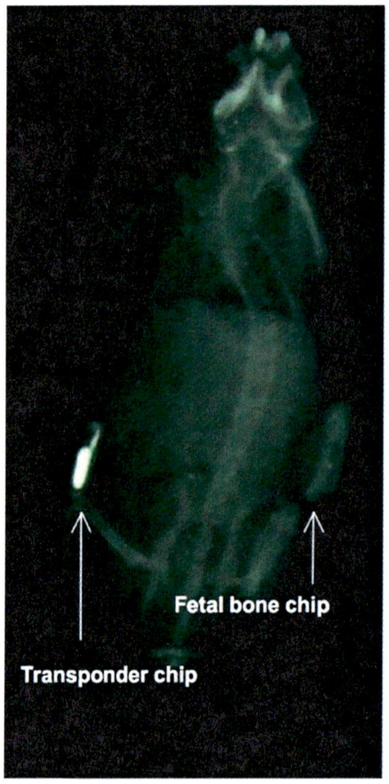

Fig. (1). SCID-hu MM model.

Overall, the SCID-hu MM model is at present the most reliable model to reproduce the human disease in mice and provides the only platform for *in vivo* investigation of the biology and therapy of human primary MM in a HuBMM. The limitation of this model is the difficult supply of fetal bone chips and the impossibility to recapitulate the development oh human disease in an adult and most importantly autologous milieu.

7. OTHER MODELS

The LAGλ-1 model has been recently described as novel clinically relevant murine model of human MM [105]. In this model, fresh whole core BM biopsies from 33 MM patients were engrafted en bloc into hind-limb muscles of SCID mice and human immunoglobulin was detected in 28 of 33 mice. Three of the mice with MM cell growth develop palpable tumors that were morphologically and immunophenotypically consistent with human MM. These cells were then serially transplanted in mice by intramuscular injections, leading to development of tumors. One of these, termed LAGλ-1, derived from cells of an IgG-λ–producing patient who had MM, was selected for further evaluation and studies. The cells of this LAGλ-1 model could lead to establishment of MM lesions after intramuscular, subcutaneous, or intravenous injection, and were tested for their *in vivo* response to established anti-MM agents, including Melphalan, doxorubicin, and bortezomib [105].

8. CONCLUSIONS AND FUTURE PERSPECTIVES

We reviewed here the most known *in vivo* models of human MM and we highlighted both related advantages and limitations. Since *in vitro* models can only address limited issues of preclinical investigation on MM pathogenesis and anti-tumor activity of novel therapeutics, animal models of MM represent an important step that has undoubtedly led to major advances in the treatment of this still incurable disease. In the past, a variety of mouse models have been developed and the *in vivo* validation of novel agents has been mostly carried out using models of murine MM, such as the 5T series, or by conventional sc or disseminated xenograft models of human MM cell lines in immunocompromised mice. Engineered mouse models constitute a relevant advancement but are not capable to recapitulate the genetic heterogeneity of human disease. The recent availability of preclinical SCID-hu models recapitulating the HuBMM provides a novel powerful and essential support to explore new drugs against the human disease in its biological human milieu. These systems represent ideal models in which drug-related manipulation of the HuBMM may be analysed by molecular technologies for identification of new therapeutic targets. The opportunity to recapitulate *ex vivo* the human disease in a HuBMM produces a novel platform where preclinical and clinical findings can be definitively integrated. However, novel models able to totally recapitulate the HuBMM and easy to reproduce are still needed. The fulfilment of these requirements in novel preclinical models will provide a fundamental support for the modern translational research which implies not only the transfer of information from bench to bedside but also the design of preclinical research on the basis of information gained from clinical studies.

ACKNOWLEDGEMENTS

This work is supported by the Italian Association for Cancer Research (AIRC) (P.T. project 2007-2009) and (P.N. project 2008-2010), Milan, and PRIN (P.T. 2007-2008), Italy.

REFERENCES

[1] Mitsiades Cs, Mitsiades N, Munshi NC, Anderson KC. Focus on multiple myeloma. Cancer Cell 2004; 6: 439-444.

[2] Potter M. Neoplastic development in plasma cells. Immunol Rev 2003; 194: 177-195.

[3] Gado K, Silva S, Paloczi K, Domjan G, Falus A. Mouse plasmacytoma: an experimental model of human multiple myeloma. Haematologica 2001; 86: 227-236.

[4] Macor P, Secco E, Zorzet S, *et al.* An update on the xenograft and mouse models suitable for investigating new therapeutic compounds for the treatment of B-cell malignancies. Curr Pharm Des 2008; 14: 2023-2039.

[5] Lubet Ra, Zhang Z, Wang Y, You M. Chemoprevention of lung cancer in transgenic mice. Chest 2004; 125: 144S-147S.

[6] Pattengale PK, Taylor CR. Experimental models of lymphoproliferative disease. The mouse as a model for human non-Hodgkin's lymphomas and related leukemias. Am J Pathol 1983; 113: 237-265.

[7] Pattengale PK, Frith CH. Immunomorphologic classification of spontaneous lymphoid cell neoplasms occurring in female BALB/c mice. J Natl Cancer Inst 1983; 70: 169-179.

[8] Di Bisceglie Am, Osmack P, Brunt Em. Chemoprevention of hepatocellular carcinoma: use of tamoxifen in an animal model of hepatocarcinogenesis. J Lab Clin Med 2005; 145: 134-138.

[9] Nagao M, Ushijima T, Toyota M, Inoue R, Sugimura T. Genetic changes induced by heterocyclic amines. Mutat Res 1997; 376: 161-167.

[10] Sugiyama T, Osaka M, Koami K, Maeda S, Ueda N. 7,12-DMBA-induced rat leukemia: a review with insights into future research. Leuk Res 2002; 26: 1053-1068.

[11] Abate-Shen C, Shen MM. Mouse models of prostate carcinogenesis. Trends Genet 2002; 18: S1-5.

[12] Jamerson MH, Johnson MD, Dickson RB. Of mice and Myc: c-Myc and mammary tumorigenesis. J Mammary Gland Biol Neoplasia 2004; 9: 27-37.

[13] Kelland LR. Of mice and men: values and liabilities of the athymic nude mouse model in anticancer drug development. Eur J Cancer 2004; 40: 827-836.

[14] Peterson JK, Houghton PJ. Integrating pharmacology and *in vivo* cancer models in preclinical and clinical drug development. Eur J Cancer 2004; 40: 837-844.

[15] Feo-Zuppardi FJ, Taylor CW, Iwato K, *et al.* Long-term engraftment of fresh human myeloma cells in SCID mice. Blood 1992; 80: 2843-2850.

[16] Tassone P, Neri P, Carrasco DR, *et al.* A clinically relevant SCID-hu *in vivo* model of human multiple myeloma. Blood 2005; 106: 713-716.

[17] Tassone P, Neri P, Kutok JL, *et al.* A SCID-hu *in vivo* model of human Waldenstrom macroglobulinemia. Blood 2005; 106: 1341-1345.

[18] Menu E, Asosingh K, Van Riet I, *et al.* Myeloma cells (5TMM) and their interactions with the marrow microenvironment. Blood Cells Mol Dis 2004; 33: 111-119.

[19] Mitsiades CS, Anderson KC, Carrasco DR. Mouse models of human myeloma. Hematol Oncol Clin North Am 2007; 21: 1051-1069, viii.

[20] Radl J, Hollander CF, Van Den Berg P, De Glopper E. Idiopathic paraproteinaemia. I. Studies in an animal model--the ageing C57BL/KaLwRij mouse. Clin Exp Immunol 1978; 33: 395-402.

[21] Radl J. Age-related monoclonal gammapathies: clinical lessons from the aging C57BL mouse. Immunol Today 1990; 11: 234-236.

[22] Asosingh K, Radl J, Van Riet I, Van Camp B, Vanderkerken K. The 5TMM series: a useful *in vivo* mouse model of human multiple myeloma. Hematol J 2000; 1: 351-356.

[23] Garrett Ir, Dallas S, Radl J, Mundy Gr. A murine model of human myeloma bone disease. Bone 1997; 20: 515-520.

[24] Vanderkerken K, De Raeve H, Goes E, *et al.* Organ involvement and phenotypic adhesion profile of 5T2 and 5T33 myeloma cells in the C57BL/KaLwRij mouse. Br J Cancer 1997; 76: 451-460.

[25] Asosingh K, Gunthert U, De Raeve H, *et al.* A unique pathway in the homing of murine multiple myeloma cells: CD44v10 mediates binding to bone marrow endothelium. Cancer Res 2001; 61: 2862-2865.

[26] Vanderkerken K, Asosingh K, Willems A, *et al.* The 5T2MM murine model of multiple myeloma: maintenance and analysis. Methods Mol Med 2005; 113: 191-205.

[27] Vanderkerken K, De Greef C, Asosingh K, *et al.* Selective initial *in vivo* homing pattern of 5T2 multiple myeloma cells in the C57BL/KalwRij mouse. Br J Cancer 2000; 82: 953-959.

[28] Libouban H, Moreau MF, Basle MF, Bataille R, Chappard D. Increased bone remodeling due to ovariectomy dramatically increases tumoral growth in the 5T2 multiple myeloma mouse model. Bone 2003; 33: 283-292.

[29] Croucher PI, De Hendrik R, Perry MJ, *et al.* Zoledronic acid treatment of 5T2MM-bearing mice inhibits the development of myeloma bone disease: evidence for decreased osteolysis, tumor burden and angiogenesis, and increased survival. J Bone Miner Res 2003; 18: 482-492.

[30] Vanderkerken K, Asosingh K, Croucher P, Van Camp B. Multiple myeloma biology: lessons from the 5TMM models. Immunol Rev 2003; 194: 196-206.

[31] Croucher PI, Shipman CM, Van Camp B, Vanderkerken K. Bisphosphonates and osteoprotegerin as inhibitors of myeloma bone disease. Cancer 2003; 97: 818-824.

[32] Asosingh K, Menu E, Van Valckenborgh E, *et al.* Mechanisms involved in the differential bone marrow homing of CD45 subsets in 5T murine models of myeloma. Clin Exp Metastasis 2002; 19: 583-591.

[33] Menu E, De Leenheer E, De Raeve H, *et al.* Role of CCR1 and CCR5 in homing and growth of multiple myeloma and in the development of osteolytic lesions: a study in the 5TMM model. Clin Exp Metastasis 2006; 23: 291-300.

[34] Vanderkerken K, Vande Broek I, Eizirik DL, *et al.* Monocyte chemoattractant protein-1 (MCP-1), secreted by bone marrow endothelial cells, induces chemoattraction of 5T multiple myeloma cells. Clin Exp Metastasis 2002; 19: 87-90.

[35] Menu E, Jernberg-Wiklund H, Stromberg T, *et al.* Inhibiting the IGF-1 receptor tyrosine kinase with the cyclolignan PPP: an *in vitro* and *in vivo* study in the 5T33MM mouse model. Blood 2006; 107: 655-660.

[36] Menu E, Asosingh K, Indraccolo S, *et al.* The involvement of stromal derived factor 1alpha in homing and progression of multiple myeloma in the 5TMM model. Haematologica 2006; 91: 605-612.

[37] Van Valckenborgh E, Bakkus M, Munaut C, *et al.* Upregulation of matrix metalloproteinase-9 in murine 5T33 multiple myeloma cells by interaction with bone marrow endothelial cells. Int J Cancer 2002; 101: 512-518.

[38] Van Valckenborgh E, De Raeve H, Devy L, *et al.* Murine 5T multiple myeloma cells induce angiogenesis *in vitro* and *in vivo*. Br J Cancer 2002; 86: 796-802.

[39] Asosingh K, De Raeve H, De Ridder M, *et al.* Role of the hypoxic bone marrow microenvironment in 5T2MM murine myeloma tumor progression. Haematologica 2005; 90: 810-817.

[40] Deleu S, Lemaire M, Arts J, *et al.* The effects of JNJ-26481585, a novel hydroxamate-based histone deacetylase inhibitor, on the development of multiple myeloma in the 5T2MM and 5T33MM murine models. Leukemia 2009; 23: 1894-1903.

[41] Mittelman M, Neumann D, Peled A, Kanter P, Haran-Ghera N. Erythropoietin induces tumor regression and antitumor immune responses in murine myeloma models. Proc Natl Acad Sci U S A 2001; 98: 5181-5186.

[42] Henry JM, Morley AA, Sykes PJ. Purging of myeloma cells using all-trans retinoic acid in a mouse model. Exp Hematol 2001; 29: 315-321.

[43] Vanderkerken K, Asosingh K, Braet F, Van Riet I, Van Camp B. Insulin-like growth factor-1 acts as a chemoattractant factor for 5T2 multiple myeloma cells. Blood 1999; 93: 235-241.

[44] Radl J, Punt YA, Van Den Enden-Vieveen MH, *et al.* The 5T mouse multiple myeloma model: absence of c-myc oncogene rearrangement in early transplant generations. Br J Cancer 1990; 61: 276-278.

[45] Kuehl WM, Bergsagel PL. Multiple myeloma: evolving genetic events and host interactions. Nat Rev Cancer 2002; 2: 175-187.

[46] Hansen K, Khanna C. Spontaneous and genetically engineered animal models; use in preclinical cancer drug development. Eur J Cancer 2004; 40: 858-880.

[47] Bernardi R, Grisendi S, Pandolfi PP. Modelling haematopoietic malignancies in the mouse and therapeutical implications. Oncogene 2002; 21: 3445-3458.

[48] Soma T, Dunbar CE. *In vivo* models for studying the role of autocrine or paracrine growth factors in hematologic malignancies. Exp Hematol 1995; 23: 385-388.

[49] Suematsu S, Matsusaka T, Matsuda T, *et al.* Generation of plasmacytomas with the chromosomal translocation t(12;15) in interleukin 6 transgenic mice. Proc Natl Acad Sci U S A 1992; 89: 232-235.

[50] Fattori E, Della Rocca C, Costa P, *et al.* Development of progressive kidney damage and myeloma kidney in interleukin 6 transgenic mice. Blood 1994; 83: 2570-2579.

[51] Rosenbaum H, Harris Aw, Bath Ml, *et al.* An E mu-v-abl transgene elicits plasmacytomas in concert with an activated myc gene. EMBO J 1990; 9: 897-905.

[52] Strasser A, Harris AW, Cory S. E mu-bcl-2 transgene facilitates spontaneous transformation of early pre-B and immunoglobulin-secreting cells but not T cells. Oncogene 1993; 8: 1-9.

[53] Kovalchuk AL, Kim JS, Park SS, *et al.* IL-6 transgenic mouse model for extraosseous plasmacytoma. Proc Natl Acad Sci U S A 2002; 99: 1509-1514.

[54] Lange K, Uckert W, Blankenstein T, *et al.* Overexpression of NPM-ALK induces different types of malignant lymphomas in IL-9 transgenic mice. Oncogene 2003; 22: 517-527.

[55] Cheung WC, Kim JS, Linden M, *et al.* Novel targeted deregulation of c-Myc cooperates with Bcl-X(L) to cause plasma cell neoplasms in mice. J Clin Invest 2004; 113: 1763-1773.

[56] Boylan KL, Gosse MA, Staggs SE, *et al.* A transgenic mouse model of plasma cell malignancy shows phenotypic, cytogenetic, and gene expression heterogeneity similar to human multiple myeloma. Cancer Res 2007; 67: 4069-4078.

[57] Chesi M, Robbiani DF, Sebag M, *et al.* AID-dependent activation of a MYC transgene induces multiple myeloma in a conditional mouse model of post-germinal center malignancies. Cancer Cell 2008; 13: 167-180.

[58] Carrasco DR, Sukhdeo K, Protopopova M, *et al.* The differentiation and stress response factor XBP-1 drives multiple myeloma pathogenesis. Cancer Cell 2007; 11: 349-360.

[59] Iwakoshi NN, Lee AH, Vallabhajosyula P, *et al.* Plasma cell differentiation and the unfolded protein response intersect at the transcription factor XBP-1. Nat Immunol 2003; 4: 321-329.

[60] Feo-Zuppardi FJ, Taylor CW, Iwato K, *et al.* Long-term engraftment of fresh human myeloma cells in SCID mice. Blood 1992; 80: 2843-2850.

[61] Tong Aw, Huang YW, Zhang BQ, *et al.* Heterotransplantation of human multiple myeloma cell lines in severe combined immunodeficiency (SCID) mice. Anticancer Res 1993; 13: 593-597.

[62] Bosma GC, Custer RP, Bosma MJ. A severe combined immunodeficiency mutation in the mouse. Nature 1983; 301: 527-530.

[63] Mccune JM, Namikawa R, Kaneshima H, *et al.* The SCID-hu mouse: murine model for the analysis of human hematolymphoid differentiation and function. Science 1988; 241: 1632-1639.

[64] Bankert RB, Egilmez NK, Hess SD. Human-SCID mouse chimeric models for the evaluation of anti-cancer therapies. Trends Immunol 2001; 22: 386-393.

[65] Tai Yt, Fulciniti M, Hideshima T, *et al.* Targeting MEK induces myeloma-cell cytotoxicity and inhibits osteoclastogenesis. Blood 2007; 110: 1656-1663.

[66] Chauhan D, Neri P, Velankar M, *et al.* Targeting mitochondrial factor Smac/DIABLO as therapy for multiple myeloma (MM). Blood 2007; 109: 1220-1227.

[67] Tassone P, Goldmacher Vs, Neri P, *et al.* Cytotoxic activity of the maytansinoid immunoconjugate B-B4-DM1 against CD138+ multiple myeloma cells. Blood 2004; 104: 3688-3696.

[68] Tassone P, Gozzini A, Goldmacher V, *et al. In vitro* and *in vivo* activity of the maytansinoid immunoconjugate huN901-N2'-deacetyl-N2'-(3-mercapto-1-oxopropyl)-maytansine against CD56+ multiple myeloma cells. Cancer Res 2004; 64: 4629-4636.

[69] Leblanc R, Catley LP, Hideshima T, *et al.* Proteasome inhibitor PS-341 inhibits human myeloma cell growth *in vivo* and prolongs survival in a murine model. Cancer Res 2002; 62: 4996-5000.

[70] Chauhan D, Hideshima T, Anderson KC. A novel proteasome inhibitor NPI-0052 as an anticancer therapy. Br J Cancer 2006; 95: 961-965.

[71] Lentzsch S, Rogers Ms, Leblanc R, *et al.* S-3-Amino-phthalimido-glutarimide inhibits angiogenesis and growth of B-cell neoplasias in mice. Cancer Res 2002; 62: 2300-2305.

[72] Bergsagel PL, Kuehl WM. Critical roles for immunoglobulin translocations and cyclin D dysregulation in multiple myeloma. Immunol Rev 2003; 194: 96-104.

[73] Dalton W, Anderson KC. Synopsis of a roundtable on validating novel therapeutics for multiple myeloma. Clin Cancer Res 2006; 12: 6603-6610.

[74] Hideshima T, Bergsagel PL, Kuehl WM, Anderson KC. Advances in biology of multiple myeloma: clinical applications. Blood 2004; 104: 607-618.

[75] Damiano JS, Cress AE, Hazlehurst LA, Shtil AA, Dalton WS. Cell adhesion mediated drug resistance (CAM-DR): role of integrins and resistance to apoptosis in human myeloma cell lines. Blood 1999; 93: 1658-1667.

[76] Shain KH, Landowski TH, Dalton WS. The tumor microenvironment as a determinant of cancer cell survival: a possible mechanism for de novo drug resistance. Curr Opin Oncol 2000; 12: 557-563.

[77] Dedera DA, Urashima M, Chauhan D, *et al.* Interleukin-6 is required for pristane-induced plasma cell hyperplasia in mice. Br J Haematol 1996; 94: 53-61.

[78] Podar K, Tai YT, Davies FE, *et al.* Vascular endothelial growth factor triggers signaling cascades mediating multiple myeloma cell growth and migration. Blood 2001; 98: 428-435.

[79] Hideshima T, Anderson KC. Molecular mechanisms of novel therapeutic approaches for multiple myeloma. Nat Rev Cancer 2002; 2: 927-937.

[80] Valeriote F, Grates H. MOPC-315 murine plasmacytoma as a model anticancer screen for human multiple myeloma. J Natl Cancer Inst 1986; 76: 61-65.

[81] Huang YW, Richardson JA, Tong AW, *et al.* Disseminated growth of a human multiple myeloma cell line in mice with severe combined immunodeficiency disease. Cancer Res 1993; 53: 1392-1396.

[82] Burk KH, Drewinko B, Turjillo Jm, Ahearn MJ. Establishment of a human plasma cell line *in vitro*. Cancer Res 1978; 38: 2508-2513.

[83] Drewinko B, Mars W, Stragand JJ, *et al.* ARH-77, an established human IgG-producing myeloma cell line. II. Growth kinetics, clonogenic capacity, chalone production, xenogeneic transplantations, and response to Melphalan. Cancer 1984; 54: 1893-1903.

[84] Huang YW, Richardson JA, Vitetta ES. Anti-CD54 (ICAM-1) has antitumor activity in SCID mice with human myeloma cells. Cancer Res 1995; 55: 610-616.

[85] Alsina M, Boyce B, Devlin RD, *et al.* Development of an *in vivo* model of human multiple myeloma bone disease. Blood 1996; 87: 1495-1501.

[86] Pilarski LM, Hipperson G, Seeberger K, *et al.* Myeloma progenitors in the blood of patients with aggressive or minimal disease: engraftment and self-renewal of primary human myeloma in the bone marrow of NOD SCID mice. Blood 2000; 95: 1056-1065.

[87] Pilarski LM, Belch AR. Clonotypic myeloma cells able to xenograft myeloma to nonobese diabetic severe combined immunodeficient mice copurify with CD34 (+) hematopoietic progenitors. Clin Cancer Res 2002; 8: 3198-3204.

[88] Mitsiades CS, Mitsiades NS, Bronson RT, *et al.* Fluorescence imaging of multiple myeloma cells in a clinically relevant SCID/NOD *in vivo* model: biologic and clinical implications. Cancer Res 2003; 63: 6689-6696.

[89] Oyajobi BO, Munoz S, Kakonen R, *et al.* Detection of myeloma in skeleton of mice by whole-body optical fluorescence imaging. Mol Cancer Ther 2007; 6: 1701-1708.

[90] Mitsiades CS, Mitsiades NS, McMullan CJ, *et al.* Antimyeloma activity of heat shock protein-90 inhibition. Blood 2006; 107: 1092-1100.

[91] Kyoizumi S, Murray LJ, Namikawa R. Preclinical analysis of cytokine therapy in the SCID-hu mouse. Blood 1993; 81: 1479-1488.

[92] Akkina RK, Rosenblatt JD, Campbell AG, Chen IS, Zack JA. Modeling human lymphoid precursor cell gene therapy in the SCID-hu mouse. Blood 1994; 84: 1393-1398.

[93] Namikawa R, Ueda R, Kyoizumi S. Growth of human myeloid leukemias in the human marrow environment of SCID-hu mice. Blood 1993; 82: 2526-2536.

[94] Urashima M, Chen BP, Chen S, *et al.* The development of a model for the homing of multiple myeloma cells to human bone marrow. Blood 1997; 90: 754-765.

[95] Yaccoby S, Barlogie B, Epstein J. Primary myeloma cells growing in SCID-hu mice: a model for studying the biology and treatment of myeloma and its manifestations. Blood 1998; 92: 2908-2913.

[96] Yaccoby S, Johnson CL, Mahaffey SC, *et al.* Antimyeloma efficacy of thalidomide in the SCID-hu model. Blood 2002; 100: 4162-4168.

[97] Hideshima T, Neri P, Tassone P, *et al.* MLN120B, a novel IkappaB kinase beta inhibitor, blocks multiple myeloma cell growth *in vitro* and *in vivo*. Clin Cancer Res 2006; 12: 5887-5894.

[98] Neri P, Tassone P, Shammas M, *et al.* Biological pathways and *in vivo* antitumor activity induced by Atiprimod in myeloma. Leukemia 2007; 21: 2519-2526.

[99] Neri P, Kumar S, Fulciniti MT, *et al.* Neutralizing B-cell activating factor antibody improves survival and inhibits osteoclastogenesis in a severe combined immunodeficient human multiple myeloma model. Clin Cancer Res 2007; 13: 5903-5909.

[100] Fulciniti M, Tassone P, Hideshima T, *et al.* Anti-DKK1 mAb (BHQ880) as a potential therapeutic agent for multiple myeloma. Blood 2009; 114: 371-379.

[101] Fulciniti M, Hideshima T, Vermot-Desroches C, *et al.* A high-affinity fully human anti-IL-6 mAb, 1339, for the treatment of multiple myeloma. Clin Cancer Res 2009; 15: 7144-7152.

[102] Tassone P, Neri P, Burger R, *et al.* Combination therapy with interleukin-6 receptor superantagonist Sant7 and dexamethasone induces antitumor effects in a novel SCID-hu *In vivo* model of human multiple myeloma. Clin Cancer Res 2005; 11: 4251-4258.

[103] Ikeda H, Hideshima T, Fulciniti MT, *et al.* The monoclonal antibody nBT062 conjugated to cytotoxic Maytansinoids has selective cytotoxicity against CD138-positive multiple myeloma cells *in vitro* and *in vivo*. Clin Cancer Res 2009; 15: 4028-4037.

[104] Shammas MA, Koley H, Bertheau RC, *et al.* Telomerase inhibitor GRN163L inhibits myeloma cell growth *in vitro* and *in vivo*. Leukemia 2008; 22: 1410-1418.

[105] Campbell RA, Manyak SJ, Yang HH, *et al.* LAGlambda-1: a clinically relevant drug resistant human multiple myeloma tumor murine model that enables rapid evaluation of treatments for multiple myeloma. Int J Oncol 2006; 28: 1409-1417.

CHAPTER 12

New Therapeutic Strategies in Multiple Myeloma

Klaus Podar[1,2*], Teru Hideshima[1], Dharminder Chauhan[1] and Kenneth C. Anderson[1]

[1]Department of Medical Oncology, Dana-Farber Cancer Institute, Harvard Medical School, Boston, MA 02115, USA; [2]National Center for Tumor Diseases (NCT)/ University of Heidelberg, Heidelberg, Germany

Abstract: The development of multiple myeloma (MM) is a complex multi-step process involving both early and late genetic changes in the tumor cell as well as selective supportive conditions by the bone marrow (BM) microenvironment. Based predominantly on our understanding of the functional importance of the MM BM microenvironment and its interrelation with the MM cell, which triggers tumor cell homing, seeding, proliferation, and survival, a multitude of new molecular targets have been identified. The clinical approval of four derived agents, thalidomide, its immunomodulatory derivative Len, the proteasome inhibitor bortezomib and pegylated liposomal doxorubicin have fundamentally changed treatment regimens in MM during the last decade. Moreover, based on a pathophysiologic rationale a multitude of additional agents, most prominently carfilzomib, pomalidomide, vorinostat, and perifosine have demonstrated promising preclinical and early/ advanced clinical activity indicating the evolvement of further treatment advancements in near future.

Keywords: Bone marrow microenvironment, thalidomide, bortezomib, ubiquitin-proteasome system (UPR), salinosporamidine A (NPI-0052), nutilins, aggresomes, signaling pathways, IL-6. VEGF, TNFα, SDF-1, CD40, BAFF/ APRIL, IGF-1, Ras/ MEK/ MAPK, PI3K/ Akt, STAT/ Jak, NFκB, Wnt.

1. INTRODUCTION

The finding that only few genetic differences distinguish monoclonal gammopathy of unknown significance (MGUS) from MM [1,2,3] highlights the essential role of the bone marrow (BM) microenvironment in MM development, maintenance and progression. Specifically, direct and indirect interactions with other cells and the extracellular matrix (ECM) within the liquid milieu of the BM environment mediate MM cell growth, survival, migration, and drug resistance. The complexity of growth factor/ cytokine-and cell-cell/ ECM adhesion-induced signaling sequelae is not only based on the initiation linear pathways including the Ras/Raf/MEK/MAPK-pathway, PI3K/ Akt-pathway, the JAK/ Stat3-pathway, the NFκB-pathway, and the Wnt-pathway but also on co-stimulatory events within the BM microenvironment. Several approaches to target *surface receptors* (*e.g.* receptor tyrosine kinases (RTKs), integrins, cadherins, selectins, syndecans, and the immunoglobulin superfamily of cell adhesion molecules including syndecan-1 (CD138), H-CAM (CD44), VLA-4 (CD49d/ CD29), ICAM-1 (CD54), N-CAM (CD56), LFA-3 (CD58), αvβ3, CD56, CD74, HM1.24, VLA-5 (CD49e/ CD29), VLA-6, and CD51, as well as CD2 subset-1 (CS-1), HLA-A, and β2-microglobulin [4,5,6,7,8,9,10,11], to neutralize their respective *ligands* (*e.g. cytokines and growth factors* including IL-6, VEGF, IGF-1, TNF-α, SDF-1α, and CD40; as well as TGF-β, bFGF, MIP-1α, SCF, HGF, IL-1β, IL-3, IL-10, IL-15, and IL-21 [12,13,14], and to inhibit the activation of downstream *intracellular molecules* are under investigation.

In summary, novel biologically-based treatment regimens aim to target not only MM cells alone but also MM cell-stromal cell interactions and the BM milieu. Below, we will briefly present up-to-date knowledge on MM pathophysiology and subsequently focus on derived new therapeutic strategies involving thalidomide, the IMiDs, inhibitors of the ubiquitin-proteasome system and a variety of targeted small molecule inhibitors (Fig. **1**). The pathophysiologic relevance of the BM microenvironment in MM including the role of the bone, BM angiogenesis, and the role of immune cells in MM will be discussed in more detail in Chapters 6 and Chapters 9 to 10, therapeutic approaches involving vaccines and therapeutic antibodies will be discussed in Chapter 13.

***Address correspondence to Klaus Podar:** National Center for Tumor Diseases, Im Neuenheimer Feld #410, phone: ++49 06221 (0) 56-38689; Fax: ++49 06221 (0) 56-8815, E-mails: klaus.podar@med.uni-heidelberg.de or klaus_podar@dfci.harvard.edu

Klaus Podar and Kenneth C. Anderson (Eds)

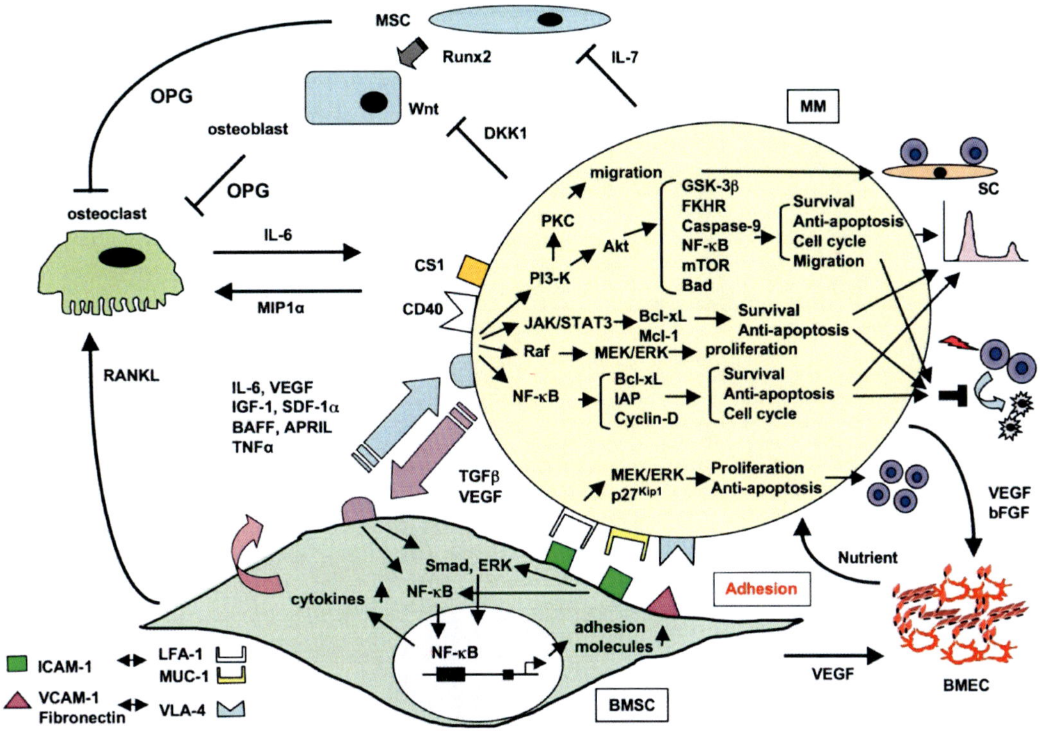

Fig. (1): Interaction of MM cells and the BM microenvironment: potential therapeutic targets. Adhesion of MM cells to BMSCs triggers cytokine-mediated tumor cell growth, survival, drug resistance, and migration *via* their receptors. Moreover, MM cell binding to BMSCs upregulates cytokine secretion from both BMSCs and MM cells. These cytokines activate major signaling pathways including Raf/MEK/ERK, JAK2/STAT3, PI3-K/Akt and NFκB. Their downstream targets include IL-6, IGF-1, and VEGF; anti-apoptotic proteins, such as Bcl-xL, inhibitor of apoptosis proteins (IAPs), MCL-1; and cell cycle modulators (ie, cyclin D). Adhesion mediated activation of NFkB upregulates adhesion molecules such as ICAM-1 and VCAM1 on both MM cells and BMSCs, thereby further increasing the binding of MM cells to BMSCs. Secretion of angiogenic factors, such as VEGF and bFGF and hepatocyte growth factor (HGF), from MM cells and BMSCs stimulates neoangiogenesis. Receptor Activator of NF-κB ligand (RANKL) and osteoprotegerin ligand (OPGL) produced by BMSCs, and macrophage inflammatory protein-1α (MIP-1α) produced by MM cells, stimulate osteoclastogenesis. In contrast, OPG secreted from BMSCs inhibits osteoclastogenesis. Osteoblastogenesis is inhibited by MM cells *via* secretion of IL-3 and Dickkopf 1 (DKK1) from MM cells and HGF from BMSCs. Stimulation of osteoclastogenesis and inhibition of osteoblastogenesis promote osteolysis.

2. THERAPEUTIC STRATEGIES TO TARGET THE CELLULAR MM BM COMPARTMENT

The **cellular BM compartment** is composed of ***hematopoietic cells*** including hematopoietic stem cells (HSCs); hematopoietic and mesenchymal progenitor and precursor cells; BM-derived circulating endothelial precursors (CEPs); immune cells (B lymphocytes, T lymphocytes, NK cells, macrophages, monocytes, NKT cells); erythrocytes; megakaryocytes and platelets; and ***non-hematopoietic*** *cells* including fibroblasts/ BMSCs; endothelial cells (ECs); as well as cells involved in bone homeostasis including chondroclasts, osteoclasts (OCs), and osteoblasts (OBs). The intimate functional interaction between these bone marrow (BM) compartments is of critical importance for finely tuned physiologic functions: the regulation of hematopoiesis; the mobilization of blood cells into the blood stream; as well as the homing of mature cells to selective sites within the BM. In MM, tumor cells impact the BM and disrupt the balanced homeostasis of MM cell-stromal cell interactions and liquid factors (cytokines, growth factors).

Targeting MM-BMSC Interactions

BMSC-associated pathophysiologic sequelae (*e.g.* tumor cell proliferation, survival, and drug resistance) are triggered directly, *via* integrin-mediated interactions of MM cells with BMSCs; or indirectly, *via* cytokines and growth factors (*e.g.* IL-6, VEGF, TNFα and IL-1) released by either tumor cells or BMSCs [15].

Key integrins mediating MM cell -ECM adhesion are β1 (CD29)-and αvβ3-integrin. MM cell adhesion to fibronectin is predominantly mediated *via* β1-integrin and directly protects tumor cells from DNA damaging drugs (*e.g.* anthracyclines and alkylating agents) *via* induction of cell-adhesion-mediated drug resistance (CAM-DR), [16,17]. MM cell adhesion to vitronectin and fibronectin is predominantly mediated *via* αvβ3-integrin binding and promotes tumor cell invasion and spreading [18]. Thal, Len, and Bort exert their anti-MM activity, at least in part, by inhibition of MM cell binding to ECM proteins as well as stromal cells. Ongoing studies are evaluating small molecule inhibitors and mAbs including the αvβ3-and the αvβ5-inhibitor cilengitide, as well as the β1-inhibitor volociximab to specifically inhibit adhesive interactions of MM cells with ECM proteins and stromal cells in the BM microenvironment in order to induce sensitization or overcome resistance to therapy [19].

Besides autocrine/ paracrine stimulation within the BM, cytokine/ growth factor secretion is mediated by CD40 activation of tumor cells (*e.g.* TNFα and IL-1). A clinical phase II study evaluating the CD40 antibody SGN-40 [20] has now been completed, a clinical trial using SGN-40 together with Len, which augments antibody-dependent cellular cytotoxicity (ADCC) [21], is ongoing. In addition to integrins and CD40/CD40L, BMSC -MM cell interaction is also mediated *via* Notch, in particular Notch ligands Jagged-1, Jagged-2 and DLL-1, in particular [22-24]. Upon Notch -Notch ligand interaction, Notch signaling pathways are activated both in MM cells as well as in BMSCs, with induction of IL-6, VEGF, and IGF-1 secretion and associated MM cell proliferation and survival [25-27]. Therefore, inhibition of Notch-1 was suggested as a new therapeutic approach to overcome resistance to chemotherapy, *e.g.* Melphalan and mitoxantrone, in MM [25]. In contrast to these data, Zweidler-McKay *et al.* reported that Notch signaling is a strong inducer of growth arrest and apoptosis in a wide range of B-cell malignancies including MM, and suggest the therapeutic potential of therapies activating Notch [28]. Further studies are required to define the potential benefits of strategies to either inhibit or promote Notch signaling. Although suggested by some authors, the existence of MM-specific abnormal BMSCs is still controversial. For example, Zdzisinska *et al.* report in a recent study that production of MMP-1, MMP-2 and TIMP-2 is significantly increased in BMSCs of MM patients vs. healthy controls [29]. Further studies are required to verify these data, to identify specific targets, and to design derived compounds.

Targeting Endothelial Cells, Osteoclasts, Osteoblasts, Immune Cells and Stem Cells within the MM BM Microenvironment

Other cellular therapeutic targets within the MM BM microenvironment include endothelial cells, osteoblasts and osteoclasts, immune cells *e.g.* T and B cells, as well as dendritic cells *e.g.* plasmacytoid dendritic cells, mesenchymal stem cells and MM stem cells. In MM, both tumor cells and BMSCs prolong survival of BM endothelial cells (ECs) both by increased secretion of EC survival factors, such as VEGF [30-32], and by decreased secretion of anti-angiogenic factors. Triggered by this imbalance of angiogenic regulators, the "angiogenic switch" accounts not only for a rapid increase of tumor vessels to support tumor growth, but also for their abnormal structure and formation of mosaic blood vessels. These mosaic vessels consist of ECs as well as highly proliferating CEPs/angioblasts, HSCs, progenitor cells, monocytes, macrophages, and tumor cells (vasculogenic mimicry) [33-35]. Moreover, recent studies suggest the existence of MM-specific ECs [32,36,37]. Functionally, tumor-associated vasculature causes chaotic and variable blood flow as well as vessel leakiness, resulting in lowered drug delivery and further selection of more malignant tumor cells. Importantly, the anti-MM activity of Thal, Bort, and Len is, at least in part, also due to their anti-angiogenic effects [38]. The clinical success of anti-angiogenic agents like bevacizumab (Avastin) suggests that their activity likely depends on tumor stage, prior treatment, and their combination with other anti-cancer agents. Indeed, although preclinical studies demonstrated a significant anti-MM effect of the VEGF receptor inhibitor pazopanib [39], a clinical phase 2 trial of pazopanib monotherapy in relapsed or refractory MM did not show any therapeutic effect [40]. Therefore similarly to treatment strategies in solid tumors anti-angiogenic therapies in MM are now being evaluated in combination with conventional or novel anti-MM therapies [41].

Osteolytic bone ("punch-out") lesions associated with bone pain, pathologic fractures, and diffuse osteoporosis in the central skeleton, the skull, and long bones are a typical clinical feature in almost all MM patients. Functionally, these defects are triggered by increased OC formation and activity in the vicinity of MM cells, as well as lower numbers of OBs and decreased bone formation [42,43]. A variety of OC-activating factors (OAFs), produced by both tumor as well as stromal cells, trigger increased OC activity [43,44]. OC activity in turn modulates MM cell growth and survival [43,44]. Conversely, lower numbers of OBs and decreased bone formation in MM are associated with dysregulation of several signaling molecules including Runx2/Cbfa1, Wnt, and IL-3 [42,43,44]. Importantly, the Wnt-signaling antagonist dickkopf-1 (DKK1), an inhibitor of OB differentiation, is significantly overexpressed in patients with MM who present with lytic bone lesions. DKK1-induced inhibition of OB precursors shifts the balance towards OCs and blocks establishment of the BM microenvironment required for HSC differentiation. Consequently, impaired differentiation also contributes to immunosuppression and anemia in MM patients. Consequently, administration of a polyclonal DKK1 antibody ameliorates the bone-specific morbidity of MM [45]; and immunodepletion of secreted frizzled-related protein (sFRP)-2, which prevents binding of Wnt proteins to their receptors and thereby inhibits OB function, significantly restores bone mineralization *in vitro* [46]. Although the main therapy used for treatment of bone disease in MM, with additional direct effects on tumor cells, is amino bisphosphonates [47], *in vivo* studies have demonstrated both a decrease in osteolysis, as well as an indirect anti-MM effect, using RANKL: Fc or OPG: Fc [42-44], the recombinant OPG construct AMGN-0007 [48], the HDAC inhibitor PXD101 [49], the MEK inhibitor AZD6244 (ARRY-142886) [50], Resveratrol [51], the CCR1 inhibitor MLN3897 [52], the Cox inhibitor SDX-308 [53], IMiD CC-4047 [54], and Bort, which additionally increases OB activity [44-46].

Both T and B cells show significant impairment of their functions in MM. While T cells are hyperactive [57], B cell-driven antibody responses are deficient. Both impairment of the global T cell receptor diversity as well as decreased numbers and function of suppressive CD25 (high) FOXP3(+)CD4(+) Treg cells in MM may, at least in part, account for the dysfunctional T cell response [57,58]. Importantly cytokines, including IL-6 abrogate generation of Treg cells [59]. Besides adverse immunologic effects, dysregulated T cell response also contributes to MM bone disease (see below). Several ongoing preclinical and clinical studies are evaluating strategies to normalize T and B cell function.

DCs of MM patients are functionally defective due, at least in part, to IL-6-, VEGF-or β2-microglobulin-triggered inhibition of DC maturation [60-63]. Direct MM cell-DC interaction enhances MM clonogenicity [64]. Moreover, plasmacytoid dendritic cells (pDCs) promote MM cell growth, survival, and drug resistance. Importantly, although pDCs are resistant to novel therapies, targeting toll-like receptors with CpG oligodeoxynucleotides both restores pDC immune function and abrogates pDC-induced MM cell growth therefore indicating the potential therapeutic value of targeting pDC-MM interactions to overcome drug resistance in MM [65]. Ongoing preclinical studies are evaluating a variety of anti-MM agents for their ability to normalize DC function and inhibit their supportive role on MM cell growth. For example, Bort enhances DC-mediated induction of immunity to MM *via* exposure of cell surface HSP-90 on dying tumor cells [66]; but also disrupts tumor-DC interactions in MM and lymphoma [67]. HSP-90-mediated protein folding within DCs is additionally required for DC-specific function. Conversely, HSP90 inhibition disrupts DC function [68].

MM stem cells (MMSCs) [69-71] represent a very small subset of cells within the tumor cell population with the capacity for self-renewal and differentiation. They reside in either the osteoblastic or the vascular niche. Similar to HSCs [72-74], it is hypothesized that the trabecular bone surface of the osteoblastic niche provides the quiescent microenvironment for MMSCs, while the sinusoids of the vascular niche facilitate their egress from the BM. Ongoing research aims to identify compounds that specifically modify the stem cell niche in order to block MM stem cell engraftment while still enabling HSC development.

Mesenchymal stem/ progenitor cells (MSCs), which differentiate in a context-specific manner into muscle, bone, fat, and other cell types, represent another potential therapeutic target in MM. BM MSCs isolated from MM patients, as compared to normal MSCs, produce high levels of IL-6, DKK1, as well as factors associated with angiogenesis and osteogenic differentiation [75]. Moreover they have decreased ability to inhibit T-cell proliferation [76]. Bort induces MSCs to preferentially undergo osteoblastic differentiation in mice, in part by modulation of the bone-specifying transcription factor Runt-related transcription factor 2

(Runx-2). Mice implanted with MSCs showed increased ectopic ossicle and bone formation after treatment with Bort. Bort treatment increased bone formation and rescued bone loss in a mouse model of osteoporosis [77]. These results are consistent with the therapeutic benefits of Bort on MM bone disease [78].

Thalidomide and the IMiDs

Several compounds have been tested to inhibit the supportive effects of non-tumor cells, *e.g.* BMSCs, on MM cell growth, survival, migration, and drug resistance. Most prominently, Thal, the IMiDs, and Bort, and have already significantly changed treatment strategies in MM during the last 5 years. Empirically tested for its anti-angiogenic activity in MM patients with refractory relapsed disease Thal achieved remarkable responses in one third of cases [79]. Indeed, Thal and the more potent immunomodulatory drugs (IMiDs) Lenalidomide (Len; IMiD CC-5013, Revlimid) and Pomalidomide (Pom; IMiD CC4047) overcome MM cell growth and survival advantage conferred by the BM milieu. Based upon a phase III clinical trial demonstrating increased response of Thal/ Dex vs. Dex, this combination was FDA approved in 2006 for treatment of patients with newly diagnosed MM [80]. Moreover, it has been combined with Melphalan and prednisone and achieved prolonged extent and frequency of response, as well as prolonged progression-free and overall survival, as initial therapy for elderly patients with MM [81,82]. IMiDs additionally co-stimulate T cells, enhance anti-tumor immunity mediated by IFNγ and IL-2, and augment NK cell cytotoxicity [83]. The use of Len in a phase I dose-escalation trial in patients with relapsed and refractory MM demonstrated either response or stabilization of disease in 79% cases [84,85]. These data were confirmed by two clinical phase II trials, which achieved complete responses even in heavily pretreated patients with favorable side effect profiles. Two clinical phase III trials demonstrated that Len plus Dex is more effective than high-dose Dex alone in relapsed or refractory MM [86,87], and Len was FDA approved in 2006 for use in combination with Dex to treat in patients with MM who have received one prior therapy. As with Thal, Len has been combined with Dex and with Melphalan and achieved promising results in newly diagnosed transplant candidates and elderly patients, respectively [88,89,90]. More than 100 clinical studies with Thal or Len combined with other agents are currently recruiting or ongoing. Similar to Len plus Dex, a recent study evaluated the therapeutic potential of Pom plus Dex. Excitingly, 63% of MM patients with relapsed disease treated with the combination achieved confirmed response including 5% CR, 28% VGPR, and 30% PR. Importantly, responses were also seen in 40% of lenalidomide-refractory patients, 37% of thalidomide-refractory patients, and 60% of bortezomib-refractory patients. The median progression-free survival time was 11.6 months and was not significantly different in patients with high-risk disease compared with patients with standard-risk disease [91].

Targeting the Ubiquitin-Proteasome System

Bort (previously denoted PS341), a dipeptide boronic acid inhibits the function of the 26S proteasome complex thereby leading to accumulation of misfolded/ damaged proteins, subsequent ER stress and cell apoptosis; as well as blockade of the unfolded protein response (UPR) by preventing stress-induced phosphorylation of IRE1 and the resultant splicing of Xbp-1 [92]. Inhibition of NFκB *via* accumulation of IκB is thought to play a key role in this process, which both inhibits MM cell growth, survival, and migration, and targets the MM microenvironment. Molecular mechanisms mediating anti-MM effects of Bort also include phosphorylation of both p53 protein and JNK, cleavage of DNA-PKcs and ATM, caspase-dependent downregulation of gp130, blockade of IL-6-triggered phosphorylation of ERK, and antiangiogenesis. Indeed, Bort: (1) downregulates caveolin-1 expression and inhibits caveolin-1 tyrosine phosphorylation, which are required for VEGF-mediated MM cell migration on fibronectin; and (2) blocks VEGF-induced tyrosine phosphorylation of caveolin-1 in HUVECs, thereby inhibiting ERK-dependent endothelial cell proliferation [5,93,94]. Moreover, Bort disrupts tumor-DC interactions and enhances DC-mediated immunity *via* exposure of cell surface HSP 90 [66,67].

Approved for therapy of relapsed and refractory MM (SUMMIT trial) in 2003 [95] and for progressive MM in 2004 (APEX trial), bortezomib was also approved for initial MM treatment in June 2008 as part of the MPV regimen (VISTA trial) [96]. Despite its success, 65% of patients with relapsed or refractory MM do not respond to Bort. Several preclinical and more than 130 clinical studies which use Bort in combination with other conventional and novel therapies are ongoing aiming to further improve the activity of Bort and overcome development of drug resistance. For example Bort-based targeted combination therapies include: Len or IMiD; Flavopiridol (NSC649890) which targets CDK; Sorafenib (BAY43-9006), a small-molecule inhibitor which targets a multitude of kinase (*e.g.* Raf, VEGFR1, VEGFR2); Bevacizumab which targets VEGF; Perifosine which predominantly targets Akt; ATN-224 which targets superoxide dismutase 1; tipifarnib (R115777), a FTI; CNTO 328, which targets IL-6; Mapatumumab, which targets TRAIL receptor; 17AAG, which targets HSP90; CCI-779/ temsirolimus which targets rapamycin; and HDAC inhibitors, which block aggresomal degradation of proteins [5]. Of note Bort has been combined with Dex and with Melphalan and prednisone as initial therapy for transplant candidates and elderly patients, respectively, and achieved enhanced extent and frequency of response, as well as prolonged survival [96,97].

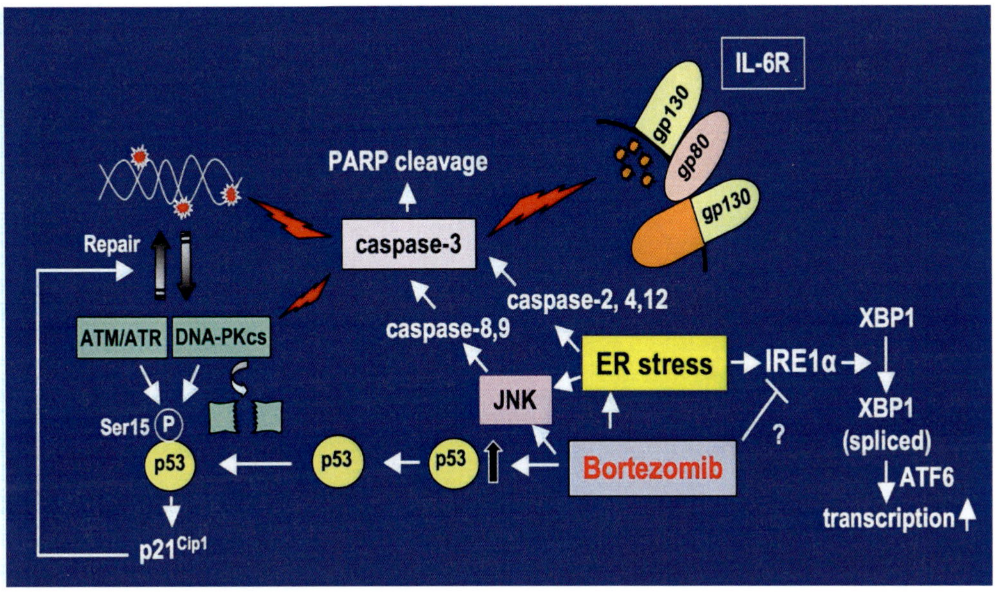

Fig. (2). Molecular mechanisms of action of anti-MM activity of bortezomib. Bortezomib induces unfolded protein response triggering ER stress and JNK activation followed by caspase-4/12 and caspase8/9 activation, respectively. ER stress activates IRE1α which subsequently induces XBP-1 splicing (active form) followed by transcription activity of ATF6. Activated caspase-3 cleaves DNA-PKcs and ATM/ATR proteins, resulting in impaired DNA repair; and induces gp130 cleavage, which inactivates IL-6 mediated signaling cascades, thereby sensitizing MM cells to apoptotic stimuli in the BM microenvironment.

Based on the clinical success of Bort in MM, the potential therapeutic activity of other proteasome inhibitors was subsequently evaluated with the aim to further increase potency, while decreasing adverse side effects and facilitating the route of administration. The epoxyketone carfilzomib, former PR-171 (Proteolix, USA), is a potent irreversible inhibitor of the CT-L activity of the proteasome. Based on promising preclinical data [98-100], and good tolerability in a phase I trial [101], several clinical trials have now been initiated testing carfilzomib, alone or in combination with Len and Dex, in relapsed/ and or refractory MM and relapsed solid tumors (http://clinicaltrials.gov). Salinosporamidine A (NPI-0052) is an orally bioavailable inhibitor of all three catalytic activities of the proteasome [102,103]. Importantly, Bort and Salinosporamidine A induce synergistic anti-MM activity *in vitro* against both MM cell lines or patient CD138+ MN cells, as well as *in vivo* in a human plasmocytome xenograft mouse model [104]. Salinosporamidine A is now being investigated in patients with relapsed or relapsed/ refractory MM, as well as in patients with advanced solid or hematologic malignancies (http://clinicaltrials.gov).

Importantly, our increased knowledge has provided the basis for new therapeutic strategies that are not only aiming to block selective proteasomal catalytic activities, but also specifically target: (1) molecular mechanisms that are involved in the assembly of the proteasome; (2) the recognition of specific substrate proteins; (3) de-ubiquitination of specific substrate proteins by the 19S base; and (4) translocation of de-ubiquitinated substrate proteins. Inhibitors of E3 ligases, E1, and de-ubiquitinating enzymes; as well as drugs that target Ubl modifiers are already under intense preclinical and clinical evaluation [105,106].

E3 ligases mediating ubiquitin conjugation play a key role in cancer development, *e.g.* RING-type E3 enzyme Mdm2, a negative regulator of p53; and the multisubunit SCF ligases. The small molecule HLI98 inhibits E3 ligase activity of Mdm2 and thereby selectively blocks p53 ubiquitination [107]. Importantly, dependent on substrate specificity, E3 ligases not only act as tumor promoters, but also on suppressors. For example, agonists of SCF (Fbxw7/hCdc4), which functions as interchangeable substrate recognition component of the SCF ubiquitin ligases, trigger increased proteasomal degradation of c-Myc, c-Jun, cyclin E1, and Notch [108].

Nutlins and *reactivation of p53 and induction of tumor cell apoptosis* (RITA, 2,5-bis(5-hydroxy-methyl-2-thienyl)furan) target protein-protein interactions between p53 and Mdm2, rather than influence their enzymatic function. Specifically, nutlins (nutlin-1, -2, -3) are cis-imidazoline analogs discovered by screening a chemical library, which was designed to identify compounds that bind Mdm2 in the p53-binding pocket. Consequently, nutlins activate the p53-pathway and induce cell cycle arrest, apoptosis, and growth inhibition in p53-wildtype cancer cells *in vitro* and *in vivo* [109]. Nutlin-3 in particular has demonstrated promising preclinical activity [110]. RITA binds the amino terminus of p53, thereby promoting growth arrest [111].

Deubiquitinating enzymes (DUBs) recognize ubiquitinated proteins and remove their ubiquitin tag. Forming five subfamilies (ubiquitin-specific proteases, Usp; ubiquitin carboxy-terminal hydrolases, UCH; ovarian tumor-like proteases, OTU; JAMM/ MPN metalloproteases; and Machado-Jakob-disease proteases, MJD), DUBs are highly investigated as another class of targets for novel compounds [112,113]. Indeed, poor prognosis of MM patients overexpressing deubiquitinase USP9X may at least in part be due to USP9X-mediated stabilization of Mcl1 and associated tumor cell survival [114].

Another therapeutic and likely the most challenging approach is to modulate the binding of ubiquitin and ubiquitin-binding domains (UBDs), small modular domains which recognize different types of ubiquitin modifications (monoubiquitination, and polyubiquitination of distinct lenghts and linkage types). For example, ubistatins inhibit proteasome-dependent degradation by binding the ubiquitin chain. Moreover, they prevent the recognition of ubiquitinated substrates by UBDs present in the proteasome receptors RPN10 and RPN13, as well as the shuttling receptor RAD23 [115,116].

In summary, efforts to identify inhibitors/ modulators of protein-protein interaction systems including ubiquitin ligases, DUBs, and UBDs hold great promise to increase drug specificity and thereby decrease adverse side effect profiles of current compounds.

Targeting the Aggresome

The aggresome represents an alternative mechanism to the proteasome for breakdown of ubiqitinated proteins. Specifically, ubiquitinated proteins are delivered by dynein-dependent retrograde transport of microtubules to the aggresomes, whereas HDAC6 inhibitors such as Tubacin and type 2 HDAC inhibitors SAHA [117] and LBH589 [118] bind both polyubiquitinated proteins and dynein motors to inhibit transport of ubiquitinated proteins to aggresomes. Importantly, Tubacin, SAHA and LBH589 combined with Bort induces synergistic cytotoxicity in MM cells, providing the preclinical rationale for clinical protocols using these combinations [117,118]. Clinical trials of SAHA and Bort in relapsed/ refractory MM are promising. Specifically, Badros, *et al.* report in a total of 16 evaluable patients 1nCR and 7PR (overall response rate 50%), 6SD and 3PD. Similarly, Weber, *et al.* report in a total of 17 evaluable patients 4PR, 2 minimal responses, and 11SD [119,120]. A clinical phase IA/II trial investigating the oral HDAC inhibitor LBH589 in advanced hematologic malignancies including MM alone and in combination with Bort is ongoing.

3. THERAPEUTIC STRATEGIES TO TARGET THE NON-CELLULAR BM COMPARTMENT

The **non-cellular BM compartment** is composed of the *ECM* including fibronectin, laminin, collagen, osteopontin, proteoglycans, glycosaminoglycans; and the *liquid* milieu.

IL-6-Induced Signaling Pathways in MM

The production and secretion of the key growth and survival factor IL-6 in MM [121,122] by BMSCs and OBs [14,42] correlates with MM tumor cell mass, disease stage, and prognosis. Moreover, IL-6 is also involved in plasma cell/ MM cell differentiation *via* induction of a the transcription factor Xbp-1 [123,124,125,126,127]. IL-6 triggers caveolin-1/ Hck/ Gab1/2-dependent activation of MEK/ MAPK-, and PI3K/ Akt-signaling pathways [5,14,128,129,130]. IL-6 triggered JAK/ STAT3-pathway induces up-regulation/ activation of anti-apoptotic proteins Mcl-1 and Bcl_{XL}, Pim1 as well as c-Myc. Conversely, blockade of IL-6 induces up-regulation of the pro-apoptotic BH3-only protein Bim concomitant with Mcl-1 downregulation and activation of Bax, thereby inducing MM cell apoptosis [14,131]. Besides MM cell growth and survival, IL-6 also triggers drug-resistance, Dex-resistance in particular [132,133].

Compounds targeting IL-6 signaling pathways include antibodies against IL-6 and IL-6 receptor, *e.g.* CNTO 328; IL-6 antisense oligonucleotides; and IL-6 superantagonist Sant7 [14] (Table **1**). However, many MM cell lines grow independently of IL-6. Moreover, binding of MM cells to BMSCs triggers survival even after inhibition of the IL-6/ gp130/ STAT3 pathway, suggesting MM growth mechanisms other than IL-6. These findings may also explain why therapeutic approaches targeting IL-6 have not induced responses in phase I clinical trials [14]. Taken together, these data show that IL-6 is a crucial, but not sole, factor in MM pathogenesis. Clinical trials are now evaluating the safety and efficacy of CNTO 328, both alone or in combination, in patients with relapsed or refractory MM.

VEGF-Induced Signaling Pathways in MM

VEGF is secreted by several MM cell lines and present in patient MM BM plasma. VEGFR-1 is highly expressed by MM cells, consistent with autocrine signaling [32]. VEGF induces: (1) a caveolin-1/ PI3K/ PKCα-dependent cascade mediating MM cell migration on fibronectin; (2) a MEK/ ERK-pathway mediating MM cell proliferation; and (3) survival signaling *via* upregulation of Mcl-1 and survivin [32,36,37]. In addition to MM cells and ECs, VEGF also affects OBs, NK cells, monocytes, and endothelial progenitors [32,41].

The most successful approach to date to therapeutically target VEGF in cancer is the use of a humanized monoclonal antibody against VEGF, bevacizumab (Avastin) (*Genentech, Inc.*, CA), especially in combination with conventional chemotherapies [134,135]. Several ongoing clinical trials in MM are testing the effects of bevacizumab used in combination with other agents including Len, dexamethasone or bortezomib. In addition to bevacizumab a multitude of other VEGF-targeting compounds are under preclinical and clinical investigation in MM including VEGF trap, ZD6474, SCIO-469, sorafenib, and sunitinib. A clinical phase II trial using the VEGF receptor tyrosine kinase inhibitor PTK787/ ZK222584 [136] as post-transplant maintenance therapy has now been completed.

However, even when given in combination with conventional chemotherapies, the activity of VEGF inhibitors is only transient due to the development of resistance and disease progression. Recent mechanistic insights have delineated unique modes of resistance to angiogenesis inhibitors [137]. Importantly, novel agents and/ or improved treatment strategies are directed to overcome these mechanisms and include vascular-disrupting agents (VDAs), which selectively destroy existing tumor vessels, and drugs which target molecular mechanisms leading to vessel branching. These agents have promise to overcome resistance to current anti-angiogenesis inhibitors, and thereby improve patient outcome.

TNF-α Superfamily-Induced Signaling Pathways in MM

The TNF-α superfamily includes SDF-1α, CD40, BAFF, and APRIL. In MM, SDF-1α and its G-protein linked cognate receptor CXCR4 (CD184) are expressed in the BM of MM patients. SDF-1α is primarily produced by BMSCs, but also by MM cells.

Functionally, *SDF-1α*: (1) rapidly and transiently up-regulates VLA-4-mediated MM cell adhesion to both the CS-1 region of fibronectin and VCAM-1; (2) promotes proliferation, induces migration and homing, and protects against Dex-induced apoptosis in MM cells; and (3) up-regulates secretion of IL-6 and VEGF in BM stromal cells [138,139,140]. The CXCR4 inhibitor AMD3100 (Genzyme, Cambridge, MA) [141,142] and bicyclam molecule reversibly block SDF-1 binding to CXCR4 and inhibit MM cell homing in *preclinical* models [139]. Its *clinical* role in the inhibition of MM cell homing is under investigation.

CD40 is expressed by antigen presenting cells, T cells, as well as B-cell malignancies including MM. Functionally, it (1) mediates p53-dependent increases in MM cell growth; (2) induces PI3K / Akt/ NFκB-dependent MM cell migration; (3) triggers VEGF secretion; (4) induces membrane translocation of Ku86 and Ku70 proteins involved in IgH class switching; and (5) protects against apoptosis triggered by irradiation and doxorubicin [20,143]. Clinical phase I/II trials using dacetuzumab (SGN-40), the humanized anti-CD40 monoclonal antibody, in patients with refractory and relapsed MM have now been completed [144, 145] and a combination trial with Len, which augments ADCC [146], is ongoing.

TNFα, secreted mainly by macrophages: (1) triggers only modest MM cell proliferation, survival, and drug resistance; (2) however, markedly upregulates (5-fold) secretion of IL-6 in BMSCs and induces NFκB-dependent expression of CD11a/ LFA-1, CD54/ ICAM-1, CD106/ VCAM-1, CD49d/ VLA-4, and/or MUC-1 on MM cell lines; as well as CD106/ VCAM-1 and CD54/ ICAM-1 expression on BMSCs. Agents that target TNFα (*i.e.* Bort, Thal, and IMiDs) therefore, at least in part, abrogate the paracrine growth and survival advantage conferred by MM cell adhesion in the BM microenvironment [147].

BAFF or B lymphocyte Stimulator (BLyS) is normally expressed by monocytes, macrophages, DCs, T cells, and BMSCs, and exists both as a membrane-bound and a cleaved soluble protein. In addition, high levels of BAFF and APRIL are also produced by OCs. In MM, both tumor cells and BMSCs express high levels of BAFF and APRIL, as well as levels of their receptors [148,149]. BAFF secretion by BMSCs is further augmented upon adhesion to MM cells [150]. Functionally, BAFF and APRIL protect MM cells from apoptosis induced by IL-6 deprivation and Dex and promote MM cell growth as well as adhesion to BMSCs [148-151]. Microarray analysis defined two patient groups based on TACI expression: MM patients with high TACI expression (TACI (hi)) display mature plasma cell gene signature indicating dependence on the BM environment; and MM patients with low TACI expression (TACI (lo)) display a gene signature of plasmablasts, suggesting an attenuated dependence on the BM microenvironment. These data identify a group of patients who may benefit most from treatment with BAFF/ APRIL inhibitors [152] and strongly suggest the therapeutic value of antibodies or small molecule inhibitors which target BAFF/ APRIL-induced signaling pathways.

Insulin-Like Growth Factor-1 (IGF-1)-Induced Signaling Pathways in MM

In MM, IGF-1 induces tumor cell growth, survival, and migration. Moreover, a positive relation of baseline body mass in Dex (BMI) and MM was recently reported on two large prospective cohorts, the Nurses'Health Study and the Health Professionals follow-up Study [153], further supporting an important role of IGF-1 in MM pathophysiology (see Chapter 2). Functionally, IGF-1 promotes proliferation, migration, invasion and drug resistance in MM cells [5,14,94]; at least in part *via* cross-activation of IGF-1 and IL-6 receptors by the close proximity of these two receptors at lipid rafts on the plasma membrane [154]. Consequently, inhibition of IGF-1 receptor using NVP-ADW742 also blocks IL-6 triggered response in MM cells [155]. A clinical trial using the mAb IMC-A12 (cixutumumab) in combination with temsirolimus is now ongoing.

4. THERAPEUTIC STRATEGIES TO TARGET PATHWAYS WITHIN MM CELLS

Ras/ MEK/ MAPK Pathway in MM

Several cytokines and growth factors within the MM BM microenvironment including IL-6, IGF-1, and VEGF, as well as direct cell-cell contact *via* integrins trigger MM cell growth, survival and drug resistance by inducing the Ras/ MEK/ MAPK pathway.

MM patients with mutant Ras have a shortened survival and are less likely to respond to chemotherapy [5,14]. A clinical phase II trial demonstrated that the farnesyl transferase inhibitor (FTI) Tipifarnib was well tolerated, induced stabilization of disease, and inhibited farnesylation and tumor survival pathways in patients with advanced MM [156]. Based on preclinical data demonstrating that the combination of bortezomib (Bort) with Tipifarnib induces synergistic MM cell apoptosis *via* downregulation of HDAC6 and inhibition of aggresome formation [157], an ongoing clinical trial is testing the efficacy of Tipifarnib together with Bort [158]. However the transfer of farnesyl groups, and therefore the effect of FTIs, on Ras may not be specific since FTI Tipifarnib (R115777) also induces MM cell apoptosis *via* Ras-independent pathways [159].

Based on its preclinical efficacy BAY 43-9006/ sorafenib/ Nexavar (Bayer Pharmaceuticals) [160], the first oral multikinase inhibitor (PDGFR, VEGFR-1,-2,-3 and c-Kit) that targets Raf-1 and affects tumor signaling and tumor vasculature is now clinically tested in MM alone or in combination with novel or conventional therapies.

Finally, significant preclinical anti-MM activity has also been demonstrated for the MEK1/2 inhibitor AZD6244 (ARRY-142886) [50,161]. A clinical trial with AZD6244 is planned.

PI3K/ Akt Pathway in MM

PI3K/ Akt plays a pivotal role in IL-6, IGF-1, VEGF, and integrin-triggered pathways in MM cells. Perifosine/ KRX-0401 inhibits Akt phosphorylation; triggers JNK activation followed by caspase-8/9 and poly (ADP)-ribose polymerase cleavage; triggers the formation of the death-inducing signaling complex (DISC) as well as the recruitment of TRAIL-R1/DR4, TRAIL-R2/DR5, and Bid in lipid rafts; induces apoptosis *via* cytochrome-c release as well as downregulation of survivin; and increases ERK phosphorylation [162-164]. Importantly, MEK inhibitors *e.g.* AZD-6244 (see above) or exogenous TRAIL synergistically enhance Perifosine-induced cytotoxicity in MM cells [50,165]. Clinical studies using Perifosine in combination with Bort and/ or with Dexamethasone (Dex) or Len with Dex are now ongoing. Other PI3K-inhibitors include SF1126, and NVP-BEZ235 [166-168].

Finally, several preclinical studies demonstrate promising results targeting mTOR, a molecule downstream of PI3K [5,14]. Clinical phase I/II trials testing sorafenib and everolimus or panobinostat and everolimus in relapsed or refractory MM are now recruiting. A clinical phase I trial testing AP23573/ ridaforolimus in advanced, refractory or recurrent MM has been completed. A clinical phase I trial testing temsirolimus (CCI-779) in combination with Len (CC-5013) in previously treated MM patients is ongoing. In contrast, a recent study demonstrated that the deregulated overexpression of the mTOR interacting mTOR-inhibitor DEPTOR in a subset of MM patients harboring cyclin D1/D3 or c-Maf/MAFB translocations represents a mechanism to activate PI3K/Akt signaling and promote cell survival [169].

Stat Signaling Pathways in MM

Dysregulated cytokine, *e.g.* IL-6, signaling triggers constitutive Stat3 activation in at least 50% of primary MM samples [170], as well as bone marrow stromal cells (BMSCs) from MM patients [171]. Inhibition of Stat3 activity by compounds including curcumin, atripimod, the JAK2 tyrosine kinase inhibitor AG490, and the pan-JAK inhibitor pyridone 6 is associated with inhibition of IL-6-induced MM cell survival [172-176]. Moreover, inhibition of constitutive Stat3 activity sensitizes MM cells to apoptosis induced by conventional chemotherapy [177]. Importantly, in the presence of BMSCs combined disruption of both the MEK/ ERK and the IL-6R/ Stat3 pathways is required to induce MM cell apoptosis [178]. A recent study demonstrated that boswellic acid blocks Stat3 signaling, proliferation, and survival of MM *via* the protein tyrosine phosphatase SHP-1 [179]. Ongoing studies are further investigating the potential role of inhibitors of Stat3 and other members of the Stat family within MM.

NFκB Signaling Pathway in MM

Mutations involving either the classical and/ or alternative NFκB pathway are present in at least 17% of MM tumors and 40% of MM cell lines and enable MM tumors to become less dependent on extrinsic BM signals that activate NFκB [180]. Two recent studies demonstrate genetic (mutation, deletion) or epigenetic alterations in a high percentage of MM cells leading to increased expression and activation of molecules within both the canonical and the non-canonical pathway[181-183]. Furthermore, NFκB signaling pathways not only play an important role within MM cells, but also trigger the production of IL-6, BAFF, or APRIL within several types of stromal cells [150,184]. Taken together, these studies further validate the therapeutic potential of NFκB inhibitors.

Over 750 inhibitors of the NFκB pathway have been identified including antioxidants, peptides, small RNA/ DNA, microbial and viral proteins, small molecules, and engineered dominant-negative or constitutively active polypeptides. Some of these inhibitors appear to target multiple steps in the NFκB pathway [185]. Importantly, anti-MM effects of bortezomib are strongly attributed to its inhibitory effect on NFκB signaling sequelae. Moreover, several recent studies strongly indicate the therapeutic potential of IKKβ inhibitors in MM: specific blockade of IKKβ decreased both growth and survival in MM cells, alone and when co-cultured with BMSCs [186-188].

However, in contrast to the initial rationale, our recent studies demonstrate that although inhibiting *induced* NFκB activity, bortezomib paradoxically enhances *constitutive* NFκB activity. Consequently, these results indicate that bortezomib-induced cytotoxicity cannot be fully attributed to inhibition of canonical NFκB activity in MM cells [189].

Wnt-Signaling Pathways in MM

The canonical Wnt/β-catenin and the alternative Wnt/ RhoA signaling pathways have recently been implicated in MM pathogenesis. Specifically, N-terminally unphosphorylated β-catenin is overexpressed in MM cells and stimulation with Wnt3a additionally increases both accumulation and nuclear localization of β-catenin and thereby MM cell proliferation [190]. Indeed, Wnt-signaling is constitutively activated in MM, correlates with hypermethylation and hence silencing of Wnt antagonist genes. Consequently, demethylation of methylated Wnt inhibitors downregulates Wnt-signaling and associated MM cell proliferation [191]. In addition to cell proliferation, Wnt-signaling pathways induce integrin α6β1 (VLA-6) and RhoA-Rho kinase-dependent cell-adhesion mediated drug resistance (CAM-DR) [192]; and also play a key role in MM bone disease. For example, aberrant expression of the Wnt pathway component BCL9 was recently observed in human MM and correlates with tumor proliferation, metastasis and angiogenesis [193]. Moreover, a functional link involved in MM progression was recently demonstrated between beta-catenin and Aurora kinase [194]. Furthermore, elevated levels of the Wnt-signaling antagonist dickkopf1 (DKK1) in the BM plasma and peripheral blood correlate with DKK1 gene expression patterns in MM patients with MRI and/ or radiograph positive bone lesions but not with control subjects or MM patients without bone lesions [45]. Indeed, DKK1 disrupts Wnt-regulated osteoprotegerin and RANKL production by osteoblasts thereby contributing to osteolytic bone lesions in MM [195]. Conversely, DKK1 inhibition removed suppression of bone formation and prevented the development of osteolytic bone disease in MM [196].

The small molecule PKF115-584, identified by high-throughput ELISA screening, efficiently blocks the formation of the β-catenin/ TCF transcriptional complex and thereby expression of Wnt target genes inducing cytotoxicity in both patient MM cells and MM cell lines [197]. The anti-DKK1 mAb BHQ880 inhibits MM growth and improves bone disease [198]. Additional strategies to target Wnt-signaling pathways include the use of small-molecule inhibitors which block interaction of β-catenin with CREB-binding protein, siRNAs, and antibodies directed against WNTs [199].

Table 1. Novel therapeutic targets; in grey: clinically far advanced therapeutic agents

target	agent	company	references
Targeting signaling events in tumor cell development			
FGFR3	SU5402	Sugen Inc.	Paterson, *et al.* 2004
	SU10991	Sugen Inc.	Grand, *et al.* 2004
	PD173074	Pfizer	Trudel, *et al.* 2004
	CHIR-258	Novartis/ Chiron	Trudel, *et al.* 2005
	PRO-001 (hu-anti-FGFR3 Fab)	ProChon Biotech Ltd.	Trudel, *et al.* 2006

Table 1. cont….

HDAC	vorinostat (suberoylanilide hydroxamic acid, SAHA)	Merck	Mitsiades, *et al.* 2003; Richardson, *et al.* 2008; Badros, *et al.* 2009
	NVP-LAQ824	Novartis	Catley, *et al.* 2003
	LBH 589	Novartis	Catley, *et al.* 2006; Badros, 2007 (ASCO); Weber, 2007 (ASCO)
	romidepsin (depsipeptide, FK228)	Gloucester Pharm.	Khan, *et al.* 2004
	ITF2357	Italfarmaco	Golay, *et al.* 2007
	PXD101/ belinostat	CuraGen	Feng, *et al.* 2007; Gimsing, *et al.*, 2008
	MS-275/ SNDX-275	Bayer Schering, Syndax	Miller, *et al.* 2007
	KD-5170	Kalypsys, Inc.	Feng, *et al.* 2008
HDAC6	tubacin	Broad Institute	Hideshima, *et al.* 2005
telomerase	GRN163	Geron Corp.	Akiyama, *et al.* 2003; Wang, *et al.* 2004
	TMPyP4		Shammas, *et al.* 2003
	telomestatin		Shammas, *et al.* 2004
CDKs	flavopiridol/ alvocidib	NCI	Semenov, *et al.* 2002
	PD 0332991	Pfizer	Baughn, *et al.* 2006; Menu, *et al.* 2008
	CYC202/ seliciclib/ R-roscovitine	Cyclacel Ltd	MacCallum, *et al.* 2005; Raje, *et al.* 2005
microtubules	Epothilone D (KOS-862)	Novartis	Lin, *et al.* 2005
Targeting the cell membrane			
HMG-CoA	statins:	Merck	
	lovastatin		Holmberg, *et al.* 1994; van de Donk, *et al.* 2002
	fluvastatin		Baulch-Brown, *et al.* 2007
	simvastatin		Otsuki, *et al.* 2004; Schmidmaier, *et al.* 2004
CD56	CD-56-DM	Immunogen	Tassone, *et al.* 2004
CD138	CD138-DM	Biotest	Tassone, *et al.* 2004
CS-1	HuLuc63	POL	Tai, *et al.* 2007; His, *et al.* 2008
Targeting cytokines, growth factors and their receptors			
IL-6	CNT328	Centocor	Levy, *et al.* 1991; Sporeno, *et al.* 1996;
	Sant7	Sigma-Tau	Tassone, *et al.* 2000&2002; Voorhees, 2007; Zaki, 2004; Trikha, 2003
VEGF	PTK787/ ZK222584 (Vatalanib)	Novartis	Lin, *et al.* 2002; Thomas, *et al.* 2003
	pazopanib (GW786034B)	GlaxoSmithKline	Podar, *et al.* 2006; Prince, *et al.* 2009
	Sorafenib (BAY43-9006/ Nexavar)	Bayer & Onyx	Rini, *et al.* 2006
	Avastin	Genentech	Ferrara, *et al.* 2004; Yang, *et al.* 2003
	ZD6474	Astra Zeneca	Bates, *et al.* 2003; Kovacs, *et al.* 2006
	Su-11248 Sugen	Sugen, Inc.	Sakamoto, *et al.* 2004
	Sunitinib (SU011248)	Pfizer	Ikezoe, *et al.* 2006
	PI-88	Progen	Ferro, *et al.* 2007
FGF, VEGF	BIBF100	Boehringer Ingelheim	Bisping, *et al.* 2006
SDF-1	AMD3100/ perixafor/ JM3100	Genzyme	Hideshima, *et al.* 2002; Alsayed, *et al.* 2007; Menu, *et al.* 2006
CD40	SGN-40	Seattle Genetics	Tai *et al.* 2004
	Chir12.12	Chiron	Tai, *et al.* 2005
TRAIL-R1	HGS-ETR1	Human Genoma	Menoret, *et al.* 2006

Table 1. cont....

TACI-Ig	Atacicept (TACI-Ig)	ZymoGenetics	Yaccoby, *et al.* 2008
IGF-1	NVP-ADW742	Novartis	Mitsiades, *et al.* 2004
	CP-571871	Pfizer	Lacy, *et al.*, 2008
	JB-1	Chiron	
Targeting MM cells and the MM BM microenvironment			
	thalidomide	Celgene	Singhal, *et al.* 1999; San-Miguel, *et al.* 2008; Vallet, *et al.* 2008
IMiD	lenalidomide (CC-5013)	Celgene	Thomas, *et al.* 2007
	Actimid/ pomalidomide (CC-4047)	Celgene	Aragon-Chin, *et al.* 2007; Lacy, *et al.* 2009 & 2010
proteasome	PS-341/ bortezomib/ Velcade	Millenium	Hideshima, *et al.* 2001; Richardson, *et al.* 2008
	NPI-0052	Nereus	Chauhan, *et al.* 2005 & 2008
	Carfilzomib (PR-171)	Proteolix	Demo, *et al.* 2007; Kuhn, *et al.* 2007;Parlati, *et al.* 2009; O'Connor, *et al.* 2009
	CEP-18770	Cephalon	Piva, *et al.* 2008
Targeting MM BM microenvironment			
IKK	PS-1145	Millenium	Hideshima, *et al.*, 2002
	Bay 11-7082	Bayer	Annunziata, *et al.*, 2007
	AS602868		Jourdan, *et al.*, 2007; Romagnoli, *et al.* 2007
	MLN120B	Millenium	Jourdan, *et al.* 2007; Romagnoli, *et al.* 2007
p38	VX-745	Vertex Pharmaceuticals	Hideshima, *et al.* 2003
	SCIO-469	SCIOS Inc./ J&J	Hideshima, *et al.* 2004
TGFbeta	SD-208	SCIOS Inc./ J&J	Hayashi, *et al.* 2004
Targeting downstream signaling pathway			
FT	R115777 (Tipifarnib/ Zarnestra)	J&J	Beaupre, *et al.* 2004; Alsina, *et al.* 2004; Armand, *et al.* 1993
	SCH66336 (Lonafarnib)	Schering-Plough	David, *et al.* 2005
Raf-1	Sorafenib (BAY43-9006/ Nexavar)	Bayer	Burton, *et al.* 2006; Ramakrishnan, *et al.* 2009
MEK1/2	AZD6244 (ARRY-14886)	Astra Zeneca	Tai, *et al.* 2007
Akt	Perifosine (KRX-0401)	Keryx	Hideshima, *et al.* 2005 & 2007; Gajate, *et al.* 2007
mTOR	rapamycin, P70S6	Genentech	Raje, *et al.* 2004
	CCI-779 (temsirolimus)	Wyeth	Hamasaki, *et al.* 2005
	RAD001 (Everolimus)	Novartis	Bharti, *et al.* 2003
	AP23573 (Deforolimus)	Ariad	De Vos, *et al.* 2000
JAK/ Stat	atiprimod	Callisto Pharm.	Pedranzini, *et al.* 2006
SAPK/ JNK	aplidin (plitidepsin)	PharmaMar	Amit-Vazina, *et al.* 2005
p38	SCIO-469	SCIOS Inc./ J&J	Hideshima, *et al.* 2004
NFkB, IkK	PS-1145	Millenium/ Takeda	Hideshima, *et al.* 2002 & 2006; Sanda, *et al.* 2005
	BAY11-7082	Biomol	Dai, *et al.* 2004
	RTA 402 (CDDO-Me)	Reata	Ikeda, *et al.* 2004; Chauhan, *et al.* 2004
	AS602868	Merck	Jourdan, *et al.* 2007; Romagnoli, *et al.* 2007

Table 1. cont….

	MLN120B	Millenium/ Takeda	Jourdan, *et al.* 2007; Romagnoli, *et al.* 2007
	ACHP	Bayer	Sanda, *et al.* 2005
	SDX-308 (CEP-18082)	Cephalon, Inc.	Yasui, *et al.* 2007; Feng, *et al.* 2007
Wnt	PKF115-584	Novartis	Sukhedo, *et al.* 2007
PKC	Enzastaurin	Eli Lilly	Podar, *et al.* 2007 & 2007
	Midostaurin (PKC412)	Novartis	Sharkey, *et al.* 2007
HSP90	Tanespimycin (KOS-953)	Kosan Biosciences/ BMS	Anderson, *et al.* 2007
	Geldanamycin (17-AAG)	Kosan Biosciences/ BMS	Mitsiades, *et al.* 2007
Inducing MM cell apoptosis			
Smac agonists	LBW242	Novartis	Chauhan, *et al.* 2007
SOD	2ME2	EntreMed	Chauhan, *et al.* 2002
Bcl2	B3139 (Genasense)/ oblimersen	Genta Incorp.	van de Donk, *et al.* 2003
Treating MM bone disease			
RANKL: Fc	RANKL: Fc		Pearse, *et al.* 2001
OPG: Fc	OPG: Fc		Croucher, *et al.* 2001
OPG	AMGN-0007	Amgen	Body, *et al.* 2003
HDAC	PXD101	CuraGen and TopoTarget	Feng, *et al.* 2007
MEK	AZD6244/ARRY-142886	Astra Zeneca	Tai, *et al.* 2007; Breitkreutz, *et al.* 2007
-	Resveratrol	Genentech	Boissy, *et al.* 2005
CCR1	MLN3897	Millenium/ Takeda	Vallet, *et al.* 2007
COX	SDX-308	Novartis	Feng, *et al.* 2007
IMiDs	IMiDs: CC-4047, lenalidomide	Cellgene	v. Metzler, *et al.* 2007; Terpos, *et al.* 2007; Breitkreutz, *et al.* 2008
proteasome	bortezomib	Millenium/ Takeda	Hideshima, *et al.* 2001
NFkB	SDX-308 (CEP-18082)	Cephalon, Inc.	Yasui, *et al.* 2007; Feng, *et al.* 2007
DKK-1			Tian, *et al.* 2003

PKC Signaling Pathways in MM

Recent studies have also identified members of the intracellular PKC family of serine/ threonine kinases as potential therapeutic targets in MM. Functionally, PKCs are: (1) involved in MM cell apoptosis; (2) required for VEGF-and Wnt-induced MM cell migration; and (3) associated with the control of IL-6 receptor α shedding. Importantly, the unique gene signature of MM patients with the adverse prognostic t(4;14)(p16;q32) translocation shows marked up-regulation of PKCβ [200]. Pre-clinical and clinical studies using the macrocyclic bisindolylmaleimide Enzastaurin or the *N*-benzylstaurosporine Midostaurin/ PKC412 to target PKC pathways demonstrate promising activity in a variety of tumors including MM and Waldenstrom's Macroglobulinemia (WM) [200-203].

Directly and Indirectly Targeting Heat Shock Proteins

Promising intracellular therapeutic targets in MM also include heat shock proteins (HSPs), Hsp27, Hsp70, and Hsp90 in particular. Specifically, overexpression of Hsp27 is associated with resistance to Dex, which is mediated *via* inhibition of second mitochondria-derived activator of caspase (Smac) release. In contrast, significant upregulation of Hsp27, Hsp70, and Hsp90 is also observed in MM cells treated with Bort, indicative of a stress and protective effect. Importantly, blocking both Hsp27 and Hsp90 enhances Bort-induced death of MM cells and provides the preclinical rationale for treatment strategies combining agents to target heat shock protein sequelae (*i.e.* p38 inhibitors and Smac mimetics) with Bort [5,14,132]. Pleiotropic effects of Hsp90 inhibitors were observed on key elements of MM pathogenesis, including suppression of IGF-1 and IL-6 signaling sequelae, as well as proteasome, telomerase, and HIF-1α activities [5,204]. Clinical trials evaluating the efficacy of Hsp inhibitor Tanespimycin (KOS-953), both alone and combined with Bort, are ongoing.

CONCLUSIONS

Based on our enhanced knowledge of MM cell biology in the BM microenvironment which defined a supportive role of stromal cells (BMSCs, endothelial cells, osteoblasts and osteoclasts, immune cells) and ECM proteins, a variety of new therapeutic targets and derived agents were identified. Significant therapeutic benefits have already been achieved with thalidomide, lenalidomide, and bortezomib, especially when combined with conventional or novel therapies to treat patients both at earlier disease stages, as well as relapsed and refractory disease, or when used together with stem cell transplantation strategies. Nevertheless MM still remains incurable, and next-generation more potent and selective drugs targeting tumor cells within the BM microenvironment are urgently needed to both overcome drug resistance and improve patient outcome. Agents with promising clinical activity likely to enter clinical practice in near future include the proteasomal inhibitor carfilzomib, the IMiD pomalidomide, the AKT inhibitor perifosine, and the histone deacetylase inhibitor vorinostat. Several others agents demonstrate promising preclinical activity.

DISCLOSURES

Part of information included in this chapter has been previously published in "Leukemia. 2009 Jan; 23(1):10-24".

REFERENCES

[1] Fonseca R, Bailey RJ, Ahmann GJ, *et al.* Genomic abnormalities in monoclonal gammopathy of undetermined significance. Blood 2002; 100: 1417-1424.

[2] Zhan F, Hardin J, Kordsmeier B, *et al.* Global gene expression profiling of multiple myeloma, monoclonal gammopathy of undetermined significance, and normal bone marrow plasma cells. Blood 2002; 99: 1745-1757.

[3] Keats JJ, Reiman T, Belch AR, Pilarski LM. Ten years and counting: so what do we know about t(4;14)(p16;q32) multiple myeloma. Leuk Lymphoma 2006; 47: 2289-2300.

[4] Hazlehurst LA, Landowski TH, Dalton WS. Role of the tumor microenvironment in mediating de novo resistance to drugs and physiological mediators of cell death. Oncogene 2003; 22: 7396-7402.

[5] Hideshima T, Mitsiades C, Tonon G, Richardson PG, Anderson KC. Understanding multiple myeloma pathogenesis in the bone marrow to identify new therapeutic targets. Nat Rev Cancer 2007; 7: 585-598.

[6] Tai YT, Dillon M, Song W, *et al.* Anti-CS1 humanized monoclonal antibody HuLuc63 inhibits myeloma cell adhesion and induces antibody-dependent cellular cytotoxicity in the bone marrow milieu. Blood 2008; 112: 1329-37.

[7] Hsi ED, Steinle R, Balasa B, *et al.* CS1, a potential new therapeutic antibody target for the treatment of multiple myeloma. Clin Cancer Res 2008; 14: 2775-2784.

[8] van Rhee F, Szmania SM, Dillon M, *et al.* Combinatorial efficacy of anti-CS1 monoclonal antibody elotuzumab (HuLuc63) and bortezomib against multiple myeloma. Mol Cancer Ther 2009; 8: 2616-2624.

[9] Tai YT, Soydan E, Song W, *et al.* CS1 promotes multiple myeloma cell adhesion, clonogenic growth, and tumorigenicity *via* c-maf-mediated interactions with bone marrow stromal cells. Blood 2009; 113: 4309-4318.

[10] Sekimoto E, Ozaki S, Ohshima T, *et al.* A single-chain Fv diabody against human leukocyte antigen-A molecules specifically induces myeloma cell death in the bone marrow environment. Cancer research 2007; 67: 1184-1192.

[11] Yang J, Qian J, Wezeman M, *et al.* Targeting beta2-microglobulin for induction of tumor apoptosis in human hematological malignancies. Cancer Cell 2006; 10: 295-307.

[12] Klein B. Cytokine, cytokine receptors, transduction signals, and oncogenes in human multiple myeloma. Semin Hematol 1995; 32: 4-19.

[13] Anderson KC, Lust JA. Role of cytokines in multiple myeloma. Semin Hematol 1999; 36: 14-20.

[14] Podar K, Hideshima T, Chauhan D, Anderson KC. Targeting signalling pathways for the treatment of multiple myeloma. Expert Opin Ther Targets 2005; 9: 359-381.

[15] Urashima M, Chauhan D, Hatziyanni M, *et al.* CD40 ligand triggers interleukin-6 mediated B cell differentiation. Leuk Res 1996; 20: 507-515.

[16] Damiano JS, Cress AE, Hazlehurst LA, Shtil AA, Dalton WS. Cell adhesion mediated drug resistance (CAM-DR): role of integrins and resistance to apoptosis in human myeloma cell lines. Blood 1999; 93: 1658-1667.

[17] Hazlehurst LA, Damiano JS, Buyuksal I, Pledger WJ, Dalton WS. Adhesion to fibronectin *via* beta1 integrins regulates p27kip1 levels and contributes to cell adhesion mediated drug resistance (CAM-DR). Oncogene 2000; 19: 4319-4327.

[18] Vacca A, Ria R, Presta M, *et al.* alpha(v)beta(3) integrin engagement modulates cell adhesion, proliferation, and protease secretion in human lymphoid tumor cells. Exp Hematol 2001; 29: 993-1003.

[19] Desgrosellier JS, Cheresh DA. Integrins in cancer: biological implications and therapeutic opportunities. Nature reviews 10: 9-22.

[20] Tai YT, Catley LP, Mitsiades CS, *et al.* Mechanisms by which SGN-40, a humanized anti-CD40 antibody, induces cytotoxicity in human multiple myeloma cells: clinical implications. Cancer Res 2004; 64: 2846-2852.

[21] Tai YT, Li X, Tong X, *et al.* Human anti-CD40 antagonist antibody triggers significant antitumor activity against human multiple myeloma. Cancer Res 2005; 65: 5898-5906.

[22] Radtke F, Wilson A, Ernst B, MacDonald HR. The role of Notch signaling during hematopoietic lineage commitment. Immunol Rev 2002; 187: 65-74.

[23] Radtke F, Raj K. The role of Notch in tumorigenesis: oncogene or tumour suppressor? Nat Rev Cancer 2003; 3: 756-767.

[24] Cheng P, Nefedova Y, Miele L, Osborne BA, Gabrilovich D. Notch signaling is necessary but not sufficient for differentiation of dendritic cells. Blood 2003; 102: 3980-3988.

[25] Nefedova Y, Cheng P, Alsina M, Dalton WS, Gabrilovich DI. Involvement of Notch-1 signaling in bone marrow stroma-mediated de novo drug resistance of myeloma and other malignant lymphoid cell lines. Blood 2004; 103: 3503-3510.

[26] Houde C, Li Y, Song L, *et al.* Overexpression of the NOTCH ligand JAG2 in malignant plasma cells from multiple myeloma patients and cell lines. Blood 2004; 104: 3697-3704.

[27] Jundt F, Probsting KS, Anagnostopoulos I, *et al.* Jagged1-induced Notch signaling drives proliferation of multiple myeloma cells. Blood 2004; 103: 3511-3515.

[28] Zweidler-McKay PA, He Y, Xu L, *et al.* Notch signaling is a potent inducer of growth arrest and apoptosis in a wide range of B-cell malignancies. Blood 2005; 106: 3898-3906.

[29] Zdzisinska B, Walter-Croneck A, Kandefer-Szerszen M. Matrix metalloproteinases-1 and -2, and tissue inhibitor of metalloproteinase-2 production is abnormal in bone marrow stromal cells of multiple myeloma patients. Leuk Res 2008:

[30] Heissig B, Ohki Y, Sato Y, *et al.* A role for niches in hematopoietic cell development. Hematology 2005; 10: 247-253.

[31] Kopp HG, Avecilla ST, Hooper AT, Rafii S. The bone marrow vascular niche: home of HSC differentiation and mobilization. Physiology (Bethesda) 2005; 20: 349-356.

[32] Podar K, Anderson KC. The pathophysiological role of VEGF in hematological malignancies: therapeutic implications. Blood 2005; 105: 1383-1395.

[33] Zhang H, Vakil V, Braunstein M, *et al.* Circulating endothelial progenitor cells in multiple myeloma: implications and significance. Blood 2005; 105: 3286-3294.

[34] de Bont ES, Guikema JE, Scherpen F, *et al.* Mobilized human CD34+ hematopoietic stem cells enhance tumor growth in a nonobese diabetic/severe combined immunodeficient mouse model of human non-Hodgkin's lymphoma. Cancer Res 2001; 61: 7654-7659.

[35] Scavelli C, Nico B, Cirulli T, *et al.* Vasculogenic mimicry by bone marrow macrophages in patients with multiple myeloma. Oncogene 2007:

[36] Ribatti D, Nico B, Vacca A. Importance of the bone marrow microenvironment in inducing the angiogenic response in multiple myeloma. Oncogene 2006; 25: 4257-4266.

[37] Jakob C, Sterz J, Zavrski I, *et al.* Angiogenesis in multiple myeloma. Eur J Cancer 2006; 42: 1581-1590.

[38] Folkman J. Angiogenesis: an organizing principle for drug discovery? Nat Rev Drug Discov 2007; 6: 273-286.

[39] Podar K, Tonon G, Sattler M, *et al.* The small-molecule VEGF receptor inhibitor pazopanib (GW786034B) targets both tumor and endothelial cells in multiple myeloma. Proc Natl Acad Sci U S A 2006:

[40] Prince HM, Honemann D, Spencer A, *et al.* Vascular endothelial growth factor inhibition is not an effective therapeutic strategy for relapsed or refractory multiple myeloma: a phase 2 study of pazopanib (GW786034). Blood 2009; 113: 4819-4820.

[41] Podar K, Anderson KC. Inhibition of VEGF signaling pathways in multiple myeloma and other malignancies. Cell Cycle 2007; 6: 538-542.

[42] Giuliani N, Rizzoli V, Roodman GD. Multiple myeloma bone disease: pathophysiology of osteoblast inhibition. Blood 2006; 108: 3992-6.

[43] Esteve FR, Roodman GD. Pathophysiology of myeloma bone disease. Best Pract Res Clin Haematol 2007; 20: 613-624.

[44] Terpos E, Sezer O, Croucher P, Dimopoulos MA. Myeloma bone disease and proteasome inhibition therapies. Blood 2007; 110: 1098-1104.

[45] Tian E, Zhan F, Walker R, *et al.* The role of the Wnt-signaling antagonist DKK1 in the development of osteolytic lesions in multiple myeloma. New Engl J Med 2003; 349: 2483-2494.

[46] Oshima T, Abe M, Asano J, *et al.* Myeloma cells suppress bone formation by secreting a soluble Wnt inhibitor, sFRP-2. Blood 2005; 106: 3160-3165.

[47] Berenson JR. Bone disease in myeloma. Curr Treat Options Oncol 2001; 2: 271-283.

[48] Body JJ, Greipp P, Coleman RE, *et al.* A phase I study of AMGN-0007, a recombinant osteoprotegerin construct, in patients with multiple myeloma or breast carcinoma related bone metastases. Cancer 2003; 97: 887-892.

[49] Feng R, Oton A, Mapara MY, *et al.* The histone deacetylase inhibitor, PXD101, potentiates bortezomib-induced anti-multiple myeloma effect by induction of oxidative stress and DNA damage. Br J Haematol 2007; 139: 385-397.

[50] Tai YT, Fulciniti M, Hideshima T, *et al.* Targeting MEK induces myeloma-cell cytotoxicity and inhibits osteoclastogenesis. Blood 2007; 110: 1656-1663.

[51] Boissy P, Andersen TL, Abdallah BM, *et al.* Resveratrol inhibits myeloma cell growth, prevents osteoclast formation, and promotes osteoblast differentiation. Cancer Res 2005; 65: 9943-9952.

[52] Vallet S, Raje N, Ishitsuka K, *et al.* MLN3897, a novel CCR1 inhibitor, impairs osteoclastogenesis and inhibits the interaction of multiple myeloma cells and osteoclasts. Blood 2007; 110: 3744-3752.

[53] Feng R, Anderson G, Xiao G, *et al.* SDX-308, a nonsteroidal anti-inflammatory agent, inhibits NF-kappaB activity, resulting in strong inhibition of osteoclast formation/activity and multiple myeloma cell growth. Blood 2007; 109: 2130-2138.

[54] Anderson G, Gries M, Kurihara N, *et al.* Thalidomide derivative CC-4047 inhibits osteoclast formation by down-regulation of PU.1. Blood 2006; 107: 3098-3105.

[55] von Metzler I, Krebbel H, Hecht M, *et al.* Bortezomib inhibits human osteoclastogenesis. Leukemia 2007; 21: 2025-2034.

[56] Heider U, Kaiser M, Muller C, *et al.* Bortezomib increases osteoblast activity in myeloma patients irrespective of response to treatment. Eur J Haematol 2006; 77: 233-238.

[57] Mariani S, Coscia M, Even J, *et al.* Severe and long-lasting disruption of T-cell receptor diversity in human myeloma after high-dose chemotherapy and autologous peripheral blood progenitor cell infusion. Br J Haematol 2001; 113: 1051-1059.

[58] Massaia M, Bianchi A, Attisano C, *et al.* Detection of hyperreactive T cells in multiple myeloma by multivalent cross-linking of the CD3/TCR complex. Blood 1991; 78: 1770-1780.

[59] Bettelli E, Carrier Y, Gao W, *et al.* Reciprocal developmental pathways for the generation of pathogenic effector TH17 and regulatory T cells. Nature 2006; 441: 235-238.

[60] Ratta M, Fagnoni F, Curti A, *et al.* Dendritic cells are functionally defective in multiple myeloma: the role of interleukin-6. Blood 2002; 100: 230-237.

[61] Brown RD, Pope B, Murray A, *et al.* Dendritic cells from patients with myeloma are numerically normal but functionally defective as they fail to up-regulate CD80 (B7-1) expression after huCD40LT stimulation because of inhibition by transforming growth factor-beta1 and interleukin-10. Blood 2001; 98: 2992-2998.

[62] Gabrilovich DI, Chen HL, Girgis KR, *et al.* Production of vascular endothelial growth factor by human tumors inhibits the functional maturation of dendritic cells. Nat Med 1996; 2: 1096-1103.

[63] Xie J, Wang Y, Freeman ME, 3rd, Barlogie B, Yi Q. Beta 2-microglobulin as a negative regulator of the immune system: high concentrations of the protein inhibit *in vitro* generation of functional dendritic cells. Blood 2003; 101: 4005-4012.

[64] Kukreja A, Hutchinson A, Dhodapkar K, *et al.* Enhancement of clonogenicity of human multiple myeloma by dendritic cells. J Exp Med 2006; 203: 1859-1865.

[65] Chauhan D, Singh AV, Brahmandam M, *et al.* Functional interaction of plasmacytoid dendritic cells with multiple myeloma cells: a therapeutic target. Cancer Cell 2009; 16: 309-323.

[66] Spisek R, Charalambous A, Mazumder A, *et al.* Bortezomib enhances dendritic cell (DC)-mediated induction of immunity to human myeloma *via* exposure of cell surface heat shock protein 90 on dying tumor cells: therapeutic implications. Blood 2007; 109: 4839-4845.

[67] Kukreja A, Hutchinson A, Mazumder A, *et al.* Bortezomib disrupts tumour-dendritic cell interactions in myeloma and lymphoma: therapeutic implications. Br J Haematol 2007; 136: 106-110.

[68] Bae J, Mitsiades C, Tai YT, *et al.* Phenotypic and functional effects of heat shock protein 90 inhibition on dendritic cell. J Immunol 2007; 178: 7730-7737.

[69] Matsui W, Huff CA, Wang Q, *et al.* Characterization of clonogenic multiple myeloma cells. Blood 2004; 103: 2332-2336.

[70] Peacock CD, Wang Q, Gesell GS, *et al.* Hedgehog signaling maintains a tumor stem cell compartment in multiple myeloma. Proc Natl Acad Sci U S A 2007; 104: 4048-4053.

[71] Matsui W, Wang Q, Barber JP, *et al.* Clonogenic multiple myeloma progenitors, stem cell properties, and drug resistance. Cancer Res 2008; 68: 190-197.

[72] Scadden DT. The stem-cell niche as an entity of action. Nature 2006; 441: 1075-1079.

[73] Wilson A, Trumpp A. Bone-marrow haematopoietic-stem-cell niches. Nat Rev Immunol 2006; 6: 93-106.

[74] Yin T, Li L. The stem cell niches in bone. J Clin Invest 2006; 116: 1195-1201.

[75] Corre J, Mahtouk K, Attal M, *et al.* Bone marrow mesenchymal stem cells are abnormal in multiple myeloma. Leukemia 2007; 21: 1079-1088.

[76] Arnulf B, Lecourt S, Soulier J, *et al.* Phenotypic and functional characterization of bone marrow mesenchymal stem cells derived from patients with multiple myeloma. Leukemia 2007; 21: 158-163.

[77] Mukherjee S, Raje N, Schoonmaker JA, *et al.* Pharmacologic targeting of a stem/progenitor population *in vivo* is associated with enhanced bone regeneration in mice. J Clin Invest 2008; 118: 491-504.

[78] Giuliani N, Morandi F, Tagliaferri S, *et al.* The proteasome inhibitor bortezomib affects osteoblast differentiation *in vitro* and *in vivo* in multiple myeloma patients. Blood 2007; 110: 334-338.

[79] Singhal S, Mehta J, Desikan R, *et al.* Antitumor activity of thalidomide in refractory multiple myeloma. New Engl J Med 1999; 341: 1565-1571.

[80] Rajkumar SV, Blood E, Vesole D, Fonseca R, Greipp PR. Phase III clinical trial of thalidomide plus dexamethasone compared with dexamethasone alone in newly diagnosed multiple myeloma: a clinical trial coordinated by the Eastern Cooperative Oncology Group. J Clin Oncol 2006; 24: 431-436.

[81] Palumbo A, Bringhen S, Caravita T, *et al.* Oral Melphalan and prednisone chemotherapy plus thalidomide compared with Melphalan and prednisone alone in elderly patients with multiple myeloma: randomised controlled trial. Lancet 2006; 367: 825-831.

[82] Facon T, Mary JY, Hulin C, *et al* Melphalan and prednisone plus thalidomide vs. Melphalan and prednisone alone or reduced-intensity autologous stem cell transplantation in elderly patients with multiple myeloma (IFM 99-06): a randomised trial. Lancet 2007; 370: 1209-1218.

[83] Richardson PG, Mitsiades C, Hideshima T, Anderson KC. Lenalidomide in multiple myeloma. Expert Rev Anticancer Ther 2006; 6: 1165-1173.

[84] Richardson PG, Schlossman RL, Weller E, *et al.* Immunomodulatory drug CC-5013 overcomes drug resistance and is well tolerated in patients with relapsed multiple myeloma. Blood 2002; 100: 3063-3067.

[85] Schey SA, Fields P, Bartlett JB, *et al.* Phase I study of an immunomodulatory thalidomide analog, CC-4047, in relapsed or refractory multiple myeloma. J Clin Oncol 2004; 22: 3269-3276.

[86] Dimopoulos M, Spencer A, Attal M, *et al.* Lenalidomide plus dexamethasone for relapsed or refractory multiple myeloma. The New England journal of medicine 2007; 357: 2123-2132.

[87] Weber DM, Chen C, Niesvizky R, *et al.* Lenalidomide plus dexamethasone for relapsed multiple myeloma in North America. New Engl J Med 2007; 357: 2133-2142.

[88] Rajkumar SV, Jacobus S, Callander N, *et al.* A randomized trial of lenalidomide Plus high-dose dexamethasone (RD) vs. lenalidomide plus low-dose dexamethasone (Rd) in newly diagnosed multiple myeloma (E4A03): a trial coordinated by the Eastern Cooperative Oncology Group. Blood 2007; 110: 121.

[89] Zonder JA, Crowley J, Hussein MA, *et al.* Superiority of lenalidomide (Len) plus high-dose dexamethasone (HD) compared to HD alone as treatment of newly-diagnosed multiple myeloma (NDMM): results of the randomized, double-blinded, placebo-controlled SWOG trial S0232. Blood 2007; 110: 121.

[90] Palumbo A, Falco P, Corradini P, *et al.* Melphalan, prednisone, and lenalidomide treatment for newly diagnosed myeloma: a report from the GIMEMA--Italian Multiple Myeloma Network. J Clin Oncol 2007; 25: 4459-4465.

[91] Lacy MQ, Hayman SR, Gertz MA, *et al.* Pomalidomide (CC4047) plus low-dose dexamethasone as therapy for relapsed multiple myeloma. J Clin Oncol 2009; 27: 5008-5014.

[92] Lee AH, Iwakoshi NN, Anderson KC, Glimcher LH. Proteasome inhibitors disrupt the unfolded protein response in myeloma cells. Proc Natl Acad Sci U S A 2003; 100: 9946-9951.

[93] Richardson PG, Mitsiades C, Hideshima T, Anderson KC. Bortezomib: proteasome inhibition as an effective anticancer therapy. Annu Rev Med 2006; 57: 33-47.

[94] Podar K, Anderson KC. Caveolin-1 as a potential new therapeutic target in multiple myeloma. Cancer Lett 2006; 233: 10-15.

[95] Richardson PG, Barlogie B, Berenson J, *et al.* A phase 2 study of bortezomib in relapsed, refractory myeloma. The New England journal of medicine 2003; 348: 2609-2617.

[96] San Miguel JF, Schlag R, Khuageva N, *et al.* MY-3002: a phase 3 study comparing bortezomib Melphalan prednisone (VMP) with Melphalan prednisone (MP) in newly diagnosed multiple myeloma. Blood 2007; 110: 121.

[97] Harousseau JL, Attal M, Coiteux V, *et al.* Bortezomib (VELCADE®) plus dexamethasone as induction treatment prior to autologous stem cell transplantation in patients with newly diagnosed multiple myeloma: preliminary results of an IFM Phase II study. J Clin Oncol, 2005 ASCO Annual Meeting Proceedings 2005; 23: 2005: 6653.

[98] Demo SD, Kirk CJ, Aujay MA, *et al.* Antitumor activity of PR-171, a novel irreversible inhibitor of the proteasome. Cancer Res 2007; 67: 6383-6391.

[99] Kuhn DJ, Chen Q, Voorhees PM, *et al.* Potent activity of carfilzomib, a novel, irreversible inhibitor of the ubiquitin-proteasome pathway, against preclinical models of multiple myeloma. Blood 2007; 110: 3281-3290.

[100] Parlati F, Lee SJ, Aujay M, *et al.* Carfilzomib can induce tumor cell death through selective inhibition of the chymotrypsin-like activity of the proteasome. Blood 2009; 114: 3439-3447.

[101] O'Connor OA, Stewart AK, Vallone M, *et al.* A phase 1 dose escalation study of the safety and pharmacokinetics of the novel proteasome inhibitor carfilzomib (PR-171) in patients with hematologic malignancies. Clin Cancer Res 2009; 15: 7085-7091.

[102] Macherla VR, Mitchell SS, Manam RR, *et al.* Structure-activity relationship studies of salinosporamide A (NPI-0052), a novel marine derived proteasome inhibitor. J Med Chem 2005; 48: 3684-3687.

[103] Chauhan D, Catley L, Li G, *et al.* A novel orally active proteasome inhibitor induces apoptosis in multiple myeloma cells with mechanisms distinct from Bortezomib. Cancer Cell 2005; 8: 407-419.

[104] Chauhan D, Singh A, Brahmandam M, *et al.* Combination of proteasome inhibitors bortezomib and NPI-0052 trigger *in vivo* synergistic cytotoxicity in multiple myeloma. Blood 2008; 111: 1654-1664.

[105] Hoeller D, Hecker CM, Dikic I. Ubiquitin and ubiquitin-like proteins in cancer pathogenesis. Nature Reviews 2006; 6: 776-788.

[106] Nalepa G, Rolfe M, Harper JW. Drug discovery in the ubiquitin-proteasome system. Nat Rev Drug Discov 2006; 5: 596-613.

[107] Yang Y, Ludwig RL, Jensen JP, *et al.* Small molecule inhibitors of HDM2 ubiquitin ligase activity stabilize and activate p53 in cells. Cancer Cell 2005; 7: 547-559.

[108] Cardozo T, Pagano M. The SCF ubiquitin ligase: insights into a molecular machine. Nat Rev Mol Cell Biol 2004; 5: 739-751.

[109] Vassilev LT, Vu BT, Graves B, *et al.* *In vivo* activation of the p53 pathway by small-molecule antagonists of MDM2. Science 2004; 303: 844-848.

[110] Shangary S, Wang S. Small-molecule inhibitors of the MDM2-p53 protein-protein interaction to reactivate p53 function: a novel approach for cancer therapy. Ann Rev Pharmacol Toxicol 2009; 49: 223-241.

[111] Issaeva N, Bozko P, Enge M, *et al.* Small molecule RITA binds to p53, blocks p53-HDM-2 interaction and activates p53 function in tumors. Nat Med 2004; 10: 1321-1328.

[112] Hussain S, Zhang Y, Galardy PJ. DUBs and cancer: the role of deubiquitinating enzymes as oncogenes, non-oncogenes and tumor suppressors. Cell Cycle 2009; 8: 1688-1697.

[113] Komander D, Clague MJ, Urbe S. Breaking the chains: structure and function of the deubiquitinases. Nat Rev Mol Cell Biol 2009; 10: 550-563.

[114] Schwickart M, Huang X, Lill JR, *et al.* Deubiquitinase USP9X stabilizes MCL1 and promotes tumour cell survival. Nature 2010; 463: 103-107.

[115] Husnjak K, Elsasser S, Zhang N, *et al.* Proteasome subunit Rpn13 is a novel ubiquitin receptor. Nature 2008; 453: 481-488.

[116] Schreiner P, Chen X, Husnjak K, *et al.* Ubiquitin docking at the proteasome through a novel pleckstrin-homology domain interaction. Nature 2008; 453: 548-552.
[117] Mitsiades N, Mitsiades CS, Richardson PG, *et al.* Molecular sequelae of histone deacetylase inhibition in human malignant B cells. Blood 2003; 101: 4055-4062.
[118] Catley L, Weisberg E, Kiziltepe T, *et al.* Aggresome induction by proteasome inhibitor bortezomib and alpha-tubulin hyperacetylation by tubulin deacetylase (TDAC) inhibitor LBH589 are synergistic in myeloma cells. Blood 2006; 108: 3441-3449.
[119] Badros A, Philip S, Niesvizky R, *et al.* Phase I trial of suberoylanilide hydroxamic acid (SAHA) plus bortezomib (Bort) in relapsed multiple myeloma (MM) patients (pts). Blood 2007; 110: 354a.
[120] Weber DM, Jagannath S, Mazumder A, *et al.* Phase I trial of oral vorinostat (suberoylanilide hydroxamic acid, SAHA) in combination with bortezomib in patients with advanced multiple myeloma. Blood 2007; 110: 355a, abstract 1172.
[121] Kawano M, Hirano T, Matsuda T, *et al.* Autocrine generation and requirement of BSF-2/IL-6 for human multiple myelomas. Nature 1988; 332: 83-85.
[122] Klein B, Zhang XG, Lu ZY, Bataille R. Interleukin-6 in human multiple myeloma. Blood 1995; 85: 863-872.
[123] Wen XY, Stewart AK, Sooknanan RR, *et al.* Identification of c-myc promoter-binding protein and X-box binding protein 1 as interleukin-6 target genes in human multiple myeloma cells. Int J Oncol 1999; 15: 173-178.
[124] Chauhan D, Li G, Auclair D, *et al.* Identification of genes regulated by 2-methoxyestradiol (2ME2) in multiple myeloma cells using oligonucleotide arrays. Blood 2003; 101: 3606-3614.
[125] Reimold AM, Iwakoshi NN, Manis J, *et al.* Plasma cell differentiation requires the transcription factor XBP-1. Nature 2001; 412: 300-307.
[126] Iwakoshi NN, Lee AH, Vallabhajosyula P, *et al.* Plasma cell differentiation and the unfolded protein response intersect at the transcription factor XBP-1. Nat Immunol 2003; 4: 321-329.
[127] Carrasco DR, Sukhdeo K, Protopopova M, *et al.* The differentiation and stress response factor XBP-1 drives multiple myeloma pathogenesis. Cancer Cell 2007; 11: 349-360.
[128] Ernst M, Gearing DP, Dunn AR. Functional and biochemical association of Hck with the LIF/IL-6 receptor signal transducing subunit gp130 in embryonic stem cells. Embo J 1994; 13: 1574-1584.
[129] Schaeffer M, Schneiderbauer M, Weidler S, *et al.* Signaling through a novel domain of gp130 mediates cell proliferation and activation of Hck and Erk kinases. Mol Cell Biol 2001; 21: 8068-8081.
[130] Podar K, Mostoslavsky G, Sattler M, *et al.* Critical role for Hck-mediated phosphorylation of Gab1 and Gab2 docking proteins in IL-6-induced proliferation and survival of MM cells. J Biol Chem 2004; 279: 21658-21665.
[131] Le Gouill S, Podar K, Harousseau JL, Anderson KC. Mcl-1 Regulation and its Role in Multiple Myeloma. Cell Cycle 2004; 3:
[132] Chauhan D, Anderson KC. Mechanisms of cell death and survival in multiple myeloma (MM): Therapeutic implications. Apoptosis 2003; 8: 337-343.
[133] Chauhan D, Neri P, Velankar M, *et al.* Targeting mitochondrial factor Smac/DIABLO as therapy for multiple myeloma (MM). Blood 2007; 109: 1220-1227.
[134] Ferrara N, Hillan KJ, Gerber HP, Novotny W. Discovery and development of bevacizumab, an anti-VEGF antibody for treating cancer. Nat Rev Drug Discov 2004; 3: 391-400.
[135] Yang JC, Haworth L, Sherry RM, *et al.* A randomized trial of bevacizumab, an anti-vascular endothelial growth factor antibody, for metastatic renal cancer. New Engl J Med 2003; 349: 427-434.
[136] Lin B, Podar K, Gupta D, *et al.* The vascular endothelial growth factor receptor tyrosine kinase inhibitor PTK787/ZK222584 inhibits growth and migration of multiple myeloma cells in the bone marrow microenvironment. Cancer research 2002; 62: 5019-5026.
[137] Bergers G, Hanahan D. Modes of resistance to anti-angiogenic therapy. Nature Reviews 2008; 8: 592-603.
[138] Aggarwal R, Ghobrial IM, Roodman GD. Chemokines in multiple myeloma. Exp Hematol 2006; 34: 1289-1295.
[139] Alsayed Y, Ngo H, Runnels J, *et al.* Mechanisms of regulation of CXCR4/SDF-1 (CXCL12)-dependent migration and homing in multiple myeloma. Blood 2007; 109: 2708-2717.
[140] Menu E, Asosingh K, Indraccolo S, *et al.* The involvement of stromal derived factor 1alpha in homing and progression of multiple myeloma in the 5TMM model. Haematologica 2006; 91: 605-612.
[141] De Clercq E. The bicyclam AMD3100 story. Nat Rev Drug Discov 2003; 2: 581-587.
[142] Pelus LM. Peripheral blood stem cell mobilization: new regimens, new cells, where do we stand. Curr Opin Hematol 2008; 15: 285-292.
[143] Podar K, Hideshima T, Tai YT, *et al.* Emerging Therapies for Multiple Myeloma. Am J Cancer 2006; 5: 141-153.

[144] Lapalombella R, Gowda A, Joshi T, *et al.* The humanized CD40 antibody SGN-40 demonstrates pre-clinical activity that is enhanced by lenalidomide in chronic lymphocytic leukaemia. Br J Haematol 2009; 144: 848-855.

[145] Hussein M, Berenson JR, Niesvizky R, *et al.* A phase 1 multidose study of dacetuzumab (SGN-40; humanized anti-CD40 mAb) in patients with multiple myeloma. Haematologica 2010:

[146] Tai YT, Catley L, Li XF, *et al.* Immunomodulatory drug Lenalidomide (CC-5013, IMiD3) augments anti-CD40 SGN-40-induced cytotoxicity in human multiple myeloma: clinical implications. Blood 2005; 106:

[147] Hideshima T, Chauhan D, Schlossman R, Richardson P, Anderson KC. The role of tumor necrosis factor alpha in the pathophysiology of human multiple myeloma: therapeutic applications. Oncogene 2001; 20: 4519-4527.

[148] Novak AJ, Darce JR, Arendt BK, *et al.* Expression of BCMA, TACI, and BAFF-R in multiple myeloma: a mechanism for growth and survival. Blood 2004; 103: 689-694.

[149] Moreaux J, Legouffe E, Jourdan E, *et al.* BAFF and APRIL protect myeloma cells from apoptosis induced by interleukin 6 deprivation and dexamethasone. Blood 2004; 103: 3148-3157.

[150] Tai YT, Li XF, Breitkreutz I, *et al.* Role of B-cell-activating factor in adhesion and growth of human multiple myeloma cells in the bone marrow microenvironment. Cancer Res 2006; 66: 6675-6682.

[151] Moreaux J, Hose D, Jourdan M, *et al.* TACI expression is associated with a mature bone marrow plasma cell signature and C-MAF overexpression in human myeloma cell lines. Haematologica 2007; 92: 803-811.

[152] Moreaux J, Cremer FW, Reme T, *et al.* The level of TACI gene expression in myeloma cells is associated with a signature of microenvironment dependence vs. a plasmablastic signature. Blood 2005; 106: 1021-1030.

[153] Birmann BM, Giovannucci E, Rosner B, Anderson KC, Colditz GA. Body mass index, physical activity, and risk of multiple myeloma. Cancer Epidemiol Biomarkers Prev 2007; 16: 1474-1478.

[154] Abroun S, Ishikawa H, Tsuyama N, *et al.* Receptor synergy of interleukin-6 (IL-6) and insulin-like growth factor-I that highly express IL-6 receptor alpha myeloma cells. Blood 2004; 103: 2291-2298.

[155] Mitsiades CS, Mitsiades NS, McMullan CJ, *et al.* Inhibition of the insulin-like growth factor receptor-1 tyrosine kinase activity as a therapeutic strategy for multiple myeloma, other hematologic malignancies, and solid tumors. Cancer Cell 2004; 5: 221-230.

[156] Alsina M, Fonseca R, Wilson EF, *et al.* Farnesyltransferase inhibitor tipifarnib is well tolerated, induces stabilization of disease, and inhibits farnesylation and oncogenic/tumor survival pathways in patients with advanced multiple myeloma. Blood 2004; 103: 3271-3277.

[157] David E, Kaufman JL, Flowers CR, *et al.* Tipifarnib sensitizes cells to proteasome inhibition by blocking degradation of bortezomib-induced aggresomes. Blood 2010; 9;116: 5285-8.

[158] Armand JP, Burnett AK, Drach J, *et al.* The emerging role of targeted therapy for hematologic malignancies: update on bortezomib and tipifarnib. Oncologist 2007; 12: 281-290.

[159] Beaupre DM, Cepero E, Obeng EA, Boise LH, Lichtenheld MG. R115777 induces Ras-independent apoptosis of myeloma cells *via* multiple intrinsic pathways. Mol Cancer Ther 2004; 3: 179-186.

[160] Ramakrishnan V, Timm M, Haug JL, *et al.* Sorafenib, a dual Raf kinase/vascular endothelial growth factor receptor inhibitor has significant anti-myeloma activity and synergizes with common anti-myeloma drugs. Oncogene 2009:

[161] Breitkreutz I, Raab MS, Vallet S, *et al.* Targeting MEK1/2 blocks osteoclast differentiation, function and cytokine secretion in multiple myeloma. Br J Haematol 2007; 139: 55-63.

[162] Hideshima T, Catley L, Yasui H, *et al.* Perifosine, an oral bioactive novel alkyl-phospholipid, inhibits Akt and induces *in vitro* and *In vivo* cytotoxicity in human multiple myeloma (MM) cells. Blood 2005; 106: 128.

[163] Hideshima T, Catley L, Raje N, *et al.* Inhibition of Akt induces significant downregulation of survivin and cytotoxicity in human multiple myeloma cells. Br J Haematol 2007; 138: 783-791.

[164] Gajate C, Mollinedo F. Edelfosine and perifosine induce selective apoptosis in multiple myeloma by recruitment of death receptors and downstream signaling molecules into lipid rafts. Blood 2007; 109: 711-719.

[165] David E, Sinha R, Kaufman JL, Lonial S. Perifosine induces DR4/DR5 expression leading to apoptosis that can be enhanced with exogenous TRAIL, and blocked with strategies directed at DR4/DR5 inhibition. Blood 2006; 108, abstract #3446

[166] De P, Peng Q, Dey N, *et al.* A vascular targeted pan PI-3 kinase inhibitor, SF1126 with activity against multiple myeloma *in vivo*. Blood 2006:

[167] Baumann P, Mandl-Weber S, Oduncu F, Schmidmaier R. The novel orally bioavailable inhibitor of phosphoinositol-3-kinase and mammalian target of rapamycin, NVP-BEZ235, inhibits growth and proliferation in multiple myeloma. Exp Cell Res 2009; 315: 485-497.

[168] McMillin DW, Ooi M, Delmore J, *et al.* Antimyeloma activity of the orally bioavailable dual phosphatidylinositol 3-kinase/mammalian target of rapamycin inhibitor NVP-BEZ235. Cancer Res 2009; 69: 5835-5842.

[169] Peterson TR, Laplante M, Thoreen CC, *et al.* DEPTOR is an mTOR inhibitor frequently overexpressed in multiple myeloma cells and required for their survival. Cell 2009; 137: 873-886.

[170] Bharti AC, Shishodia S, Reuben JM, *et al.* Nuclear factor-kappaB and STAT3 are constitutively active in CD138+ cells derived from multiple myeloma patients, and suppression of these transcription factors leads to apoptosis. Blood 2004; 103: 3175-3184.

[171] Catlett-Falcone R, Landowski TH, Oshiro MM, *et al.* Constitutive activation of Stat3 signaling confers resistance to apoptosis in human U266 myeloma cells. Immunity 1999; 10: 105-115.

[172] Bharti AC, Donato N, Aggarwal BB. Curcumin (diferuloylmethane) inhibits constitutive and IL-6-inducible STAT3 phosphorylation in human multiple myeloma cells. J Immunol 2003; 171: 3863-3871.

[173] Amit-Vazina M, Shishodia S, Harris D, *et al.* Atiprimod blocks STAT3 phosphorylation and induces apoptosis in multiple myeloma cells. Br J Cancer 2005; 93: 70-80.

[174] Hamasaki M, Hideshima T, Tassone P, *et al.* Azaspirane (N-N-diethyl-8,8-dipropyl-2-azaspiro[4.5] decane-2-propanamine) inhibits human multiple myeloma cell growth in the bone marrow milieu *in vitro* and *in vivo*. Blood 2005; 105: 4470-4476.

[175] De Vos J, Jourdan M, Tarte K, Jasmin C, Klein B. JAK2 tyrosine kinase inhibitor tyrphostin AG490 downregulates the mitogen-activated protein kinase (MAPK) and signal transducer and activator of transcription (STAT) pathways and induces apoptosis in myeloma cells. Br J Haematol 2000; 109: 823-828.

[176] Pedranzini L, Dechow T, Berishaj M, *et al.* Pyridone 6, a pan-Janus-activated kinase inhibitor, induces growth inhibition of multiple myeloma cells. Cancer Res 2006; 66: 9714-9721.

[177] Alas S, Bonavida B. Inhibition of constitutive STAT3 activity sensitizes resistant non-Hodgkin's lymphoma and multiple myeloma to chemotherapeutic drug-mediated apoptosis. Clin Cancer Res 2003; 9: 316-326.

[178] Chatterjee M, Stuhmer T, Herrmann P, *et al.* Combined disruption of both the MEK/ERK and the IL-6R/STAT3 pathways is required to induce apoptosis of multiple myeloma cells in the presence of bone marrow stromal cells. Blood 2004; 104: 3712-3721.

[179] Kunnumakkara AB, Nair AS, Sung B, Pandey MK, Aggarwal BB. Boswellic acid blocks signal transducers and activators of transcription 3 signaling, proliferation, and survival of multiple myeloma *via* the protein tyrosine phosphatase SHP-1. Mol Cancer Res 2009; 7: 118-128.

[180] Demchenko YN, Glebov OK, Zingone A, *et al.* Classical and/or alternative NF {kappa}B pathway activation in multiple myeloma. Blood 2010:

[181] Gilmore TD. Introduction to NF-kappaB: players, pathways, perspectives. Oncogene 2006; 25: 6680-6684.

[182] Annunziata CM, Davis RE, Demchenko Y, *et al.* Frequent engagement of the classical and alternative NF-kappaB pathways by diverse genetic abnormalities in multiple myeloma. Cancer Cell 2007; 12: 115-130.

[183] Keats JJ, Fonseca R, Chesi M, *et al.* Promiscuous mutations activate the noncanonical NF-kappaB pathway in multiple myeloma. Cancer Cell 2007; 12: 131-144.

[184] Chauhan D, Uchiyama H, Akbarali Y, *et al.* Multiple myeloma cell adhesion-induced interleukin-6 expression in bone marrow stromal cells involves activation of NF-kappa B. Blood 1996; 87: 1104-1112.

[185] Gilmore TD, Herscovitch M. Inhibitors of NF-kappaB signaling: 785 and counting. Oncogene 2006; 25: 6887-6899.

[186] Hideshima T, Chauhan D, Richardson P, *et al.* NF-kappa B as a therapeutic target in multiple myeloma. J Biol Chem 2002; 277: 16639-16647.

[187] Hideshima T, Neri P, Tassone P, *et al.* MLN120B, a novel IkappaB kinase beta inhibitor, blocks multiple myeloma cell growth *in vitro* and *in vivo*. Clin Cancer Res 2006; 12: 5887-5894.

[188] Sanda T, Iida S, Ogura H, *et al.* Growth inhibition of multiple myeloma cells by a novel IkappaB kinase inhibitor. Clin Cancer Res 2005; 11: 1974-1982.

[189] Hideshima T, Ikeda H, Chauhan D, *et al.* Bortezomib induces canonical nuclear factor-kappaB activation in multiple myeloma cells. Blood 2009; 114: 1046-1052.

[190] Derksen PW, Tjin E, Meijer HP, *et al.* Illegitimate WNT signaling promotes proliferation of multiple myeloma cells. Proc Natl Acad Sci U S A 2004; 101: 6122-6127.

[191] Chim CS, Pang R, Fung TK, Choi CL, Liang R. Epigenetic dysregulation of Wnt signaling pathway in multiple myeloma. Leukemia 2007; 21: 2527-36.

[192] Kobune M, Chiba H, Kato J, *et al.* Wnt3/RhoA/ROCK signaling pathway is involved in adhesion-mediated drug resistance of multiple myeloma in an autocrine mechanism. Mol Cancer Ther 2007; 6: 1774-1784.

[193] Mani M, Carrasco DE, Zhang Y, *et al.* BCL9 promotes tumor progression by conferring enhanced proliferative, metastatic, and angiogenic properties to cancer cells. Cancer Res 2009; 69: 7577-7586.

[194] Dutta-Simmons J, Zhang Y, Gorgun G, *et al.* Aurora kinase A is a target of Wnt/beta-catenin involved in multiple myeloma disease progression. Blood 2009; 114: 2699-2708.

[195] Qiang YW, Chen Y, Stephens O, *et al.* Myeloma-derived Dickkopf-1 disrupts Wnt-regulated osteoprotegerin and RANKL production by osteoblasts: a potential mechanism underlying osteolytic bone lesions in multiple myeloma. Blood 2008:

[196] Heath DJ, Chantry AD, Buckle CH, *et al.* Inhibiting Dickkopf-1 (Dkk1) removes suppression of bone formation and prevents the development of osteolytic bone disease in multiple myeloma. J Bone Miner Res 2009; 24: 425-436.

[197] Sukhdeo K, Mani M, Zhang Y, *et al.* Targeting the beta-catenin/TCF transcriptional complex in the treatment of multiple myeloma. Proc Natl Acad Sci U S A 2007; 104: 7516-7521.

[198] Fulciniti M, Tassone P, Hideshima T, *et al.* Anti-DKK1 mAb (BHQ880) as a potential therapeutic agent for multiple myeloma. Blood 2009; 114: 371-379.

[199] Lepourcelet M, Chen YN, France DS, *et al.* Small-molecule antagonists of the oncogenic Tcf/beta-catenin protein complex. Cancer Cell 2004; 5: 91-102.

[200] Podar K, Raab MS, Chauhan D, Anderson KC. The therapeutic role of targeting protein kinase C in solid and hematologic malignancies. Expert Opin Investig Drugs 2007; 16: 1693-1707.

[201] Sharkey J, Khong T, Spencer A. PKC412 demonstrates JNK-dependent activity against human multiple myeloma cells. Blood 2007; 109: 1712-1719.

[202] Podar K, Raab MS, Zhang J, *et al.* Targeting PKC in multiple myeloma: *in vitro* and *in vivo* effects of the novel, orally available small-molecule inhibitor enzastaurin (LY317615.HCl). Blood 2007; 109: 1669-1677.

[203] Moreau AS, Jia X, Ngo HT, *et al.* Protein kinase C inhibitor enzastaurin induces *in vitro* and *in vivo* antitumor activity in Waldenstrom macroglobulinemia. Blood 2007; 109: 4964-4972.

[204] Mitsiades CS, Hayden PJ, Anderson KC, Richardson PG. From the bench to the bedside: emerging new treatments in multiple myeloma. Best Pract Res Clin Haematol 2007; 20: 797-816.

CHAPTER 13

Antibody-based Therapies in Multiple Myeloma

Yu-Tzu Tai*

Department of Medical Oncology, Dana-Farber Cancer Institute, Harvard Medical School, Boston, USA

Abstract: The unmet need for improved multiple myeloma (MM) therapy has stimulated clinical development of monoclonal antibodies (mAbs) targeting either MM cells or cells of the bone marrow (BM) microenvironment. In contrast to small-molecule inhibitors, therapeutic mAbs present the potential to specifically target tumor cells and directly induce an immune response to lyse tumor cells. Unique immune-effector mechanisms are only triggered by therapeutic mAbs but not by small molecule targeting agents. Although therapeutic murine mAbs or chimeric mAbs can cause immunogenicity, the advancement of genetic recombination for humanizing rodent mAbs has allowed large-scale production and designation of mAbs with better affinities, efficient selection, decreasing immunogenicity, and improved effector functions. These advancements of antibody engineering technologies has largely overcome the critical obstacle of antibody immunogenicity and enabled the development and subsequent Food and Drug Administration (FDA) approval of therapeutic Abs for cancer and other diseases.

Keywords: Rituximab, tocilizumab, elotuzumab, HuLuc63, daratumumab, anti-HM1.24 mAb, mapatumumab, milatuzumab, CNTO 328, denosumab, BHQ880, ACE-011, atacicept, bevacizumab.

1. INTRODUCTION

Despite the landmark approval of the anti-CD20 mAb rituximab for the treatment of B cell malignancies, to date, no mAb-based therapy has been approved for MM treatment. The development of effective cytotoxic mAb therapies in MM has been hindered by the lack of uniquely and constitutively expressed target molecules on all MM cells. Indeed, studies in early 2000 demonstrated only minimal activity of anti-CD20 rituximab and antibodies against plasma cell-specific CD38 antibodies in MM[1-4]. However, numerous efforts to identify new targets on MM cells including gene expression profiling and oncogenomic studies are under way. Derived mAbs (*e.g.* against CD40, HM1.24, IGF-1R, CD56, CS1, CD138, CD74, IL-6R, CD38, TRAIL-R1, and the activin receptor type IIA (ActRIIA)) have already demonstrated promising preclinical as well as early clinical activity (Table **1**).

Given the importance of the bone marrow (BM) microenvironment for MM cell growth, survival, and drug resistance, mAbs have been additionally designed to functionally block both autocrine and paracrine secreted cytokines and growth factors as well as molecules mediating MM-stromal cell interaction. For example, mAbs targeting interleukin-6 (IL-6), vascular endothelial growth factor (VEGF), Receptor Activator of NFκB ligand (RANKL) (also known as osteoprotegerin ligand (OPGL)), and Dickkopf homolog 1 (DKK1) are among those under clinical evaluation. Specifically, targeting bone-MM cell interactions *via* bone biology modulating factors such as DKK1, and RANKL are likely to trigger anti-MM effects but also improve bone disease thereby improving both patient survival as well as patient's quality of life.

In the coming years, the preclinical progress in defining novel MM markers will be continued and subsequently advance the clinical development of therapeutic mAbs, alone or in combination with other anti-MM agents, to improve patient outcome in MM.

2. MECHANISMS OF ACTION OF THERAPEUTIC MONOCLONAL ANTIBODIES

Antibodies of IgG, the most commonly used immunoglobulin form in cancer therapy, are unique proteins with dual functionality. Therapeutic mAbs use one or more following mechanisms to reduce tumor burden

***Address correspondence to Yu-Tzu Tai:** Dana-Farber Cancer Institute, Department of Medical Oncology, Jerome Lipper Multiple Myeloma Center, 44 Binney Street, Boston, MA 02115: E-mail: yu-tzu_tai@dfci.harvard.edu

Klaus Podar and Kenneth C. Anderson (Eds)

in patients. They can be categorized into direct and indirect actions. Three modes of action could be further subcategorized from the direct action of mAb-based cancer therapy, including blocking the function of target signaling molecules or receptors, stimulating apoptosis signaling cascades, and targeting function to selectively target tumor cells and deliver toxins. The receptor functional blocking can occur by inhibiting ligand binding to inhibit cell cycle progression, DNA repair, or angiogenesis. It could also occur by increasing internalization of receptors or decreasing proteolytic cleavage of receptors. In the case of targeting function, mAbs could be conjugated with immunotoxins, *i.e.* anti-tubulin agents (DM1/DM4, auristatin), doxorubicin, radioisotopes, or other chemotherapeutic drugs, thus selectively targeting and killing tumor cells. Indirect action of mAb therapy is mediated by the immune system. The elimination of tumor cells using mAbs depend on Ig-mediated mechanisms, including andtibody-dependent cellular cytotoxicity (ADCC) and complement dependent cytotoxicity (CDC), to activate immune effector cells to lyse target tumor cells These two mechanisms are believed to have the greatest impact, although there are conflicting views of which of these two pathways contributes the most to the response. ADCC involves the recognition of the Ab by immune cells that engage the Ab-marked cells and either through their direct action, or through the recruitment of other cell types, led to the tagged-cell's death. CDC is a process where a cascade of different complement proteins become activated, usually when several IgGs are in close proximity to each other, either with one direct outcome being cell lysis, or one indirect outcome being attracting other immune cells to this location for effector cell function.

3. ANTIBODIES TARGETING CELL SURFACE PROTEIN ON MM CELLS

Several mAbs directed against MM cell surface are being investigated as potential therapy in MM[96]. Listed below are mAbs against receptor antigens that are currently under clinical development or investigation in MM.

3.1. Limited Clinical Benefit from Anti-CD20 mAb Rituximab in MM

MM is usually not considered as a disease suitable for anti-CD20 therapy due to weak CD20 expression in the majority of patients. For example, results from a clinical phase II trial in relapsed MM showed that Rituximab treatment yielded significant reductions in circulating B cells and serum IgM levels but had no beneficial clinical effect [5].

Moreover, rituximab was investigated for maintenance therapy in MM following autologous hematopoietic stem cell transplantation (SCT) [2]. Although the number of MM patients was too low to draw definitive conclusions, the use of rituximab in this setting was associated with an unexpectedly high rate of early relapse. The authors therefore hypothesized a possible role for rituximab in provoking a further decrease in the residual, normal B-cell activity within the context of the complex network of anti-tumor immune response. Taken together, the resistance of MM cells against rituximab could be due to the level of CD20 expression, dissociated action of CDC and ADCC, polymorphism in FGCR3 (CD16) receptor, and an inadequate dose schedule.

In contrast, other studies demonstrated that the CD20+ phenotype is associated with patients with t(11,14)(q13;q32) and with shorter survival[6] and that occasional clinical responses have been achieved in selected patients with $CD20^{+}$ myelomatous plasma cells [7,8].

Finally, new insights suggest that circulating $CD20^{+}$ clonotypic B cells act as precursors or'neoplastic stem cells'in MM patients, representing the proliferative compartment of the disease able to play a role in determining relapse after effective treatments [9]. Thus, clinical trials using rituximab in MM may deserve further investigation.

3.2. Monoclonal Antibodies Targeting IL-6R to Overt IL-6/IL-6R Function

IL-6 is a major growth and survival factor in MM cells whose effects are mainly paracrine [10]. Various therapeutic agents which affect IL-6-mediated effects have been tested including IL-6-conjugated mAbs directed against IL-6R and IL-6 [11]. IL-6R antagonist SANT-7, in combination with Dex and all-trans retinoic acid (ATRA) or zoledronic acid, strongly inhibited growth and induced apoptosis in MM cells[12-13]. These studies suggest that overcoming IL-6-mediated cell resistance by SANT-7 potentiates the effect of glucocorticoides and bisphosphonates on MM cell growth and survival, providing a rationale for therapies using IL-6 antagonists in MM.

Tocilizumab (MRA, atlizumab, Roche Pharmaceuticals) is a humanized anti-human IL-6R mAb (rhPM-1, IgG1 class) designed by using genetic engineering technology and the first therapeutic mAb developed in Japan [15]. Tocilizumab specifically blocks IL-6 actions and ameliorates diseases associated with with IL-6 overproduction [16]. For example, besides Castleman's disease and rheumatoid arthritis (RA), tocilizumab has been shown to be effective in patients with juvenile idiopathic arthritis and Crohn's disease [17,18]. Tocilizumab treatment is generally well tolerated and safe. Moreover, blockade of IL-6R may prove effective in limiting MM cell growth. Indeed it is now evaluated in open-label Phase I (U.S.) and II (France) trials to assess its safety and efficacy as monotherapy in MM patients who are not candidates for, or who have relapsed after stem cell transplantation (SCT).

In addition, NRI, another receptor inhibitor of IL-6 genetically engineered from tocilizumab, is under preclinical evaluation [19]. NRI consists of VH and VL of tocilizumab in a single-chain fragment format dimerized by fusing to the Fc portion of human immunoglobulin G1. The binding activity to IL-6R and the biological activity of the purified NRI were found to be similar to those of parental tocilizumab. Because NRI is encoded on a single gene, it is easily applicable to a gene delivery system using virus vehicles. An adenovirus vector encoding NRI was administered to mice intraperitoneally (i.p.) and monitored for the serum NRI level and growth reduction property on the xenografted IL-6-dependent MM cell line S6B45. These findings indicate that NRI is a promising agent applicable to the therapeutic gene delivery approach for IL-6-driven diseases.

3.3. Targeting CD40 by SGN-40 or HCD122

Novel monoclonal antibodies targeting CD40 activation in MM cells, SGN-40/Dacetuzumab (Seattle Genetics, Genentech) and HCD122/ Lucatumumab (Novartis), have been investigated [20,21]. In preclinical studies, SGN-40, a humanized IgG_1 partial agonistic mAb mediates cytotoxicity against CD40-expressing MM cell lines and patient MM cells *via* suppression of IL-6–induced proliferative and anti-apoptotic effects, as well as ADCC [20]. SGN-40 also induced significant anti-tumor activity in xenograft mouse models of human MM and lymphoma [22]. HCD122 (CHIR12.12) (Novartis), a novel, fully human, IgG_1 antagonistic mAb specifically blocked CD40L-induced adhesion, cytokine secretion, and survival of MM, as well as induced marked ADCC against CD40+ MM cells [21]. *In vivo* anti-MM activity by HCD122 was demonstrated in a xenograft model of 12BM MM plasmacytoma in mice [23]. Early clinical trials have evaluated the pharmacokinetics, safety and efficacy of dacetuzumab monotherapy in patients with relapsed/refractory MM and other B-cell tumors [24,25]. Phase I data suggest both agents are well tolerated with no immunogenicity and show early evidence of single-agent clinical activity in relapsed and refractory MM and NHL [26,27]. SGN-40 Phase Ib clinical trials in combination with lenalidomide and dexamathasone/or bortezomib are planned based on enhanced anti-MM activities when combining SGN-40 with lenalidomide [28].

3.4. Targeting CS1 by HuLuc63/elotuzumab in MM

Using subtractive hybridization of naïve B-cell cDNA from memory B/plasma cell cDNA, CS1 (CD2 subset-1, CRACC, SLAMF7, CD319), a novel member of the signaling lymphocyte activating-molecule (SLAM)-related receptor family, was identified to be highly expressed in plasma cells [29,30]. Specifically, CS1 mRNA and protein are expressed in CD138-purified primary tumor cells from the majority of MM patients (>97%), but neither in major body organs nor CD34+ stem cells. To a low extent, its expression was also observed in NK cells, a subset of T-cells, activated monocytes and activated dendritic cells. CS1 may contribute to MM pathogenesis by increasing MM cell adhesion, clonogenic growth, and tumorigenicity *via* c-maf-mediated interactions with BMSCs [31]. A novel humanized ani-CS1 mAb HuLuc63 (elotuzumab) was selected for clinical development due to its potent tumor-killing activity *in vivo* and *in vitro*. Specifically, elotuzumab induced significant ADCC against MM cells even in the presence of

BMSCs. Moreover, it triggered autologous ADCC against primary MM cells resistant to conventional or novel therapies including bortezomib and HSP90 inhibitor, and markedly enhanced HuLuc63-induced MM cell lysis when pretreated with conventional or novel anti-MM drugs [29,32].

A phase I study of HuLuc63 was well tolerated in MM patients [33]. Preliminary PK data reveal that peak serum drug levels for the 0.5 mg/kg dosing cohort reached 10 mcg / mL, which was sufficient to achieve CS 1 saturation of at least 70% on the antigen rich NK cell subset. Drug levels dropped below 1 mg/mL by day 7, however, coinciding with a decrease in saturation. This indicates that the higher doses to be used in subsequent cohorts may achieve and surpass sustained concentrations in patients above this level. Enrollment is continuing to determine the MTD. Early results of clinical trials of HuLuc63 in combination with bortezomib or lenalidomide or dexamethasone were reported at the ASH meeting 2009 [34,35], suggesting that elotuzumab may enhance the activity of bortezomib and lenalidomide in treating MM with acceptable toxicity. PK analysis suggests a serum half-life of 10-11 days at higher doses (10 and 20 mg/kg). Preliminary analysis of peripheral blood mononuclear cells and and of the BM indicates that objective responses correlate well with complete saturation of CS1 sites by elotuzumab on BM plasma cells and NK cells. The combination of elotuzumab with lenalidomide and low-dose dexamethasone has a manageable adverse event profile and compared to historical data for lenalidomide and high-dose dexamethasone, the preliminary efficacy data (PR of 92%) are very encouraging.

3.5. Targeting CD56 with Immunotoxin-Conjugated mAb

HuN901 conjugated with the maytansinoid $N^{2'}$-deacetyl-$N^{2'}$-(3-mercapto-1-oxopropyl)-maytansine (DM1), a potent antimicrotubular cytotoxic agent may provide targeted delivery of the drug to CD56-expressing tumors including MM. HuN901-DM1 has significant *in vitro* and *in vivo* anti-MM activity at doses that were well tolerated in a murine model [36].

The phase I clinical study of huN901-DM1 (BB-10901) in 23 MM patients determined the MTD as 140 mg/m2/week dose and demonstrated an overall favorable safety profile [37]. Exciting single agent activity was observed in heavily pretreated MM patients, which warrant continued investigation of this novel agent in MM patients especially when used in combination with approved anti-MM agents/regimens such as lenalidomide and dexamethasone.

Table 1. Antigens targeted by antibodies in multiple myeloma in different stages of preclinical/clinical development

Target	Brand name	Company/Sponsor	Type of mAb (conjugate)	Phase	Remarks
CD138	B-B4-DM1	ImmunoGen	the maytansinoid immunoconjugate mouse IgG1 mAb B-B4	preclincial	Tassone Blood 2004 104, 3688-96.
HM1.24	humanized HM1.24	Chugai Pharmaceutical	humanized	preclincial	Ozaki Blood 1999 93,3922-3930
IL-6	OP-R003-1, 1339 Elsilimomab	OPi EUSA Pharma; Vaccinex	human IgG1	preclincial	Fulciniti Clin Cancer Res 2009
HLA-DR	1D09C3	GPC Biotech, AG	human	preclincial	Carlo-Stella Cancer Res 2007
kininogen	C11C1	Temple University School of Medicine	mouse	preclincial	Sainz Cancer Immunol Immunother 2006 C11C1 mAb inhibits its own tumor growth in vivo, slows down B38-MM growth rate when both MM are implanted together and when mAb C11C1 is injected intraperitoneally. MAb C11C1-treated-MM showed decreased MVD and kinino
HLA class I	2D7-DB	Chugai Pharmaceutical Co. Ltd.	converted from mouse IgG2b,single-	preclincial	Sekimoto Cancer Res 2007 a recombinant single-chain Fv diabody 2D7-DB

			chain Fv diabody		specifically induces multiple myeloma cell death in the bone marrow environment
b2-microglobulin	anti-b2M mAbs	MD Anderson Cancer Center	mouse	preclincial	Yang Blood 2007 & Clin Cancer Res 2009 Strong apoptotic effect on myeloma cells and low toxocity in the mice suppports potential use as therapeutic agents.
CD38	MOR202	MorphoSys AG	human	preclincial	Stevenson Mol Med 2006 Tesar Journal of Clinical Oncology, 2007 ASCO Annual Meeting Proceedings Part I. Vol 25, No. 18S (June 20 Supplement), 2007: 8106
CD32B	MGA321(2B6)	MacroGenics	humanized	preclincial	Zhou Blood 2008 humanized 2B6 MoAb may target in patients with systemic AL-amyloidosis. It blocks Fc engagement of CD32B may improve the performance of other cancer Mabs when combined with them during administration.
FGFR3	PRO-001	Prochon Biotech Ltd.	human	preclincial	Trudel Blood 2006 The inhibitory anti-FGFR3 antibody, PRO-001, is cytotoxic to t(4;14) MM cells and deserves further study for the treatment of FGFR3-expressing myeloma.
ICAM-1	cUV3	Abiogen	chimeric IgG1	preclincial	Smallshaw J Immunother 2004; Coleman J Immunother 2006 cUV3 significantly prolongs the survival of SCID/ARH-77 mice
BLyS	BLyS/rGel	Targa Therapeutics	Fusion protein of an antibody tethered to a toxin	preclincial	Lyu Mol Cancer Ther 2007
TACI	Atacicept (TACI-Ig)	ZymoGenetics Inc.	fusion protein	preclincial	Gatto Curr Opin Investig Drugs 2008; Yaccoby Leukemia 2008 22, 406–413
CD70	SGN-70	Seatle Genetics	humanized IgG1	preclincial	McEarchern Clin Cancer Res 2008 14, 7763-72
TRAIL-R2(DR5)	lexatumumab	Human Genome Sciences	human	preclincial	Menoret Blood 2006
IL-6R	NRI (engineered Tocilizumab)	Roche Pharmaceuticals	a single-chain fragment format dimerized by fusing to the Fc portion of human immunoglobulin G1	preclincial	Yoshio-Hoshino Cancer Res 2007 the NRI gene introduction combined with adenovirus gene delivery inhibited the in vivo S6B45 cell growth significantly.
BCMA	SG1	Seatle Genetics	Auristatin-BCMA mAb	preclincial	Ryan et. al. 2007
IL-6	Azintrel®	Vaccinex licensed to Glaxo Smith Kline	human IgG1	preclincial	Fulciniti, et.al., 2009 CCR 15,7144-52
CD20	Rituxan	NCI & Memorial Sloan-Kettering Cancer Center	chimeric with a human IgG1 Fc	II (ongoing)	NCT00258206 (with cyclophosphamide); NCT00505895. High-dose cyclophosphamide in combination with rituximab in patients with primary refractory, high-risk, or relapsed myeloma; also

					being studied for the treatment of peripheral neuropathy in patients with
CD20	Zevalin (yttrium Y 90 ibritumomab tiuxetan)	NCI	mouse IgG1	I (ongoing)	NCT00477815 Zevalin radioimmunotherapy with high-dose Melphalan and stem cell transplant for MM
CD40	SGN-40 (Dacetuzumab)	Seatle Genetics/Genentech	humanized IgG1	I b (ongoing)	NCT00664898, Safety and pharmacology of SGN-40 administered in combination with Bortezomib (Velcade®, PS-341) in patients with relapsed or refractory MM. NCT00525447 is the study of SGN40, lenalidodmide, and dex in MM patients.
CD40	HCD122 (Lucatumumab)	Norvatis	human IgG1	I (ongoing)	NCT00231166 Dose-finding trial of HCD122 in MM patients that is relapsed or has not responded to prior therapy
CD20	Bexxar (131-tositumomab)	GlaxoSmithKline	radioactive iodine 131 attaching to anti-CD20;muIgG2a (131)	II (ongoing)	NCT00135200 To see whether the treatment with Bexxar will decrease and possibly eliminate residual myeloma cells resistant to chemotherapy.
CD56	BB-10901 (IMGN901)	ImmunoGen, Inc.	humanized (maytansine DM1)	I (ongoing)	NCT00346255: Given as an intravenous infusion weekly for two consecutive weeks every three weeks to relapsed and relapsed refractory CD56-positive MM
RANKL	Denosumab	Amgen	human IgG2	II/III (ongoing)	NCT00259740: To determine if denosumab is effective in the treatment of relapsed or plateau-phase MM ; NCT00104650: to determine the effectiveness of AMG 162 in reducing urinary N-telopeptide in advanced cancer subjects with bone metastases; NCT00330759:
VEGF	Avastin becacizumab	Genentech	humanized	II (ongoing)	NCT00428545 (in combination with bortezomib); NCT00410605 (added with lenalidomide and dexamathasone)
CD52	Campath-1H (alemtuzumab)	NCI; Fred Hutchinson Cancer Research Institute	humanized	II (ongoing)	NCT00625144 Studying the side effects of giving fludarabine and busulfan together with alemtuzumab followed by donor stem cell transplant and to see how well it works in treating patients with hematological cancer or other disease.
IL-6	CNTO 328	Centocor, Inc	chimerized	I/II (ongoing)	NCT00401843 (in combination with bortezomib); NCT00911859 (added with Velcade-Melphalan-Prednisone); NCT00402181 (in combination with dexamethason)
IL-6	B-E8 (Elsilimomab)	Orphan Pharma International and	murine	II	Preliminary efficacy was seen but there is a limitation

		Diaclone SA			for the clinical use of a murine monoclonal antibody since it frequently induces human anti-mouse antibodies (HAMA)
TRAIL-R1(DR4)	Mapatumumab(TRM-1)	Human Genome Sciences	human	II (ongoing)	NCT00315757 (in combination with bortezomib)
EGFR	Erbitux(EMMA-1)	Imclone; Bristol Meyers-Squibb	chimerized	II (ongoing)	NCT00368121 (in combination with dexamethasone)
CS1	elotuzumab/HuLuc63	Facet Biotech; Bristol-Myers Squibb	humanized	I /II (ongoing)	NCT00742560 & NCT00726869 (in combination with bortezomib)
CD38	HuMax-CD38	Genmab	human	I/II (ongoing)	NCT00574288: To establish safety profile of HuMax-CD38 when given as monotherapy in patients with MM relapsed or refractory to at least 2 different cytoreductive therapies and without further established treatment options.
DKK	BHQ880	Novartis	human IgG1	I/II (ongoing)	NCT00741377: in combination with Zoledronic Acid in relapsed/refractory myeloma.
CD138	BT062	Biotest; ImmunoGen	chimeric (B-B4-maytansinoid DM4)	I (ongoing)	NCT00723359
KIR	IPH 2101	Innate Pharma	human IgG4	I/IIa (ongoing)	NCT00552396 (ASCO May 30 2009 abstract 09-AB-3032 safety and tolerability study for patients with relapsed/refractory MM. Pre-clinical characterization of 1-7F9, a novel human anti-KIR therapeutic antibody that augments NK-mediated killing of tumor cells
ActRIIA*	ACE-011	Acceleron Pharma, Inc	human IgG1	I/IIa (ongoing)	NCT00747123 (in patients with osteolytic lesions with MM)
IGF-1R	AVE1642	Sanofi-Aventis	humanized	I/II (ongoing)	Descamps et al. 2009; Anti-IGF-1R Monoclonal Antibody combined with bortezomib for patients with rel/ref MM
Ganglioside GM2	BIW-8962	BioWa, Incorporated	humanized	I/II (ongoing)	Dosing study of anti-GM-2 ganglioside (expressed at high levels on the surface of mm cells) followed by efficacy study.
CD74 (variant MHC II)	milatuzumab (hLL1, IMMU-110)	Immunomedics, Inc.	humanized or humanized doxorubucin conjugate	I/II (ongoing)	NCT00421525, in patients with recurrent or refractory multiple myeloma who have failed at least two prior standard systemic treatments. Its isotope, drug, and toxin conjugates have high antitumor activity in non-Hodgkin's lymphoma and multiple myeloma in
Alpha-4 integrin	natalizumab (Tysabri®)	Biogen Idec	humanized IgG4	I/II (ongoing)	NCT00675428, patients with relapsed or refractory multiple myeloma.

MHC II (HLA-DR)	1D09C3	GPC Biotech	human IgG4	I	Carlo-Stella et al. 2007 showed that IFN-gamma-induced up-regulation of HLA-DR results in a potent enhancement of the in vivo antimyeloma activity of 1D09C3 in mice. Initial clinical testing with 1D09C3 has not raised any unexpected or unacceptable safet
IGF-1R	CP-751,871/figitumumab	Pfizer	human IgG2	I	Lacy et al. 2008 reported that CP-751,871 is well tolerated and may constitute a novel agent in the treatment of multiple myeloma.

Every effort has been made to obtain reliable data from multiple sources including http://clinicaltrials.gov, company, and other web sites, but accuracy cannot be guaranteed.

* the activin receptor type IIA (ActRIIA)

3.6. Targeting CD38 in MM

The CD38 molecule is expressed on cell surfaces in a majority of lymphoid tumors, notably MM [38,39]. However, early studies using anti-CD38 mAb with or without an immunotoxin (ricin) have not led to useful clinical applications [4,40].

Recently, a human anti-CD38 IgG_1 HuMax-CD38 (Daratumumab) was raised after immunizing transgenic mice (HuMax-Mouse®) possessing human, but not mouse, Ig genes. Preclinical studies indicated that HuMax-CD38 was effective in killing primary CD38+CD138+ patient MM cells and a range of MM/ lymphoid cell lines by both ADCC and CDC [41]. In SCID mouse animal models, using sensitive bioluminescence imaging, treatment with Hu

Max-CD38 inhibited CD38+ tumor cell growth in both preventive and therapeutic settings. In addition, HuMax-CD38 inhibits the CD38 ADP-ribosyl cyclase activity in target cells, which may contribute to the effectiveness of HuMax-CD38 in killing both primary MM and plasma cell leukemia cells.

Similarly, MOR202 (MorphoSysAG), a fully human anti-CD38 IgG_1 mAb produced by a human combinatorial antibody library (HuCAL) platform, also efficiently triggers ADCC against CD38+ MM cell lines and patient MM cells *in vitro* as well as *in vivo* in a xenograft mouse model [39,42]. One practical problem in applying anti-CD38 therapy is the wide expression on lymphoid, myeloid, and epithelial cells, especially following cell activation. However, mAbs specifically blocking CD38 might still provide a new approach for interfering with deleterious growth circuits, therefore increasing the susceptibility of MM and leukemic cells to conventional chemotherapy.

3.7. Targeting HM1.24 on MM cells

HM1.24 (CD137) was originally identified as a cell surface protein differentially overexpressed on MM cells [43] and later was found to be identical to bone stromal cell antigen 2 (BST-2). A role of HM1.24 in trafficking and signaling between the intracellular and cell surface of MM cells was suggested since it is one of the important activators of NF-kappaB pathway [44]. The humanized anti-HM1.24 mAb (IgG1/kappa, AHM, Chugai Pharmaceutical Co., Ltd.) is able to effectively induce ADCC against some human myeloma cells in the presence of human PBMCs as effectively as a chimeric anti-HM1.24 mAb [45]. Single intravenous injection of AHM significantly inhibited tumor growth in both orthotopic and ectopic human MM xenograft models [46]. Although limited, the only one phase I/II clinical study reported that a humanized anti-HM1.24 mAb did not cause any serious toxicity when administered to patients with relapsed or refractory MM [46].

Most recently, we characterized XmAb®5592, a novel Fc-engineered and humanized anti-HM1.24 mAb, and studied mechanisms of its anti-MM activity [47]. XmAb®5592, with double amino acid substitution in Fc region of the wild type IgG1, has approximately 40-fold and 10-fold increases in affinity for Fc gamma receptor III (FcRIIIa) and (FcRIIa), respectively, expressed on effector cells including NK cells. It triggers 10-100-fold higher ADCC against these MM cell lines than a native/non Fc-engineered version (anti-HM1.24 IgG1) of the Ab. XmAb5592 also induced more potent anti-MM activity in murine subcutaneous xenograft murine models using RPMI 8226 cells. These results suggest that XmAb5592 is a promising next-generation immunotherapeutic for MM.

3.8. Targeting TRAIL Death Signaling Pathway

Two human agonistic mAbs directed against TRAILR1 (HGS-ETR1, TRM-1, Mapatumumab) and TRAILR2 (HGS-ETR2) killed 68% and 45% of MM cell lines, respectively [48]. Only 18% of MM cell lines are resistant to either antibody. There is no correlation between TRAILR expression level and sensitivity to TRAIL-R1 or TRAIL-R2 triggering. Both the extrinsic (caspase 8, Bid) and the intrinsic (caspase 9) pathways are activated by anti-TRAIL mAbs. Mapatumumab is well tolerated in a phase I study in patients with advanced solid malignancies (n=41) and 12 patients had stable disease for 1.9 to 29.4 months [49]. These studies encouraged clinical trials of anti–TRAILR1 mAb in MM. In addition, based on enhanced cytotoxicity when combining mapatumumab with bortezomib in preclinical experiments [50], a randomized phase II study was recently started comparing TRM-1 plus bortezomib (Velcade®) versus bortezomib alone in patients with relapsed or refractory MM.

3.9. Targeting CD74 with Milatuzumab

CD74 is an integral membrane protein that functions as a MHC class II chaperone. Milatuzumab is a humanized anti-CD74 mAb constructed using the same human backbone as epratuzumab (anti-CD22), whose safety has been demonstrated in clinical trials of patients with B-cell malignancies and autoimmune disorders [51,52]. MM cell lines express CD74 (~60% of samples) and milatuzumab caused growth inhibition and induction of apoptosis in CD74-expressing MM cell lines when cross-linked with an anti-human immunoglobulin G secondary antibody [53]. Moreover milatuzumab demonstrated promising therapeutic activity in a CAG-SCID mouse model of disseminated disease for MM when used alone or in combination with doxorubicin, dexamethasone, bortezomib, or lenalidomide [54,55]. In a phase I trial, milatuzumab showed no severe adverse effects in patients with relapsed/refractory MM and it stabilized the disease in some patients for up to 12 weeks [51]. Supporting the data in MM ongoing clinical trials testing different treatment schedules of milatuzumab in chronic lymphocytic leukemia, non-Hodgkin's lymphoma and MM indicate that milatuzumab shows no severe adverse effects in humans.

4. ANTIBODIES TARGETING MM CELLS IN THE BONE MARROW MICROENVIRONMENT

MM cells are highly dependent on the BM microenvironment for growth and survival through interactions particularly with BM stromal cells (BMSCs) and osteoclasts, which secrete important MM growth factors and cytokines. Importantly, these factors/cytokines are further induced from BMSCs when MM cells adhere to BMSCs [10]. Thus, mAbs designed to block the binding of MM cell growth and survival factors to their cognate receptors have been under intensive development.

4.1. Blockage of IL-6 Binding to MM Cells

Early work in developing mAb-based immunotherapies for MM has been focused on the blockade of IL-6 secretion from BM microenvironment because of its key role in promoting MM cell growth and survival. Initial studies of mouse mAb to IL-6 (murine BE-4 and BE-8) demonstrated a transient tumor cytostasis and reduction in toxicities from IL-6 [56]. The potential of combination therapy, including BE-8 (250 mg), Dex (49 mg/day), and high-dose Melphalan [220 mg/m^2 (HDM220)], followed by autologous SCT was demonstrated for the treatment of 16 patients with advanced MM. Overall, 13 of 16 patients (81.3%) exhibited a response, with a complete response (CR) seen in 6 patients (37.5%) without any toxic or allergic reactions. However, the incidence of thrombocytopenia and neutropenia increased. Subsequent clinical trials of BE-8 concluded that limitations of this regimen are first the amount of BE-8 that can be injected due to its short half-life (3–4 days); and second the continued production of IL-6 *in vivo*. Most recently, a high-affinity fully human version of BE-8, OP-R003-1(or 1339, Azintrel®), was selected through ActivMAb antibody discovery technology. Indeed, it enhanced cytotoxicity induced by dexamethasone, as well as bortezomib, lenalidomide, and perifosine, in a synergistic fashion [57]. Importantly, Azintrel® also blocked bone turnover in SCID-hu mouse model of MM, providing an additional rationale for its use in MM.

Despite overcoming the safety concerns of human anti-mouse antibodies associated with murine anti-IL-6 mAb and a long half-life (17.8 days) in circulation, the chimeric mouse mAb to IL-6 CNTO 328 has been ineffective in producing a meaningful response in MM [58,59]. Nevertheless, due to enhanced anti-MM activities of combined CNTO 328 and bortezomib/or dexamethasone in preclinical models, ongoing studies are investigating these regimens for their clinical value in treating MM [60,61]. Specifically, results of a small safety analysis (n=21) done as a run-in to a larger ongoing Phase II trial showed promising preliminary efficacy of CNTO 328 in combination with bortezomib in relapsed/refractory MM. CNTO 328 is also being evaluated as part of a combination therapy for initial treatment of MM in a Phase II trial which compares the safety and effectiveness of CNTO 328 plus Velcade-Melphalan-prednisone (VMP) with VMP alone.

4.2. Targeting MM-Induced Bone Lesion

4.2.1. Targeting RANK/RANKL/OPG axis using denosumab for MM-associated bone destruction

Receptor activator of nuclear factor-kappaB ligand (RANKL) is a cytokine member of the tumor necrosis factor family that is the principal mediator of osteoclastic bone resorption [62]. Osteoprotegerin (OPG), a natural soluble decoy receptor of RANKL, modulates the effect of RANKL and is able to prevent excessive bone resorption in the normal state. RANKL expression is elevated in patients with MM [63,64]. Denosumab (AMG 162, Amgen Inc., Thousand Oaks, CA) is an investigational fully human mAb with high affinity and specificity for RANKL that mimics the natural bone-protecting actions of OPG [65]. A phase 1 clinical trial in patients with MM (n=25) or breast cancer with bone metastases (n=29) showed that following a single s.c. dose of denosumab ((0.1, 0.3, 1.0, or 3.0 mg/kg), levels of urinary and serum N-telopeptide decreased within 1 day, and this decrease lasted through 84 days at the higher denosumab doses [66]. Mean half-lives of denosumab were 33.3 and 46.3 days for the two highest dosages. Larger trials are ongoing to investigate the effect of denosumab for the treatment of cancer-induced bone disease and other bone loss disorders [67].

4.2.2. Targeting the Wnt inhibitor Dickkopf-1 (DKK-1)

Dickkopf-1 (DKK1), a soluble inhibitor of wingless (Wnt) signaling secreted by MM cells contributes to osteolytic bone disease by inhibiting the differentiation of osteoblasts. The effect of anti-DKK1 mAb on bone metabolism and tumor growth in a SCID-rab system has been evaluated [68]. The implants of control animals showed signs of MM-induced resorption, whereas mice treated with anti-DKK1 antibodies blunted resorption and improved the bone mineral density of the implants. Histologic examination revealed that myelomatous bones of anti-DKK1-treated mice had increased numbers of osteocalcin-expressing osteoblasts and reduced number of multinucleated TRAP-expressing osteoclasts. The bone anabolic effect of anti-DKK1 was associated with reduced MM burden ($P < .04$). Anti-DKK1 also significantly increased BMD of the implanted bone and murine femur in non-myelomatous SCID-rab mice, suggesting that DKK1 is physiologically an important regulator of bone remodeling in adults. Anti-DKK1 agents including BHQ880 (Novartis) may therefore represent the next generation of therapeutic options for the enhancement of bone repair in some malignant and degenerative bone diseases including MM [69,70]. Although BHQ880 had no direct effect on MM cell growth, BHQ880 increased osteoblast differentiation, neutralized the negative effect of MM cells on osteoblastogenesis, and reduced IL-6 secretion. Furthermore, in a SCID-hu murine model of human MM, BHQ880 treatment led to a significant increase in osteoblast number, serum human osteocalcin level, and trabecular bone. Preliminary results from a phase I/II trial in MM where BHQ880 was given IV for 28 days was well tolerated when given in combination with zoledronic acid.

4.2.3. Targeting the Activin Receptor Type IIA (ActRIIA)

ACE-011, a novel bone anabolic agent currently in a Phase 2 clinical trial in MM, is a protein therapeutic based on the activin receptor IIA. In numerous preclinical models of bone loss, ACE-011 has demonstrated beneficial effects on both trabecular and cortical bone [71,72]. ACE-011 increased bone mineral density, improved bone architecture, increased the mineral apposition and bone formation rates and improved bone mechanical strength [73]. Results of the Phase 1 study in postmenopausal women demonstrated that a single dose of ACE-011 caused a rapid, sustained, dose-dependent increase in serum levels of bone-specific alkaline phosphatase (BSAP), a marker of bone formation, while a marker of bone resorption, C-terminal type 1 collagen telopeptide (CTX), decreased. In MM an ongoing multi-center Phase 2 trial is conducted in Russian patients which are treated with Melphalan, prednisone and thalidomide and randomized to receive either monthly doses of ACE-011 or placebo for up to three months. Preliminary results show clinical significant increases in biomarkers of bone formation, improvement in skeletal metastases, decreases in bone pain, as well as anti-tumor activity [54]. In summary, these data indicate that ACE-011 is well-tolerated and has significant hematologic activity in MM patients receiving myelosuppressive chemotherapy.

Moreover, ACE-011 has potential as a novel therapy for chemotherapy-induced anemia and may be an effective alternative to erythropoietin (EPO)-based treatments.

4.3. Targeting Angiogenesis by VEGF Inhibitor Bevacizumab (Avastin)

Vascular endothelial factor (VEGF) is important for the formation of new blood vessels and plays a key role not only in solid tumors but also in hematologic malignancies, including MM [74]. Bevacizumab targets and blocks VEGF and VEGF's binding to its receptor on the vascular endothelium [75]. Anti-VEGF Abs were active alone, and in combination with radiation in earlier preclinical studies [75,76]. It is currently being studied clinically in many solid and blood tumors including primary systemic amyloidosis and MM [77,78]. NCI's Cancer Therapy Evaluation Program is sponsoring a phase II study of bevacizumab plus thalomide in MM [78].

4.4. Targeting BAFF/ARPIL Growth and Survival Pathway by Atacicept (TACI-Ig) or BAFF Inhibitor

Recently, B-cell-activating factor of the tumor necrosis factor (TNF) family (BAFF; also known as B lymphocyte stimulator, BLyS) and a proliferation inducing ligand (APRIL), were identified as new survival factors for MM[79-81]. In addition to BMSCs, osteoclasts produce these factors to support MM cells in the BM microenvironment [81,82]. Their cognate receptors are BAFF-R/BR3, transmembrane activator and calcium modulator (TACI), and B cell maturation antigen (BCMA) with heterogeneous expression among patient MM cells. Specifically, RNA expression of BCMA and TACI is approximately >30-fold and >10-fold higher, respectively, than that of BR3 [81]. BR3 specifically bind BAFF but not APRIL, and has very limited expression in mature B cells plasma cells [83]. In fact, BCMA expression is only acquired in mature B cells and accompanied by loss of BAFF-R expression [83], suggesting a key role of BCMA in plasma cell survival. These studies provide clinical rationale to target BAFF/APRIL survival pathway in MM.

Atacicept (TACI-Ig, ZymoGenetics; Serono) acts as a decoy receptor by binding to and neutralizing soluble BAFF and APRIL, and preventing these ligands from binding to their cognate receptors on B-cell tumors, thereby enhancing cytotoxicity. An open-label, dose-escalation Phase I/II study enrolled 16 patients with refractory or relapsed MM (n=12) or active, progressive Waldenstrom's Macroglobulinemia (n=4) [84]. Atacicept was well tolerated and showed clinical and biological activity consistent with its mechanism of action. TACI was expressed heterogeneously among patient MM cells, which may explain promising results for the treatment of $TACI^{high}$ MM cells in a trial for atacicept [84,85].

In addition, the *in vivo* antitumor activity of neutralizing anti-BAFF mAb in SCID-hu model of human MM provide the preclinical rationale for its evaluation in the treatment of MM [86]. Moreover, since all MM cell lines and patient MM cells express BCMA, BCMA might be a promising target for monoclonal antibody development against MM. [87] Thus, BCMA is a target of donor B-cell immunity in patients with myeloma who respond to donor lymphocyte infusion (DLI). Antibody responses to cell-surface BCMA may contribute directly to tumor rejection *in vivo*. Indeed, BCMA antibodies show cytotoxic activity both as naked IgG and as drug conjugates, which warrant further evaluation as therapeutic candidates for plasma cell malignancies [88].

5. OTHER POTENTIAL TARGETS

Additional mAbs are directed against a variety of further MM cell targets including HLA-DR by 1D09C3,[89] HLA-class I by 2D7-DB [90], kininogen by C11C1 [91], and polyclonal rabbit anti-thymocyte globulin (rATG) [92].

Finally, since NK cells play a critical role in ADCC to lyse tumor target cells *via* therapeutic monoclonal antibodies and inhibitory-cell killer immunoglobulin-like receptors (KIRs) negatively regulate natural killer (NK) cell–mediated killing of HLA class I–expressing tumors, mAbs targeting KIR might prevents their inhibitory signaling leading to enhanced ADCC. A novel fully human anti-KIR blocking mAb, 1-7F9 (or IPH 2101), antagonizes inhibitory KIR signaling, activates NK cells and augments natural killer–mediated killing of tumor cells [93,94]. Importantly, 1-7F9 enhances patient NK cell cytotoxicity against autologous MM tumor cells *in vitro* and appears safe in an ongoing phase I clinical trial [95]. A multicenter, open label Phase IIa clinical trial (trial IPH 2101-201, in France) has started to evaluate IPH 2101 as a single agent in patients with stable measurable MM after induction therapy. Another phase II clinical trial to assess the potential of lenalidomide combined with 1-7F9 will be initiated in patients with MM.

REFERENCES

[1] Treon SP, Shima Y, Grossbard ML, *et al.* Treatment of multiple myeloma by antibody mediated immunotherapy and induction of myeloma selective antigens. Ann Oncol 2000; 11 Suppl 1: 107-111.

[2] Gemmel C, Cremer FW, Weis M, *et al.* Anti-CD20 antibody as consolidation therapy in a patient with primary plasma cell leukemia after high-dose therapy and autologous stem cell transplantation. Ann Hematol 2002; 81: 119-123.

[3] Musto P, Carella AM, Jr., Greco MM, *et al.* Short progression-free survival in myeloma patients receiving rituximab as maintenance therapy after autologous transplantation. Br J Haematol 2003; 123: 746-747.

[4] Ellis JH, Barber KA, Tutt A, *et al.* Engineered anti-CD38 monoclonal antibodies for immunotherapy of multiple myeloma. J Immunol 1995; 155: 925-937.

[5] Zojer N, Kirchbacher K, Vesely M, Hubl W, Ludwig H. Rituximab treatment provides no clinical benefit in patients with pretreated advanced multiple myeloma. Leuk Lymphoma 2006; 47: 1103-1109.

[6] Robillard N, Avet-Loiseau H, Garand R, *et al.* CD20 is associated with a small mature plasma cell morphology and t(11;14) in multiple myeloma. Blood 2003; 102: 1070-1071.

[7] Gozzetti A, Fabbri A, Lazzi S, Bocchia M, Lauria F. Reply to Rituximab activity in CD20 positive multiple myeloma. Leukemia 2007; 21: 1842-1843.

[8] Hofer S, Hunziker S, Dirnhofer S, Ludwig C. Rituximab effective in a patient with refractory autoimmune haemolytic anaemia and CD20-negative multiple myeloma. Br J Haematol 2003; 122: 690-691.

[9] Huff CA, Matsui W. Multiple myeloma cancer stem cells. J Clin Oncol 2008; 26: 2895-2900.

[10] Hideshima T, Mitsiades C, Tonon G, Richardson PG, Anderson KC. Understanding multiple myeloma pathogenesis in the bone marrow to identify new therapeutic targets. Nat Rev Cancer 2007; 7: 585-598.

[11] Trikha M, Corringham R, Klein B, Rossi JF. Targeted anti-interleukin-6 monoclonal antibody therapy for cancer: a review of the rationale and clinical evidence. Clin Cancer Res 2003; 9: 4653-4665.

[12] Honemann D, Chatterjee M, Savino R, *et al.* The IL-6 receptor antagonist SANT-7 overcomes bone marrow stromal cell-mediated drug resistance of multiple myeloma cells. Int J Cancer 2001; 93: 674-680.

[13] Tassone P, Forciniti S, Galea E, *et al.* Synergistic induction of growth arrest and apoptosis of human myeloma cells by the IL-6 super-antagonist Sant7 and Dexamethasone. Cell Death Differ 2000; 7: 327-328.

[14] Tassone P, Galea E, Forciniti S, Tagliaferri P, Venuta S. The IL-6 receptor super-antagonist Sant7 enhances antiproliferative and apoptotic effects induced by dexamethasone and zoledronic acid on multiple myeloma cells. Int J Oncol 2002; 21: 867-873.

[15] Plushner SL. Tocilizumab: an interleukin-6 receptor inhibitor for the treatment of rheumatoid arthritis. Ann Pharmacother 2008; 42: 1660-1668.

[16] Kanda J, Kawabata H, Yamaji Y, *et al.* Reversible cardiomyopathy associated with Multicentric Castleman disease: successful treatment with tocilizumab, an anti-interleukin 6 receptor antibody. Int J Hematol 2007; 85: 207-211.

[17] Nishimoto N. Clinical studies in patients with Castleman's disease, Crohn's disease, and rheumatoid arthritis in Japan. Clin Rev Allergy Immunol 2005; 28: 221-230.

[18] Woo P, Wilkinson N, Prieur AM, *et al.* Open label phase II trial of single, ascending doses of MRA in Caucasian children with severe systemic juvenile idiopathic arthritis: proof of principle of the efficacy of IL-6 receptor blockade in this type of arthritis and demonstration of prolonged clinical improvement. Arthritis Res Ther 2005; 7: R1281-1288.

[19] Yoshio-Hoshino N, Adachi Y, Aoki C, *et al.* Establishment of a new interleukin-6 (IL-6) receptor inhibitor applicable to the gene therapy for IL-6-dependent tumor. Cancer Res 2007; 67: 871-875.

[20] Tai YT, Catley LP, Mitsiades CS, *et al.* Mechanisms by which SGN-40, a humanized anti-CD40 antibody, induces cytotoxicity in human multiple myeloma cells: clinical implications. Cancer Res 2004; 64: 2846-2852.

[21] Tai YT, Li X, Tong X, *et al.* Human anti-CD40 antagonist antibody triggers significant antitumor activity against human multiple myeloma. Cancer Res 2005; 65: 5898-5906.

[22] Law CL, Gordon KA, Collier J, *et al.* Preclinical antilymphoma activity of a humanized anti-CD40 monoclonal antibody, SGN-40. Cancer Res 2005; 65: 8331-8338.

[23] Long L, Tong X, Patawaran M, *et al.* Antagonist anti-CD40 antibody CHIR-12.12 causes tumor regression and prolongs survival in multiple myeloma xenograftmodels. IMF Oral Presentation and Abstract No. 3 2005

[24] Bensinger W, Jagannath S, Becker PS, *et al.* A phase 1 dose escalation study of a fully human, antagonist anti-CD40 antibody, HCD 122 (formerly CHIR-12.12), in patients with relapsed and refractory multiple myeloma. Blood 2006; 108: Abstract 3675.

[25] Hussein MA, Berenson JR, Niesvizky R, *et al.* Results of a Phase I Trial of SGN-40 (Anti-huCD40 mAb) in Patients with Relapsed Multiple Myeloma. Blood 2006; 108: 3576.

[26] Khubchandani S, Czuczman MS, Hernandez-Ilizaliturri FJ. Dacetuzumab, a humanized mAb against CD40 for the treatment of hematological malignancies. Curr Opin Investig Drugs 2009; 10: 579-587.

[27] Advani R, Forero-Torres A, Furman RR, *et al.* Phase I study of the humanized anti-CD40 monoclonal antibody dacetuzumab in refractory or recurrent non-Hodgkin's lymphoma. J Clin Oncol 2009; 27: 4371-4377.

[28] Tai YT, Li XF, Catley L, *et al.* Immunomodulatory drug lenalidomide (CC-5013, IMiD3) augments anti-CD40 SGN-40-induced cytotoxicity in human multiple myeloma: clinical implications. Cancer Res 2005; 65: 11712-11720.

[29] Tai YT, Dillon M, Song W, *et al.* Anti-CS1 humanized monoclonal antibody HuLuc63 inhibits myeloma cell adhesion and induces antibody-dependent cellular cytotoxicity in the bone marrow milieu. Blood 2008; 112: 1329-1337.

[30] Hsi ED, Steinle R, Balasa B, *et al.* CS1, a potential new therapeutic antibody target for the treatment of multiple myeloma. Clin Cancer Res 2008; 14: 2775-2784.

[31] Tai YT, Soydan E, Song W, *et al.* CS1 promotes multiple myeloma cell adhesion, clonogenic growth, and tumorigenicity *via* c-maf-mediated interactions with bone marrow stromal cells. Blood 2009; 113: 4309-4318.

[32] van Rhee F, Szmania SM, Dillon M, *et al.* Combinatorial efficacy of anti-CS1 monoclonal antibody elotuzumab (HuLuc63) and bortezomib against multiple myeloma. Mol Cancer Ther 2009; 8: 2616-2624.

[33] Bensinger W, Zonder J, Singhal S, *et al.* Phase I Trial of HuLuc63 in Multiple Myeloma. Blood (ASH Annual Meeting Abstracts) 2007; 110:

[34] Jakubowiak AJ, Bensinger W, Siegel D, *et al.* Phase 1/2 Study of Elotuzumab in Combination with Bortezomib in Patients with Multiple Myeloma with One to Three Prior Therapies: Interim Results. Blood 2009; 114: 3876.

[35] Lonial S, Vij R, Harousseau J-L, *et al.* Phase 1/2 Study of Elotuzumab in Combination with Lenalidomide and Low Dose Dexamethasone in Relapsed or Refractory Multiple Myeloma: Interim Results. Blood 2009; 114: 432.

[36] Tassone P, Gozzini A, Goldmacher V, *et al.* *In vitro* and *in vivo* activity of the maytansinoid immunoconjugate huN901-N2'-deacetyl-N2'-(3-mercapto-1-oxopropyl)-maytansine against CD56+ multiple myeloma cells. Cancer Res 2004; 64: 4629-4636.

[37] Chanan-Khan A, Wolf J, Gharibo M, *et al.* Phase I Study of IMGN901, Used as Monotherapy, in Patients with Heavily Pre-Treated CD56-Positive Multiple Myeloma -A Preliminary Safety and Efficacy Analysis. Blood 2009; 114: 2883.

[38] Stevenson FK, Bell AJ, Cusack R, *et al.* Preliminary studies for an immunotherapeutic approach to the treatment of human myeloma using chimeric anti-CD38 antibody. Blood 1991; 77: 1071-1079.

[39] Stevenson GT. CD38 as a therapeutic target. Mol Med 2006; 12: 345-346.

[40] Goldmacher VS, Bourret LA, Levine BA, *et al.* Anti-CD38-blocked ricin: an immunotoxin for the treatment of multiple myeloma. Blood 1994; 84: 3017-3025.

[41] Tai YT, de Weers M, Li X, *et al.* Daratumumab, a Novel Potent Human Anti-CD38 Monoclonal Antibody, Induces Significant Killing of Human Multiple Myeloma Cells: Therapeutic Implication. 2009; 114: 608.

[42] Tesar M. Fully human antibody MOR202 against CD38 for the treatment of multiple myeloma and other blood-borne malignancies. J Clin Onc 2007; 25: 8106.

[43] Ozaki S, Kosaka M, Wakatsuki S, *et al.* Immunotherapy of multiple myeloma with a monoclonal antibody directed against a plasma cell-specific antigen, HM1.24. Blood 1997; 90: 3179-3186.

[44] Matsuda A, Suzuki Y, Honda G, *et al.* Large-scale identification and characterization of human genes that activate NF-kappaB and MAPK signaling pathways. Oncogene 2003; 22: 3307-3318.

[45] Ozaki S, Kosaka M, Wakahara Y, *et al.* Humanized anti-HM1.24 antibody mediates myeloma cell cytotoxicity that is enhanced by cytokine stimulation of effector cells. Blood 1999; 93: 3922-3930.

[46] Kawai S, Yoshimura Y, Iida S, *et al.* Antitumor activity of humanized monoclonal antibody against HM1.24 antigen in human myeloma xenograft models. Oncol Rep 2006; 15: 361-367.

[47] Tai YT, Muchhal U, Li X, *et al.* XmAb®5592 Fc-Engineered Humanized Anti-HM1.24 Monoclonal Antibody Has Potent *in Vitro* and *In Vivo* Efficacy against Multiple Myeloma. Blood 2009; 114: 609.

[48] Menoret E, Gomez-Bougie P, Geffroy-Luseau A, *et al.* Mcl-1L cleavage is involved in TRAIL-R1-and TRAIL-R2-mediated apoptosis induced by HGS-ETR1 and HGS-ETR2 human mAbs in myeloma cells. Blood 2006; 108: 1346-1352.

[49] Hotte SJ, Hirte HW, Chen EX, *et al.* A phase 1 study of mapatumumab (fully human monoclonal antibody to TRAIL-R1) in patients with advanced solid malignancies. Clin Cancer Res 2008; 14: 3450-3455.

[50] Smith MR, Jin F, Joshi I. Bortezomib sensitizes non-Hodgkin's lymphoma cells to apoptosis induced by antibodies to tumor necrosis factor related apoptosis-inducing ligand (TRAIL) receptors TRAIL-R1 and TRAIL-R2. Clin Cancer Res 2007; 13: 5528s-5534s.

[51] Berkova Z, Tao RH, Samaniego F. Milatuzumab -a promising new immunotherapeutic agent. Expert Opin Investig Drugs 2010; 19: 141-149.

[52] Stein R, Mattes MJ, Cardillo TM, *et al.* CD74: a new candidate target for the immunotherapy of B-cell neoplasms. Clin Cancer Res 2007; 13: 5556s-5563s.

[53] Burton JD, Ely S, Reddy PK, *et al.* CD74 is expressed by multiple myeloma and is a promising target for therapy. Clin Cancer Res 2004; 10: 6606-6611.

[54] Abdulkadyrov KM, Salogub GN, Khuazheva NK, *et al.* ACE-011, a Soluble Activin Receptor Type Iia IgG-Fc Fusion Protein, Increases Hemoglobin (Hb) and Improves Bone Lesions in Multiple Myeloma Patients Receiving Myelosuppressive Chemotherapy: Preliminary Analysis. Blood 2009; 114: 749.

[55] Stein R, Smith MR, Chen S, Zalath M, Goldenberg DM. Combining milatuzumab with bortezomib, doxorubicin, or dexamethasone improves responses in multiple myeloma cell lines. Clin Cancer Res 2009; 15: 2808-2817.

[56] Moreau P, Harousseau JL, Wijdenes J, *et al.* A combination of anti-interleukin 6 murine monoclonal antibody with dexamethasone and high-dose Melphalan induces high complete response rates in advanced multiple myeloma. Br J Haematol 2000; 109: 661-664.

[57] Fulciniti M, Hideshima T, Vermot-Desroches C, *et al.* A high-affinity fully human anti-IL-6 mAb, 1339, for the treatment of multiple myeloma. Clin Cancer Res 2009; 15: 7144-7152.

[58] Van Zaanen HC, Lokhorst HM, Aarden LA, *et al.* Blocking interleukin-6 activity with chimeric anti-IL6 monoclonal antibodies in multiple myeloma: effects on soluble IL6 receptor and soluble gp130. Leuk Lymphoma 1998; 31: 551-558.

[59] van Zaanen HC, Lokhorst HM, Aarden LA, *et al.* Chimaeric anti-interleukin 6 monoclonal antibodies in the treatment of advanced multiple myeloma: a phase I dose-escalating study. Br J Haematol 1998; 102: 783-790.

[60] Voorhees PM, Chen Q, Kuhn DJ, *et al.* Inhibition of interleukin-6 signaling with CNTO 328 enhances the activity of bortezomib in preclinical models of multiple myeloma. Clin Cancer Res 2007; 13: 6469-6478.

[61] Voorhees PM, Chen Q, Small GW, *et al.* Targeted inhibition of interleukin-6 with CNTO 328 sensitizes pre-clinical models of multiple myeloma to dexamethasone-mediated cell death. Br J Haematol 2009; 145: 481-490.

[62] Lewiecki EM. RANK ligand inhibition with denosumab for the management of osteoporosis. Expert Opin Biol Ther 2006; 6: 1041-1050.

[63] Terpos E, Szydlo R, Apperley JF, *et al.* Soluble receptor activator of nuclear factor kappaB ligand-osteoprotegerin ratio predicts survival in multiple myeloma: proposal for a novel prognostic index. Blood 2003; 102: 1064-1069.

[64] Giuliani N, Bataille R, Mancini C, Lazzaretti M, Barille S. Myeloma cells induce imbalance in the osteoprotegerin/osteoprotegerin ligand system in the human bone marrow environment. Blood 2001; 98: 3527-3533.

[65] Burkiewicz JS, Scarpace SL, Bruce SP. Denosumab in osteoporosis and oncology. Ann Pharmacother 2009; 43: 1445-1455.

[66] Body JJ, Facon T, Coleman RE, *et al.* A study of the biological receptor activator of nuclear factor-kappaB ligand inhibitor, denosumab, in patients with multiple myeloma or bone metastases from breast cancer. Clin Cancer Res 2006; 12: 1221-1228.

[67] Santini D, Fratto ME, Vincenzi B, *et al.* Denosumab: the era of targeted therapies in bone metastatic diseases. Curr Cancer Drug Targets 2009; 9: 834-842.

[68] Yaccoby S, Ling W, Zhan F, *et al.* Antibody-based inhibition of DKK1 suppresses tumor-induced bone resorption and multiple myeloma growth *in vivo*. Blood 2007; 109: 2106-2111.

[69] Heath DJ, Chantry AD, Buckle CH, *et al.* Inhibiting Dickkopf-1 (Dkk1) removes suppression of bone formation and prevents the development of osteolytic bone disease in multiple myeloma. J Bone Miner Res 2009; 24: 425-436.

[70] Fulciniti M, Tassone P, Hideshima T, *et al.* Anti-DKK1 mAb (BHQ880) as a potential therapeutic agent for multiple myeloma. Blood 2009; 114: 371-379.

[71] Lotinun S, Pearsall RS, Davies MV, *et al.* A soluble activin receptor Type IIA fusion protein (ACE-011) increases bone mass *via* a dual anabolic-antiresorptive effect in cynomolgus monkeys. Bone 2010

[72] Vallet S, Mukherjee S, Vaghela N, *et al.* Restoration of Bone Balance *Via* Activin a Inhibition Results in Anti-Myeloma Activity. Blood 2008; 114: 645.

[73] Ruckle J, Jacobs M, Kramer W, *et al.* Single-dose, randomized, double-blind, placebo-controlled study of ACE-011 (ActRIIA-IgG1) in postmenopausal women. J Bone Miner Res 2009; 24: 744-752.

[74] Podar K, Anderson KC. Inhibition of VEGF signaling pathways in multiple myeloma and other malignancies. Cell Cycle 2007; 6: 538-542.

[75] Ferrara N, Hillan KJ, Novotny W. Bevacizumab (Avastin), a humanized anti-VEGF monoclonal antibody for cancer therapy. Biochem Biophys Res Commun 2005; 333: 328-335.

[76] Gorski DH, Beckett MA, Jaskowiak NT, *et al.* Blockage of the vascular endothelial growth factor stress response increases the antitumor effects of ionizing radiation. Cancer Res 1999; 59: 3374-3378.

[77] Hoyer RJ, Leung N, Witzig TE, Lacy MQ. Treatment of diuretic refractory pleural effusions with bevacizumab in four patients with primary systemic amyloidosis. Am J Hematol 2007; 82: 409-413.

[78] Goldman B. For investigational targeted drugs, combination trials pose challenges. J Natl Cancer Inst 2003; 95: 1744-1746.

[79] Novak AJ, Darce JR, Arendt BK, *et al.* Expression of BCMA, TACI, and BAFF-R in multiple myeloma: a mechanism for growth and survival. Blood 2004; 103: 689-694.

[80] Moreaux J, Legouffe E, Jourdan E, *et al.* BAFF and APRIL protect myeloma cells from apoptosis induced by interleukin 6 deprivation and dexamethasone. Blood 2004; 103: 3148-3157.

[81] Tai YT, Li XF, Breitkreutz I, *et al.* Role of B-cell-activating factor in adhesion and growth of human multiple myeloma cells in the bone marrow microenvironment. Cancer Res 2006; 66: 6675-6682.

[82] Moreaux J, Cremer FW, Reme T, *et al.* The level of TACI gene expression in myeloma cells is associated with a signature of microenvironment dependence versus a plasmablastic signature. Blood 2005; 106: 1021-1030.

[83] Darce JR, Arendt BK, Wu X, Jelinek DF. Regulated expression of BAFF-binding receptors during human B cell differentiation. J Immunol 2007; 179: 7276-7286.

[84] Rossi JF, Moreaux J, Hose D, *et al.* Atacicept in relapsed/refractory multiple myeloma or active Waldenstrom's macroglobulinemia: a phase I study. Br J Cancer 2009; 101: 1051-1058.

[85] Yaccoby S, Pennisi A, Li X, *et al.* Atacicept (TACI-Ig) inhibits growth of TACI(high) primary myeloma cells in SCID-hu mice and in coculture with osteoclasts. Leukemia 2008; 22: 406-413.

[86] Neri P, Kumar S, Fulciniti MT, *et al.* Neutralizing B-cell activating factor antibody improves survival and inhibits osteoclastogenesis in a severe combined immunodeficient human multiple myeloma model. Clin Cancer Res 2007; 13: 5903-5909.

[87] Bellucci R, Alyea EP, Chiaretti S, *et al.* Graft-versus-tumor response in patients with multiple myeloma is associated with antibody response to BCMA, a plasma-cell membrane receptor. Blood 2005; 105: 3945-3950.

[88] Ryan MC, Hering M, Peckham D, *et al.* Antibody targeting of B-cell maturation antigen on malignant plasma cells. Mol Cancer Ther 2007; 6: 3009-3018.

[89] Carlo-Stella C, Guidetti A, Di Nicola M, *et al.* IFN-gamma enhances the antimyeloma activity of the fully human anti-human leukocyte antigen-DR monoclonal antibody 1D09C3. Cancer Res 2007; 67: 3269-3275.

[90] Sekimoto E, Ozaki S, Ohshima T, *et al.* A single-chain Fv diabody against human leukocyte antigen-A molecules specifically induces myeloma cell death in the bone marrow environment. Cancer Res 2007; 67: 1184-1192.

[91] Sainz IM, Isordia-Salas I, Espinola RG, *et al.* Multiple myeloma in a murine syngeneic model:modulation of growth and angiogenesis by a monoclonal antibody to kininogen. Cancer Immunol Immunother 2006; 55: 797-807.

[92] Zand MS, Vo T, Pellegrin T, *et al.* Apoptosis and complement-mediated lysis of myeloma cells by polyclonal rabbit antithymocyte globulin. Blood 2006; 107: 2895-2903.

[93] Johansson SE, Hejdeman B, Hinkula J, *et al.* NK cell activation by KIR-binding antibody 1-7F9 and response to HIV-infected autologous cells in viremic and controller HIV-infected patients. Clin Immunol 2009: Clin Immunol 2010 Feb;134(2):158-68.

[94] Romagne F, Andre P, Spee P, *et al.* Preclinical characterization of 1-7F9, a novel human anti-KIR receptor therapeutic antibody that augments natural killer-mediated killing of tumor cells. Blood 2009; 114: 2667-2677.

[95] Benson DM, Romagne F, Squiban P, *et al.* Novel monoclonal antibody that enhances natural killer (NK) cell cytotoxicity against multiple myeloma (MM): Preclinical data and interim phase I clinical trial results. J Clin Oncol 2009; 27: 15s: (abst.3032).

[96] Antibody-based therapies in multiple. Bone Marrow Res 2011; Article ID 924058.

INDEX

A

B

C

K

L

M

N

O

P

R

S

T

U

V

W

X

Z